Assisted Reproductive Technology Surveillance

Assisted Reproductive Technology Surveillance

Edited by

Dmitry M. Kissin
Division of Reproductive Health, U.S. Centers for Disease Control and Prevention, USA

G. David Adamson
International Committee Monitoring Assisted Reproductive Technologies, USA

Georgina M. Chambers
National Perinatal Epidemiology and Statistics Unit, University of New South Wales, Australia

Christian De Geyter
European IVF Monitoring Consortium, European Society of Human Reproduction and Embryology, Switzerland

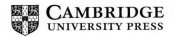
CAMBRIDGE
UNIVERSITY PRESS

CAMBRIDGE
UNIVERSITY PRESS

University Printing House, Cambridge CB2 8BS, United Kingdom

One Liberty Plaza, 20th Floor, New York, NY 10006, USA

477 Williamstown Road, Port Melbourne, VIC 3207, Australia

314–321, 3rd Floor, Plot 3, Splendor Forum, Jasola District Centre, New Delhi – 110025, India

79 Anson Road, #06–04/06, Singapore 079906

Cambridge University Press is part of the University of Cambridge.

It furthers the University's mission by disseminating knowledge in the pursuit of
education, learning, and research at the highest international levels of excellence.

www.cambridge.org
Information on this title: www.cambridge.org/9781108498586
DOI: 10.1017/9781108653763

First published 2019

Printed in the United Kingdom by TJ International Ltd. Padstow Cornwall

A catalogue record for this publication is available from the British Library.

Library of Congress Cataloging-in-Publication Data
Names: Kissin, Dmitry M., 1972– editor. | Adamson, G. David, editor. | Chambers, Georgina M., 1963– editor. |
De Geyter, Christian, editor.
Title: Assisted reproductive technology surveillance / edited by Dmitry M. Kissin, G. David Adamson,
Georgina M. Chambers, Christian De Geyter.
Description: Cambridge, United Kingdom : Cambridge University Press, [2019] | Includes bibliographical
references and index.
Identifiers: LCCN 2018059162 | ISBN 9781108498586 (hardback)
Subjects: | MESH: Reproductive Techniques, Assisted – statistics & numerical data | Pregnancy Outcome |
Population Surveillance
Classification: LCC RG133.5 | NLM WQ 208 | DDC 618.1/78–dc23
LC record available at https://lccn.loc.gov/2018059162

ISBN 978-1-108-49858-6 Hardback

....

Contents

Foreword   vii
List of Contributors   viii

Section 1 Introduction to ART Surveillance

1 **Infertility and ART**   1
Sheree L. Boulet, Anjani Chandra, Aaron Rosen and Alan DeCherney

2 **Importance and History of ART Surveillance**   12
Jacques de Mouzon, Paul Lancaster and Anders Nyboe Andersen

Section 2 General Principles of ART Surveillance

3 **ART Surveillance: Who, What, When and How?**   23
Sara Crawford, Dmitry M. Kissin and Georgina M. Chambers

4 **Future Directions for ART Surveillance and Monitoring Novel Technology**   31
Christian De Geyter and Eli Y. Adashi

Section 3 Using ART Surveillance Data

5 **Reporting ART Success Rates**   37
Georgina M. Chambers, Kevin Doody and Sara Crawford

6 **Using ART Surveillance Data in Clinical Research**   47
Valerie L. Baker, Sheree L. Boulet and Anja Bisgaard Pinborg

7 **Monitoring ART Safety and Biovigilance**   56
Luca Gianaroli, Anna Pia Ferraretti and Borut Kovačič

8 **Quality Assurance of ART Practice: Using Data to Improve Clinical Care**   69
Kevin Doody, Carlos Calhaz-Jorge and Jesper Smeenk

9 **Monitoring Long-Term Outcomes of ART: Linking ART Surveillance Data with Other Datasets**   81
Barbara Luke, Sheree L. Boulet and Anna-Karina Aaris Henningsen

10 **Use of ART Surveillance by People Experiencing Infertility**   93
Sandra K. Dill, Edgar Mocanu and Petra Thorn

Section 4 Global Variations in ART Surveillance

11 **Global ART Surveillance: The International Committee Monitoring Assisted Reproductive Technologies (ICMART)**   101
G. David Adamson

12 **Global Variations in ART Policy: Data from the International Federation of Fertility Societies (IFFS)**   116
Steven J. Ory and Kathleen Miller

13 **ART Surveillance in Africa**   124
Silke Dyer, Paversan Archary and G. David Adamson

14 **ART Surveillance in Asia** 133
Osamu Ishihara, Manish Banker and Bai Fu

15 **ART Surveillance in Australia and New Zealand** 142
Georgina M. Chambers, Paul Lancaster and Peter Illingworth

16 **ART Surveillance in Europe** 153
Christian De Geyter, Markus S. Kupka and Carlos Calhaz-Jorge

17 **ART Surveillance in the Middle East: Governance, Culture and Religion** 163
Johnny Awwad, Dalia Khalife and Ragaa Mansour

18 **ART Surveillance in North America** 172
James Patrick Toner, Andrea Lanes and Dmitry M. Kissin

19 **ART Surveillance in Latin America** 182
Fernando Zegers-Hochschild, Javier A. Crosby and Juan Enrique Schwarze

Section 5 Surveillance of Non-ART Fertility Treatments

20 **The Importance of Non-ART Fertility Treatments in Public Health** 191
Christine Wyns, Diane de Neubourg and Eli Y. Adashi

21 **Non-ART Surveillance** 200
Markus S. Kupka and Anja Bisgaard Pinborg

Appendix A ART Surveillance System Variables and Definitions 206
Appendix B International Glossary on Infertility and Fertility Care 209
Appendix C ICMART Data Collection Form 219
Index 235

Colour plates are to be found between pp. 110 and 111.

Foreword

This textbook, *Assisted Reproductive Technology Surveillance*, has been written because the editors and publisher realized that many professionals, policy makers and patients were unaware of the significant accomplishments of global ART surveillance made during the past four decades. Because management is not possible without measurement, it is important to share the international history, experience, successes, current knowledge and challenges to increase the quantity and quality of global ART data. Subsequent analysis and understanding of ART practice will lead to improved-quality patient care.

The purpose of this book is to provide: a comprehensive history since the very beginning of global ART registry development and surveillance; the principles of surveillance; a detailed description of how to collect, analyze and use surveillance data; an understanding of international similarities and differences; surveillance of non-ART fertility treatments; and standardized terminology and data collection forms. This book will provide the reader with everything they need to develop, improve, understand and use national and international ART surveillance data.

This book is written by the professionals who, over decades, have created and maintained most of the national, regional and global registries for ART surveillance. Their wealth of experience, knowledge and expertise is unparalleled. They share not only their successes, but also their failures, limitations and current challenges.

This comprehensive book on global ART surveillance is a must-read for all stakeholders in the international ART community. Understanding where we have been, where we are and where we are going will enable all of us to improve the systems of care, the evidence we use and the personalized care we give to each patient. It is important to acknowledge all the patients who provided their data, the professionals who have created the current ART surveillance systems and the readers who will continue this progress in the future.

G. David Adamson, MD, FRCSC, FACOG, FACS
November 2018

Contributors

G. David Adamson, MD, FRCSC, FACOG, FACS
Stanford University School of Medicine; University of California San Francisco; Equal3 Fertility, Cupertino, CA, USA

Eli Y. Adashi, MD, MS, CPE, FACOG
The Warren Alpert Medical School, Brown University, Providence RI, USA

Paversan Archary, FCOG, MMed
African Network and Registry for Assisted Reproductive Technology (ANARA), Reproductive Medicine Unit, Groote Schuur Hospital and Faculty of Health Sciences, University of Cape Town, Cape Town, South Africa

Johnny Awwad, MD, HCLD/TS (ABB)
Division of Reproductive Endocrinology and Infertility, AUBMC Haifa Idriss Fertility Center, Department of Obstetrics and Gynecology, American University of Beirut Medical Center, Beirut, Lebanon

Valerie L. Baker, MD
Division of Reproductive Endocrinology and Infertility, Department of Obstetrics and Gynecology, Stanford University School of Medicine, Sunnyvale, CA, USA

Manish Banker, MD
Nova IVI Fertility, Pulse Women's Hospital, Gujarat, India

Sheree L. Boulet, DrPH, MPH
Division Reproductive Health, National Center for Chronic Disease Prevention and Health Promotion, Centers for Disease Control and Prevention (CDC), Atlanta, GA, USA

Carlos Calhaz-Jorge, Prof.
Department of Obstetrics, Gynecology and Reproductive Medicine, Reproductive Medicine Unit, University Hospital – Faculdade de Medicina, Universidade de Lisboa, Lisbon, Portugal

Georgina M. Chambers, PhD, MBA
National Perinatal Epidemiology and Statistics Unit, The University of New South Wales, Sydney, Australia

Anjani Chandra, PhD
Division of Vital Statistics, National Center for Health Statistics, Centers for Disease Control and Prevention (CDC), Hyattsville, MD, USA

Sara Crawford, PhD
Division of Reproductive Health, National Center for Chronic Disease Prevention and Health Promotion, Centers for Disease Control and Prevention (CDC), Atlanta, GA, USA

Javier A. Crosby
Reproductive Medicine Unit, Clinica Las Condes, Santiago, Chile

Alan DeCherney, MD
Eunice Kennedy Shriver National Institute of Child Health and Human Development, National Institutes of Health (NIH), Bethesda, MD, USA

Christian De Geyter, Prof.
Reproductive Medicine and Gynecological Endocrinology (RME), University Hospital, University of Basle, Basle, Switzerland

Diane De Neubourg, MD, PhD, M Med Sci, Prof.
Reproductive Medicine, University of Antwerp, Antwerp, Belgium

Sandra K Dill, AM, BComm, MLS
Access Australia's National Infertility Network Ltd., Newington, NSW, Australia

Kevin Doody, MD
Center for Assisted Reproduction, Bedford, TX, USA

Silke Dyer, FCOG, MMed, PhD
African Network and Registry for Assisted
Reproductive Technology (ANARA), Department of
Obstetrics & Gynaecology, Groote Schuur Hospital
and Faculty of Health Sciences, University of Cape
Town, Cape Town, South Africa

Anna Pia Ferraretti, PhD
S.I.S.Me.R. Reproductive Medicine Unit, Bologna,
Italy

Bai Fu, MD
ART Management Department, National Center for
Women and Children's Health, Beijing, P.R. China

Luca Gianaroli, MD
S.I.S.Me.R. Reproductive Medicine Unit, Bologna, Italy

Anna-Karina Aaris Henningsen, MD
The Fertility Clinic, Rigshospitalet, University of
Copenhagen, Copenhagen, Denmark

Peter Illingworth, MD, FRCOG, FRANZCOG, CREI
IVF Australia, Sydney, Australia

Osamu Ishihara, MD, PhD
Department of Obstetrics & Gynaecology, Faculty of
Medicine, Saitama Medical University,
Moroyama, Saitama, Japan

Dalia Khalife, MD
Reproductive Endocrinology and Infertility,
Department of Obstetrics and Gynecology, American
University of Beirut Medical Center, Beirut, Lebanon

Dmitry M. Kissin, MD, MPH
Division of Reproductive Health, National Center for
Chronic Disease Prevention and Health Promotion,
Centers for Disease Control and Prevention (CDC),
Atlanta, GA, USA

Borut Kovačič, PhD
Department of Reproductive Medicine and
Gynecological Endocrinology, University Medical
Centre Maribor, Maribor, Slovenia

Markus S. Kupka, MD, PhD, Prof.
European IVF Monitoring Consortium (EIM),
European Society of Human Reproduction and
Embryology (ESHRE), German IVF Registry (DIR),
Fertility Center – Gynaekologicum, Hamburg,
Germany

Paul Lancaster, AM, MB, BS, MPH, FRACP, FAFPHM
Menzies Centre for Health Policy, School of Public
Health, University of Sydney, Sydney, Australia

Andrea Lanes, PhD
Better Outcomes Registry & Network (BORN)
Ontario, Children's Hospital of Eastern Ontario,
Ottawa, Ontario, Canada

Barbara Luke, ScD, MPH
Department of Obstetrics, Gynecology, and
Reproductive Biology, Michigan State University,
East Lansing, MI, USA

Ragaa Mansour, MD, PhD
The Egyptian IVF-ET Center, Cairo, Egypt

Kathleen Miller, DH Sc
International Federation of Fertility Societies, Mt.
Royal, NJ, USA

Edgar Mocanu, MD, FRCOG Dip Ethics
Rotunda Hospital and RCSI, Parnell Square, Dublin,
Ireland

Jacques de Mouzon, MD, MPH
International Committee Monitoring Assisted
Reproductive Technologies, Paris, France

Anders Nyboe Andersen, MD, PhD, Prof.
The Fertility Clinic, Copenhagen University Hospital,
Copenhagen, Denmark

Steven J. Ory, MD
Department of Obstetrics and Gynecology, Florida
International University; IVF Florida Reproductive
Associates, Margate, FL, USA

Anja Bisgaard Pinborg, MD, DMSc, Prof.
The Fertility Clinic, Rigshospitalet, Copenhagen
University Hospital, Copenhagen,
Denmark

Aaron Rosen, MD
Mercy Hospital and Medical Center, Department of
OB/GYN, Chicago, IL, USA

Jesper Smeenk, MD, Phd
Elisabeth-Tweesteden Hospital, Department of
Obstetrics and Gynecology,
Tilburg, the Netherlands

Juan Enrique Schwarze, MD, MSc
Reproductive Medicine Unit, Clinica Las Condes, Santiago, Chile

Petra Thorn, PhD
Private Practice for Couple and Family Therapy, Infertility Counselling, Moerfelden, Germany

James Patrick Toner, Jr, MD, PhD
Emory School of Medicine, Atlanta, GA, USA

Christine Wyns, MD, PhD, Prof.
Gynaecology & Andrology, Cliniques Universitaires Saint-Luc, Catholic University of Louvain, Brussels, Belgium

Fernando Zegers-Hochschild, MD
Reproductive Medicine Unit, Clinica Las Condes; Program of Ethics and Public Policies in Human Reproduction,
University Diego Portales,
Santiago, Chile

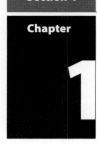

Chapter

1

Infertility and ART

Sheree L. Boulet, Anjani Chandra, Aaron Rosen and Alan DeCherney

The findings and conclusions in this report are those of the authors and do not necessarily represent the official position of the Centers for Disease Control and Prevention.

Infertility

Infertility, commonly defined as the inability to establish a clinical pregnancy after 12 months of regular, unprotected sexual intercourse [1], is a global public health issue affecting millions of women and men worldwide [2]. The absolute prevalence of infertility is difficult to estimate as it varies across populations and can be measured using different methods, depending on the purpose of the measurement. For example, clinical definitions of infertility may include women >35 years of age who attempted pregnancy for 6 months, as these women may benefit from earlier evaluation and treatment [3]. Demographic and epidemiological definitions typically aim to measure infertility among populations using standard definitions but also may vary in their approach. Demographers often define infertility as the absence of a live birth among sexually active women who are not using contraception and use longer intervals, such as 2 or 5 years, to assess infertility prevalence [4, 5, 6]. Epidemiological definitions usually measure an inability to achieve pregnancy among women who are attempting to become pregnant and are 'at risk' for conception. Varying criteria are used to identify at-risk populations, including couple status, use of contraception, frequency of unprotected intercourse, timing of last birth, breastfeeding status and the desire for a child [4, 5, 7]. Infertility can be measured over the course of a lifetime or as a current condition and is often reported separately for nulliparous women (primary infertility) and women with one or more previous live births (secondary infertility) [1].

Recurrent pregnancy loss, distinguished by the spontaneous loss of two or more pregnancies before 22 weeks' gestation, is distinct from infertility as the underlying pathology may differ [1, 3]. By definition, measures of infertility prevalence that use live birth as

an outcome include a proportion of women with recurrent pregnancy loss. Impaired fecundity is a term that has been used to describe populations that have difficulty getting pregnant and carrying a pregnancy to term [8]. Although this term is sometimes used interchangeably with infertility, it represents a broader construct that is inclusive of pregnancy loss as well as difficulty getting pregnant.

Globally, it has been estimated that approximately 2% of nulliparous women 20–44 years of age were unable to achieve a live birth after 5 years of trying, and 10% of women 20–44 years of age with at least one previous live birth were unable to have another child over a 5-year period [2]. Estimates of primary infertility were lowest in middle-income countries in Latin America (0.8–1.0%) and highest in countries in Eastern Europe, North Africa/Middle East, Oceania and sub-Saharan Africa (>3.0%). In Canada, the prevalence of current infertility (an inability to achieve pregnancy in the past 12 months among married and cohabiting couples) ranged from 11.5 to 15.7%, depending on how risk of conception was defined (e.g. whether restricted to couples reporting having intercourse in the past 12 months who were trying to become pregnant) [9]. In the United States (US), 6.7% of married women 15–44 years of age in 2011–2015 were infertile (had unprotected intercourse with the same husband for at least 12 consecutive months but did not have a pregnancy) (Table 1.1). Using the broader measure of impaired fecundity that includes pregnancy loss as well as physical difficulties conceiving a pregnancy, the prevalence of impaired fecundity was 15.5% for married women aged 15–44 in 2011–2015 and 12.1% for all women aged 15–44, regardless of marital status. In addition, the prevalence of infertility among nulliparous married women increased with age. Among all women, the prevalence of impaired fecundity increased with age.

Table 1.1 Infertility and impaired fecundity among women aged 15–44 years, by selected characteristics: US, 2011–2015

Characteristic	Infertility among married women[a]	Impaired fecundity among married women[b]	Impaired fecundity among all women[b]
	Percent (standard error)		
Total	6.7 (0.52)	15.5 (0.79)	12.1 (0.41)
Age			
15–24 years	4.6 (2.01)	15.4 (3.04)	7.8 (0.68)*
25–34 years	6.3 (0.78)	14.7 (1.18)	12.6 (0.69)
35–44 years	7.3 (0.87)	16.1 (1.22)	15.7 (0.90)
Parity and age			
No births	14.2 (1.63)**	23.6 (2.59)**	11.2 (0.74)
15–24 years	1.6 (0.98)*	15.1 (4.65)*	7.0 (0.76)*
25–34 years	11.7 (1.83)	16.3 (2.11)	12.3 (1.23)
35–44 years	24.4 (3.90)	39.6 (5.83)	28.7 (3.11)
1 or more births	4.9 (0.56)	13.5 (0.84)	12.8 (0.57)
15–24 years	7.6 (3.74)	15.7 (4.67)	11.9 (1.49)
25–34 years	4.5 (0.84)	14.1 (1.42)	12.8 (0.86)
35–44 years	4.9 (0.77)	12.9 (1.13)	13.0 (0.93)

[a] Married women are classified as infertile if they have been exposed to the risk of pregnancy (had unprotected intercourse) with the same husband for at least 12 consecutive months, but have not had a pregnancy. See reference 8 for further details on this measure.

[b] Impaired fecundity indicates physical difficulties in getting pregnant or carrying a pregnancy to live birth. See reference 8 for further details on this measure.

* Older age among nulliparous women was significantly associated with a higher percentage with the specified fertility problem ($p<0.05$).

** The percentage for women with 1 or more births was significantly higher than that for women with 0 births ($p<0.05$).

Source: CDC/NCHS, 2011–2015 National Survey of Family Growth

Advancing age (typically 35 years or older) is the most important predictor of infertility in women [10, 11]. In many developed countries, maternal age at first birth has been increasing over time as more women delay childbearing to pursue educational or employment opportunities or because of personal circumstances [12, 13, 14]. Because the number and quality of eggs decline as a woman ages, postponement of childbearing can result in couples seeking to start a family at a time when female fecundity is declining [15]. Other risk factors for female infertility include a history of sexually transmitted infections, smoking, illicit drug use, alcohol use, exposure to certain environmental factors and chronic conditions such as diabetes, obesity and cardiovascular disease [15, 16, 17, 18].

Among men, advanced paternal age is associated with decreased semen quality and increasing rates of DNA fragmentation in sperm [19, 20]. Other factors that may affect male fertility are smoking, illicit drug use, alcohol use, exposure to certain environmental factors and obesity [16, 21, 22, 23, 24, 25]. Notably, findings

from a recent meta-analysis suggest that sperm counts declined from 1973 to 2011 in North America, Europe, Australia and New Zealand [26]. The reason for the decrease is not known but may be the result of environmental exposures or lifestyle factors.

The History of Assisted Reproductive Technology as a Treatment for Infertility

In the late 1800s, the German researcher Wilhelm August Oscar Hertwig took a position in the Mediterranean studying sea urchins. During this time, he observed the fertilization of an oocyte by a sperm outside of the sea urchin's body. Despite resistance from the scientific community, he published his observations, setting the groundwork for the modern theory of chromosome continuity [27].

The study of fertilization and embryo development continued over the years, and eventually an American biologist, Gregory Pincus, with an interest

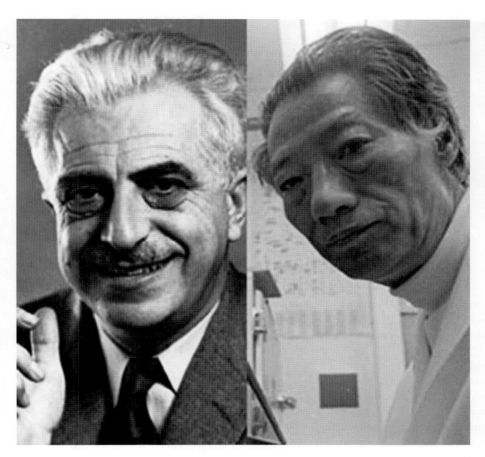

Figure 1.1 Gregory Pincus and Min Chueh Chang, early pioneers in IVF in animal studies.

in the way that hormones affected the reproductive system, began his famous work with rabbits. He removed an oocyte from a mother rabbit and succeeded in fertilizing it outside of the body, so-called Pincogenesis in vitro, and after replacing the embryo in the rabbit he published on the first birth of a mammal by in vitro fertilization (IVF) [28]. Peers had difficulty replicating his experiment until Dr Min Chueh Chang, in 1959, was able to fertilize a black rabbit's eggs with a black rabbit sperm and transfer those embryos into the womb of a white rabbit [29]. Once that rabbit birthed a litter of black rabbits, the potential for use of IVF in humans was visualized by the scientific community. Figure 1.1 contains images of both scientists.

Early use of IVF in animals rapidly caught the public's attention as well. In the classic dystopian science fiction novel *Brave New World*, author Aldous Huxley wrote about a world populated by people grown in artificial wombs through laboratory experiments. His 1932 novel introduced the public to the possibility of a 'test tube baby' [30].

Pincus' and Chang's work with mammals inspired a generation of physician scientists around the world to pursue the fertilization of the human oocyte in vitro. In the 1940s, Menken and Rock harvested oocytes from reproductive-aged women undergoing laparotomy and were the first to publish on the fertilization and cleavage of human embryos in culture [31]. Dr Robert Edwards, an English physiologist, developed the techniques to culture and mature human oocytes in the lab. In a groundbreaking *Lancet* publication, Edwards predicted the potential of IVF to circumvent tubal factor infertility with embryo transfer through the cervix. He even suggested the potential of preimplantation screening of embryos to exhibit control over sex-linked recessive conditions (Fig. 1.2) [32]. The first biochemical

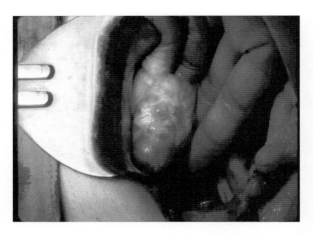

Figure1.2 Stimulated ovaries visible on laparotomy. Photo credit Dr Alan DeCherney.

pregnancy achieved through IVF was accomplished by Carl Wood, John Leeton and Alan Trounson in 1973 at Monash University; however, it resulted in an early miscarriage [33].

A British gynaecologist, Patrick Steptoe, working in the field of laparoscopy in gynaecological procedures, collaborated with Dr Edwards on the development of techniques for IVF. They successfully used hormonal medications to hyperstimulate infertile women's ovaries and used laparoscopy to collect oocytes [34]. Eventually, they used varying techniques to clean and purify sperm samples and fertilized those oocytes in a Petri dish [35]. In 1976, they successfully transplanted an embryo grown in culture into a uterus, resulting in a positive pregnancy test. Although this pregnancy was later identified as ectopic, it proved their technique was feasible [36]. They continued their pioneering work, which eventually resulted in the birth of the world's first IVF baby, Louise Brown, on 25 July 1978 in Oldham General Hospital, Manchester, United Kingdom (UK) [37].

In Australia, the Melbourne team of Wood, Leeton, Trounson and Dr Ian Johnson followed the success of Steptoe and Edwards with the birth of Candice Reed in 1980 [38]. Similar to Edwards and Steptoe, the Melbourne group had focused on natural cycle IVF for their early work.

Husband and wife team Drs Howard and Georgeanna Segar Jones further improved stimulated cycles by incorporating human menopausal gonadotropin. They established the first IVF clinic and lab in the US. Their work at the Eastern Virginia Medical School in Norfolk, Virginia, resulted in the birth of Elizabeth Jordan Carr, the first US-born IVF baby, in 1981 [39].

In France, the work of Dr Rene Frydman and Dr Jacques Testart led to the development of an assay, which could reliably predict the luteinizing hormone (LH) surge in plasma. This breakthrough allowed for improved timing of oocyte retrievals. France celebrated the birth of an IVF baby in 1982 [40].

With the field demonstrating more successes and expanding in popularity, collaboration and technology advanced. In 1976, Dr Yves Menezo developed a culture medium designed to mimic the natural environment the oocyte would be exposed to during fertilization in the fallopian tube [41]. This medium, named B2, was important in the standardization and improvement of embryology labs around the world and is still used today. From 1979–1980, the Melbourne group experimented with various catheter designs for embryo transfer and demonstrated the superiority of the Teflon-lined, open-ended catheter [42]. In 1981, Dr Robert Edwards organized an international meeting at Bourn Hall, the site of his new laboratory near Cambridge (Fig. 1.3). It was at this meeting that the superiority of stimulated cycles using clomiphene was agreed upon, thanks to the increase in oocyte yield and their ability to facilitate the timing of procedures [43]. This desire to increase the success of stimulated cycles stoked the interest of the academic community in expanding their arsenal of injectable gonadotropins.

Prior to the development of injectable gonadotropins, clomiphene was the drug of choice in ovarian stimulation. Although clomiphene was initially synthesized in 1956, it was not approved for marketing until 1967 after it was discovered that anovulatory patients taking clomiphene had higher than expected rates of pregnancy [44].

Human menopausal gonadotropins, follicle stimulating hormone (FSH) and luteinizing hormone (LH), were first extracted from the urine of postmenopausal women in 1949 and introduced into clinical practice for the management of infertility by Dr Bruno Lunenfeld in 1961 [45]. Dr Lunenfeld developed international standards for gonadotropins as well as established guidelines for classification of infertile patients and ovarian hyperstimulation syndrome resulting from infertility treatment. In 1983,

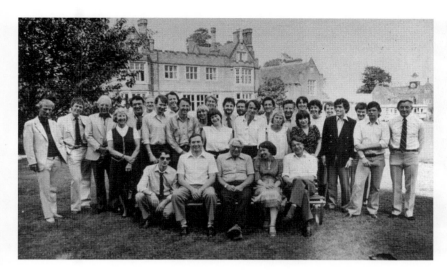

Figure 1.3 The first international meeting of IVF practitioners, organized by Dr Robert Edwards, at Bourn Hall in 1981.

high-dose human menopausal gonadotropin (hMG) was shown to be a better method for stimulation prior to oocyte retrieval and did not require serum or urinary LH monitoring because of low incidence of spontaneous ovulation [46].

Urinary preparations of LH/FSH were commonly used until more 'pure' methods were discovered using recombinant DNA/RNA technologies. Recombinant FSH and LH have since become the standard of care for use in stimulation cycles [47].

While Steptoe and Edwards had pioneered oocyte retrieval via direct visualization laparoscopy, improvements in ultrasound technology provided for safety and decreased costs incurred during the treatment of infertility. Using abdominal ultrasound, Drs Lenz and Lauritsen were able to harvest eggs percutaneously through the abdominal wall and the bladder [48]. Later, in 1983, Mount Sinai and Rush Medical Center investigators in Chicago, Illinois, demonstrated the possibility of using abdominal ultrasound with a transvaginal approach to collect human oocytes [49]. A Danish group improved on these techniques by installing a guide for the needle on the ultrasound transducer to improve visualization and subsequent yield from the procedure [50]. Dr Pierre Dellenbach, working in Strasbourg, France, was the first to demonstrate a transvaginal approach to oocyte retrieval using an abdominal ultrasound (Fig. 1.4) [51]. Following advancements in transvaginal ultrasonography, Dr David Meldrum proposed that visualization of developing oocytes was superior with the transvaginal approach and advocated for its use in oocyte retrieval [52]. Like the abdominal probes, the transducers for transvaginal ultrasound were eventually fitted with guides to aid in needle aspiration of oocytes. Transvaginal ultrasonography with transvaginal aspiration of oocytes replaced laparoscopy, resulting in decreased need for anaesthesia, decreased operative times, faster recoveries and, eventually, the ability to perform procedures in-office without the need for a traditional operating room.

Working with the Melbourne Group in Australia in 1983, Dr Trounson and his colleagues made major strides in the field of oocyte donation. Using a 42-year-old donor from whom they collected 6 oocytes, they were able to transfer an embryo into a 38-year-old recipient; the embryo implanted successfully. This pregnancy resulted in miscarriage at 10 weeks' gestation [53]; however, the same group, with the help of Dr Lutjen, used similar techniques and reported on the first baby born from oocyte donation in 1984 [54].

While treatment options for patients with absent or non-functioning ovaries were expanding, some women without a uterus began searching for options to have a genetic child of their own. In the treatment of a patient with a history of caesarean hysterectomy, a group out of Mount Sinai Medical Center in Cleveland, Ohio, was able to retrieve her oocytes and fertilize them with her husband's sperm, and later transfer an embryo into the uterus of a friend of the intended mother. The recipient of the embryo became the world's first gestational surrogate [55].

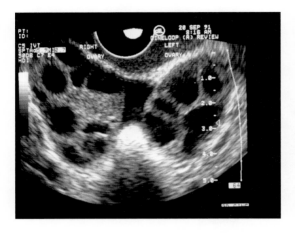

Figure 1.4 Early transvaginal ultrasound of stimulated ovaries. Photo credit Dr Alan DeCherney.

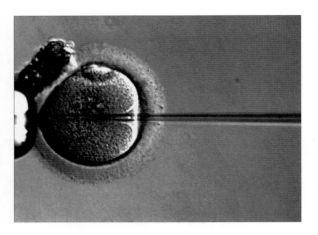

Figure 1.5 Early image of ICSI in progress. Photo credit Dr Alan DeCherney.

As oocyte retrieval procedures improved and more embryos were created in vitro, physician-scientists continued investigations into improving the implantation rate of those embryos. Jacques Cohen, an embryologist working out of Bourn Hall, noted that embryos with a thinner zona pellucida had higher implantation rates. Through this, he postulated that embryos created in the lab may have an impaired ability to hatch from the zona pellucida, an important factor in implantation, and started micromanipulating embryos to assist their ability to hatch. By making artificial defects in the zona pellucida in what would be called 'assisted hatching', they were able to improve their implantation rates from 11% to 23% [56].

As micromanipulation techniques for oocytes, spermatozoa and embryos improved, so did the treatment of male factor infertility. Efforts to bring the sperm closer to the egg, and even into the perivitelline space, under microscopy yielded mixed results. While attempting such a procedure at Vrije University in Brussels, Drs Palermo, Devroey and Van Steirteghem managed to inject spermatozoa directly into an oocyte, which eventually developed into a healthy embryo. They called this method intracytoplasmic sperm injection (ICSI) (Fig. 1.5). They published on their first successful pregnancy with this technique in 1991, which led to a successful delivery in 1992 [57]. ICSI resulted in higher fertilization rates among men with male factor infertility and rapidly became the preferred method of treating male-factor infertility.

As more techniques were developed to increase the number of embryos that were available for transfer, the need for a method of preservation became increasingly important. Using existing models of animal embryo cryopreservation, Trouson and Mohr used slow freezing and thawing techniques of 4- and 8-cell embryos to successfully store and transfer a viable embryo, which resulted in a pregnancy in 1983. The first of these pregnancies resulted in a loss secondary to premature rupture of membranes at 24 weeks' gestational age; however, one year later the group reported a successful term birth after frozen embryo transfer [58]. Vitrification, which involved the use of fast freezing and cryoprotectants to minimize damage to the embryo from ice crystal formation, was developed in 1987 [59].

Oocyte cryopreservation has gained success and popularity using similar vitrification techniques. It can be considered in patients hoping to preserve their future fertility for personal or medical reasons, including plans to undergo gonadotoxic chemotherapies. As of January 2013, the American Society for Reproductive Medicine no longer classifies oocyte cryopreservation as experimental and encourages practitioners to integrate oocyte cryopreservation into their practice [60].

With improvements in cryopreservation and the techniques of embryo micromanipulation, Edwards' theories about IVF allowing for the control over various genetic diseases have become reality. Preimplantation genetic testing (PGT) involves

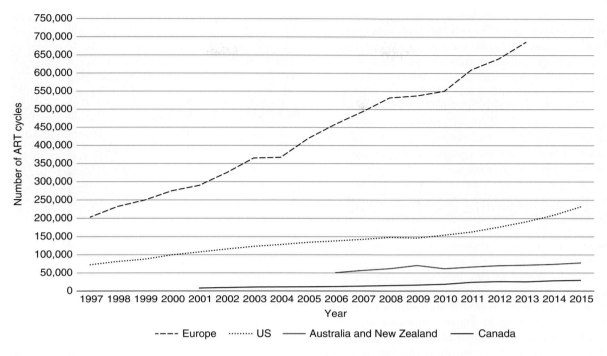

Figure 1.6 Trends in number of ART cycles in Europe, the US, Australia/New Zealand and Canada.
Sources: (1) Calhaz-Jorge C, De Geyter C, Kupka MS, et al. The European IVF-monitoring Consortium (EIM) for the European Society of Human Reproduction and Embryology (ESHRE). Assisted reproductive technology in Europe, 2013: results generated from European registers by ESHRE. *Hum Reprod*. 2017;**32**(10):1957–73; (2) www.cdc.gov/art/reports/archive.html; (3) https://npesu.unsw.edu.au/surveillance-type/annual-reports; (4) https://cfas.ca/cartr-annual-reports/.

the testing of a sample obtained from a developing embryo before embryo transfer. Techniques for the biopsy of embryos were developed in the 1980s by Wilton (cleavage stage biopsy), Verlinsky (polar body) and Muggleton-Harris (blastocyst biopsy) [53]. In 1989, Handyside et al. published on the first biopsy of a human preimplantation embryo. During their experiment, they removed a single cell from 30 embryos in the 6- to 10-cell cleavage stage and determined embryo sex via polymerase chain reaction [61]. This allowed for embryology labs and doctors treating infertility to effectively screen out sex-linked genetic disorders. They reported on the births of healthy babies from this technique in couples carrying genes for X-linked mental retardation and adrenoleukodystrophy [62]. In 1992, Munne and colleagues used fluorescence in situ hybridization (FISH) to screen for sex and ploidy status of embryos [63]. As newer technologies developed, including whole genome amplifications, microarray and next-generation sequencing, the

ability of PGT to properly screen for various genetic disorders has expanded rapidly [64].

Variations in Assisted Reproductive Technology across the Globe

The number of assisted reproductive technology (ART) cycles performed globally has increased over time (Fig. 1.6), with concurrent increases in the number of fertility clinics providing ART [67, 76, 77, 78]. Use of ART varies considerably across regions, countries and states or jurisdictions [67, 76, 77, 79]. Availability of services often depends on factors such as legal restrictions related to relationship status, sex or gender identity [67]. In high- and middle-income countries, the average cost for one fresh IVF procedure is estimated to be $4,950 (USD) and ranges from $1,800 to $13,000 per treatment cycle [80]. Lack of reimbursement of treatment costs is a barrier to accessing ART services [80, 81]; however, there are considerable differences in subsidization of fertility treatments across countries [67, 80]. In a recent surveillance report from the International Federation of Fertility Societies (IFFS), only 37 of 70 responding countries reported that insurance coverage or government funding was available for fertility treatments [67]. Moreover, funding for treatments is often limited based on fertility status (primary versus secondary), duration of infertility, income and age [67]. Likewise, certain procedures such as ICSI, assisted hatching, preimplantation genetic testing, cryopreservation of eggs or embryos and use of donor eggs or sperm or a gestational carrier may be exempt from reimbursement, depending on the patient's country of residence [67].

In addition to economic barriers to treatment, there may be other obstacles that prevent certain populations from accessing ART or policies that restrict the use of specific procedures. For example, some countries and jurisdictions have regulations or professional guidelines requiring couples to be heterosexual and/or legally married to access ART [67]. Other regulations may apply to use of egg or embryo cryopreservation for non-medical conditions, third-party reproduction (e.g. use of donor gametes, embryos or a gestational carrier), selective reduction, preimplantation genetic testing or fertility preservation [67].

Other differences in the practice of ART across countries have also been noted. For instance, there is some evidence that starting gonadotropin doses are higher in the US than in Europe [82]. In addition, while the rate of single embryo transfer (SET) has been increasing overall, country- or continent-specific SET rates are variable. In 2010, Australia/ New Zealand, Europe and Asia had the highest SET rates, while Latin America, sub-Saharan Africa and North America had the lowest rates [77]. Explanations for variations in SET rates may include reimbursement policies, implementation of clinical care guidelines and patient preference [67].

Conclusion

Infertility is an important global public health problem. In the absence of a standard definition of infertility, it is difficult to compare prevalence estimates across populations; however, it is estimated that nearly 50 million couples worldwide are infertile [2]. ART has emerged as a fundamental treatment for infertility, with a century of investigation and collaboration propelling the field of ART towards the success and popularity it currently holds. Globally, access to and utilization of ART are variable and influenced by reimbursement policies, as well as the adoption of legal restrictions and guidelines in the country or jurisdiction where the procedure takes place.

Acknowledgements

Nola Herlihy, MD, and Karissa Hammer, MD, contributed to the content of this chapter.

References

1. Zegers-Hochschild F, Adamson GD, Dyer S, Racowsky C, de Mouzon J, Sokol R, et al. The International Glossary on Infertility and Fertility Care, 2017. *Hum Reprod*. 2017;**32**(9): 1786–801.

2. Mascarenhas MN, Flaxman SR, Boerma T, Vanderpoel S, Stevens GA. National, regional, and global trends in infertility prevalence since 1990: a systematic analysis of 277 health surveys. *PLoS Med*. 2012;**9**(12):e1001356.

3. Practice Committee of American Society for Reproductive Medicine. Definitions of infertility and recurrent pregnancy loss: a committee opinion. *Fertil Steril*. 2013;**99**(1):63.

4. Larsen U. Research on infertility: which definition should we use? *Fertil Steril*. 2005;**83**(4):846–52.

5. Gurunath S, Pandian Z, Anderson RA, Bhattacharya S. Defining infertility – a systematic review of prevalence studies. *Hum Reprod Update*. 2011;**17**(5):575–88.

6. Hollos M. Infertility: demographic aspects. In JD Wright (ed.), *International Encyclopedia of the Social & Behavioral Sciences*, 2nd edn. Amsterdam: Elsevier; 2015. pp.45–9.

7. Mascarenhas MN, Cheung H, Mathers CD, Stevens GA. Measuring infertility in populations: constructing a standard definition for use with demographic and reproductive health surveys. *Popul Health Metr*. 2012;**10**(1):17.

8. Chandra A, Copen CE, Stephen EH. Infertility and impaired fecundity in the United States, 1982–2010: data from the National Survey of Family Growth. *Natl Health Stat Report*. 2013 (67):1–18.

9. Bushnik T, Cook JL, Yuzpe AA, Tough S, Collins J. Estimating the prevalence of infertility in Canada. *Hum Reprod*. 2012;**27**(3):738–46.

10. Eijkemans MJ, van Poppel F, Habbema DF, Smith KR, Leridon H, te Velde ER. Too old to have children? Lessons from natural fertility populations. *Hum Reprod*. 2014;**29**(6):1304–12.

11. Wesselink AK, Rothman KJ, Hatch EE, Mikkelsen EM, Sorensen HT, Wise LA. Age and fecundability in a North American preconception cohort study. *Am J Obstet Gynecol.* 2017;**217**(6):667 e1–e8.

12. Mathews TJ, Hamilton BE. Mean age of mothers is on the rise: United States, 2000–2014. *NCHS Data Brief.* 2016(232):1–8.

13. Milan A. *Fertility: Overview, 2009 to 2011.* Ottawa, Canada: Statistics Canada; 9 July 2013.

14. Mills M, Rindfuss RR, McDonald P, te Velde E, ESHRE Reproduction and Society Task Force. Why do people postpone parenthood? Reasons and social policy incentives. *Hum Reprod Update.* 2011;**17**(6): 848–60.

15. Practice Committee of the American Society for Reproductive Medicine in collaboration with the Society for Reproduction and Infertility. Optimizing natural fertility: a committee opinion. *Fertil Steril.* 2017;**107**(1):52–8.

16. Exposure to toxic environmental agents. ACO Committee Opinion No. 575. *Obstet Gynecol.* 2013;**122** (4):931–5.

17. Practice Committee of the American Society for Reproductive Medicine. Smoking and infertility: a committee opinion. *Fertil Steril.* 2012;**98**(6):1400–6.

18. Wiesenfeld HC, Hillier SL, Meyn LA, Amortegui AJ, Sweet RL. Subclinical pelvic inflammatory disease and infertility. *Obstet Gynecol.* 2012;**120**(1):37–43.

19. Eisenberg ML, Meldrum D. Effects of age on fertility and sexual function. *Fertil Steril.* 2017;**107**(2):301–4.

20. Sharma R, Agarwal A, Rohra VK, Assidi M, Abu-Elmagd M, Turki RF. Effects of increased paternal age on sperm quality, reproductive outcome and associated epigenetic risks to offspring. *Reprod Biol Endocrinol.* 2015;**13**:35.

21. Barratt CLR, Bjorndahl L, De Jonge CJ, Lamb DJ, Osorio Martini F, McLachlan R, et al. The diagnosis of male infertility: an analysis of the evidence to support the development of global WHO guidance-challenges and future research opportunities. *Hum Reprod Update.* 2017;**23**(6):660–80.

22. Ricci E, Al Beitawi S, Cipriani S, Candiani M, Chiaffarino F, Vigano P, et al. Semen quality and alcohol intake: a systematic review and meta-analysis. *Reprod Biomed Online.* 2017;**34**(1):38–47.

23. du Plessis SS, Agarwal A, Syriac A. Marijuana, phytocannabinoids, the endocannabinoid system, and male fertility. *J Assist Reprod Genet.* 2015;**32**(11):1575–88.

24. Harlev A, Agarwal A, Gunes SO, Shetty A, du Plessis SS. Smoking and male infertility: an evidence-based review. *World J Mens Health.* 2015;**33**(3):143–60.

25. Fronczak CM, Kim ED, Barqawi AB. The insults of illicit drug use on male fertility. *J Androl.* 2012;**33**(4): 515–28.

26. Levine H, Jorgensen N, Martino-Andrade A, Mendiola J, Weksler-Derri D, Mindlis I, et al. Temporal trends in sperm count: a systematic review and meta-regression analysis. *Hum Reprod Update.* 2017;**23**(6):646–59.

27. Brind'Amour K, Garcia B, Wilhelm August Oscar Hertwig (1849–1922). In *The Embryo Project Encyclopedia.* Tempe, AZ: The Embryo Project at Arizona State University; 2007, modified 2015. Available at: http://embryo.asu.edu/handle/10776/1707.

28. Pincus G, Enzmann EV. The comparative behavior of mammalian eggs in vivo and in vitro: I. The activation of ovarian eggs. *J Exp Med.* 1935;**62**(5):665–75.

29. Chang MC. Fertilization of rabbit ova in vitro. *Nature.* 1959;**184**(Suppl 7):466–7.

30. Huxley A. *Brave New World.* New York: Harper & Bros.; 1932.

31. Menkin MF, Rock J. In vitro fertilization and cleavage of human ovarian eggs. *Am J Obstet Gynecol.* 1948;**55** (3):440–52.

32. Edwards RG. Maturation in vitro of human ovarian oocytes. *Lancet.* 1965;**2**(7419):926–9.

33. De Kretzer D, Dennis P, Hudson B, Leeton J, Lopata A, Outch K, et al. Transfer of a human zygote. *Lancet.* 1973;**2**(7831):728–9.

34. Steptoe PC, Edwards RG. Laparoscopic recovery of preovulatory human oocytes after priming of ovaries with gonadotrophins. *Lancet.* 1970;**1**(7649):683–9.

35. Steptoe PC, Edwards RG, Purdy JM. Human blastocysts grown in culture. *Nature.* 1971;**229**(5280):132–3.

36. Steptoe PC, Edwards RG. Reimplantation of a human embryo with subsequent tubal pregnancy. *Lancet.* 1976;**1**(7965):880–2.

37. Steptoe PC, Edwards RG. Birth after the reimplantation of a human embryo. *Lancet.* 1978;**2** (8085):366.

38. Lopata A, Johnston IW, Hoult IJ, Speirs AI. Pregnancy following intrauterine implantation of an embryo obtained by in vitro fertilization of a preovulatory egg. *Fertil Steril.* 1980;**33**(2):117–20.

39. Sullivan W. 'Test-tube' baby born in US, joining successes around the world. *New York Times;* 29 December 1981.

40. Cohen J, Trounson A, Dawson K, Jones H, Hazekamp J, Nygren KG, et al. The early days of IVF outside the UK. *Hum Reprod Update.* 2005;**11**(5):439–59.

41. Menezo Y. [Synthetic medium for gamete survival and maturation and for culture of fertilized eggs]. *C R Acad*

Sci Hebd Seances Acad Sci D. 1976;**282**(22):1967–70. [In French.]

42. Leeton J, Trounson A, Jessup D, Wood C. The technique for human embryo transfer. *Fertil Steril*. 1982;**38**(2):156–61.

43. Cohen J, Jones HW, Jr. In vitro fertilization: the first three decades. In DK Gardner (ed.), *In Vitro Fertilization: A Practical Approach*. New York: CRC Press; 2006. pp.1–15.

44. Dickey RP, Holtkamp DE. Development, pharmacology and clinical experience with clomiphene citrate. *Hum Reprod Update*. 1996;**2**(6):483–506.

45. Lunenfeld B. Historical perspectives in gonadotrophin therapy. *Hum Reprod Update*. 2004;**10**(6):453–67.

46. Laufer N, DeCherney AH, Haseltine FP, Polan ML, Mezer HC, Dlugi AM, et al. The use of high-dose human menopausal gonadotropin in an in vitro fertilization program. *Fertil Steril*. 1983;**40**(6):734–41.

47. Practice Committee of American Society for Reproductive Medicine, Birmingham Alabama. Gonadotropin preparations: past, present, and future perspectives. *Fertil Steril*. 2008;**90**(Suppl 5):S13–20.

48. Lenz S, Lauritsen JG. Ultrasonically guided percutaneous aspiration of human follicles under local anesthesia: a new method of collecting oocytes for in vitro fertilization. *Fertil Steril*. 1982;**38**(6):673–7.

49. Gleicher N, Friberg J, Fullan N, Giglia RV, Mayden K, Kesky T, et al. EGG retrieval for in vitro fertilisation by sonographically controlled vaginal culdocentesis. *Lancet*. 1983;**2**(8348):508–9.

50. Wikland M, Nilsson L, Hansson R, Hamberger L, Janson PO. Collection of human oocytes by the use of sonography. *Fertil Steril*. 1983;**39**(5):603–8.

51. Dellenbach P, Nisand I, Moreau L, Feger B, Plumere C, Gerlinger P, et al. Transvaginal, sonographically controlled ovarian follicle puncture for egg retrieval. *Lancet*. 1984;**1**(8392):1467.

52. Meldrum DR, Chetkowski RJ, Steingold KA, Randle D. Transvaginal ultrasound scanning of ovarian follicles. *Fertil Steril*. 1984;**42**(5):803–5.

53. Trounson A, Leeton J, Besanko M, Wood C, Conti A. Pregnancy established in an infertile patient after transfer of a donated embryo fertilised in vitro. *Br Med J (Clin Res Ed)*. 1983;**286**(6368):835–8.

54. Lutjen P, Trounson A, Leeton J, Findlay J, Wood C, Renou P. The establishment and maintenance of pregnancy using in vitro fertilization and embryo donation in a patient with primary ovarian failure. *Nature*. 1984;**307**(5947):174–5.

55. Utian WH, Sheean L, Goldfarb JM, Kiwi R. Successful pregnancy after in vitro fertilization and embryo transfer from an infertile woman to a surrogate. *N Engl J Med*. 1985;**313**(21):1351–2.

56. Cohen J, Elsner C, Kort H, Malter H, Massey J, Mayer MP, et al. Impairment of the hatching process following IVF in the human and improvement of implantation by assisting hatching using micromanipulation. *Hum Reprod*. 1990;**5**(1):7–13.

57. Palermo G, Joris H, Devroey P, Van Steirteghem AC. Pregnancies after intracytoplasmic injection of single spermatozoon into an oocyte. *Lancet*. 1992;**340**(8810):17–18.

58. Trounson A, Mohr L. Human pregnancy following cryopreservation, thawing and transfer of an eight-cell embryo. *Nature*. 1983;**305**(5936):707–9.

59. Trounson A, Peura A, Kirby C. Ultrarapid freezing: a new low-cost and effective method of embryo cryopreservation. *Fertil Steril*. 1987;**48**(5):843–50.

60. Practice Committees of American Society for Reproductive Medicine; Society for Assisted Reproductive Technology. Mature oocyte cryopreservation: a guideline. *Fertil Steril*. 2013;**99**(1):37–43.

61. Handyside AH, Pattinson JK, Penketh RJ, Delhanty JD, Winston RM, Tuddenham EG. Biopsy of human preimplantation embryos and sexing by DNA amplification. *Lancet*. 1989;**1**(8634):347–9.

62. Handyside AH, Kontogianni EH, Hardy K, Winston RM. Pregnancies from biopsied human preimplantation embryos sexed by Y-specific DNA amplification. *Nature*. 1990;**344**(6268):768–70.

63. Munne S, Lee A, Rosenwaks Z, Grifo J, Cohen J. Diagnosis of major chromosome aneuploidies in human preimplantation embryos. *Hum Reprod*. 1993;**8**(12):2185–91.

64. Fiorentino F, Bono S, Biricik A, Nuccitelli A, Cotroneo E, Cottone G, et al. Application of next-generation sequencing technology for comprehensive aneuploidy screening of blastocysts in clinical preimplantation genetic screening cycles. *Hum Reprod*. 2014;**29**(12):2802–13.

65. Lancaster PA. Registers of in-vitro fertilization and assisted conception. *Hum Reprod*. 1996;**11**(Suppl 4):89–104; discussion 5–9.

66. International Federation of Fertility Societies International Conference. IFFS Surveillance 98. *Fertil Steril*. 1999;**71**(5 Suppl 2): 1S–34S.

67. International Federation of Fertility Societies. IFFS Surveillance 2016. *Global Reproductive Health*. 2016;**1**(e1):1–143.

68. Brown S. *ESHRE: The First 21 Years*. Grimbergen, Belgium: ESHRE; 2005.

69. European Society of Human Reproduction and Embryology. *ESHRE Annual Report 2016*. Grimbergen, Belgium, ESHRE; 2017.

70. Nygren KG, Andersen AN. Assisted reproductive technology in Europe, 1997. Results generated from European registers by ESHRE. European IVF-Monitoring Programme (EIM), for the European Society of Human Reproduction and Embryology (ESHRE). *Hum Reprod*. 2001;**16**(2):384–91.

71. Mlsna LJ. Stem cell based treatments and novel considerations for conscience clause legislation. *Indiana Health Law Review*. 2010;**8**(2):471–96.

72. President Clinton's Comments on NIH and Human Embryo Research. U.S. National Archives; 1994.

73. Dunn K. The politics of stem cells. *Nova Science Now*. 2005. Available at: www.pbs.org/wgbh/nova/science now/dispatches/050413.html.

74. Duka WED, DeCherney AH. *From the Beginning: A History of the American Fertility Society, 1944–1994*. Washington, DC: American Fertility Society; 1994.

75. Toner JP, Coddington CC, Doody K, Van Voorhis B, Seifer DB, Ball GD, et al. Society for Assisted Reproductive Technology and assisted reproductive technology in the United States: a 2016 update. *Fertil Steril*. 2016;**106**(3):541–6.

76. European IV-Monitoring Consortium, European Society of Human Reproduction and Embryology, Calhaz-Jorge C, De Geyter C, Kupka MS, et al. Assisted reproductive technology in Europe, 2013: results generated from European registers by ESHRE. *Hum Reprod*. 2017;**32**(10):1957–73.

77. Dyer S, Chambers GM, de Mouzon J, Nygren KG, Zegers-Hochschild F, Mansour R, et al. International Committee for Monitoring Assisted Reproductive Technologies world report: assisted reproductive technology 2008, 2009 and 2010. *Hum Reprod*. 2016;**31**(7):1588–609.

78. Centers for Disease Control and Prevention, American Society for Reproductive Medicine, Society for Assisted Reproductive Technology. *2015 Assisted Reproductive Technology National Summary Report*. Atlanta, GA; 2017.

79. Sunderam S, Kissin DM, Crawford SB, Folger SG, Boulet SL, Warner L, et al. Assisted reproductive technology surveillance – United States, 2015. *MMWR Surveill Summ*. 2018;**67**(3):1–28.

80. Chambers GM, Adamson GD, Eijkemans MJ. Acceptable cost for the patient and society. *Fertil Steril*. 2013;**100**(2):319–27.

81. Farley Ordovensky Staniec J, Webb NJ. Utilization of infertility services: how much does money matter? *Health Serv Res*. 2007;**42**(3 Pt 1):971–89.

82. Baker VL, Jones CE, Cometti B, Hoehler F, Salle B, Urbancsek J, et al. Factors affecting success rates in two concurrent clinical IVF trials: an examination of potential explanations for the difference in pregnancy rates between the United States and Europe. *Fertil Steril*. 2010;**94**(4):1287–91.

Chapter

2

Importance and History of ART Surveillance

Jacques de Mouzon, Paul Lancaster and Anders Nyboe Andersen

Introduction

In the 1980s it became clear that the newly developed in vitro fertilization (IVF) would rapidly be implemented in clinical practice. Professionals, patients and society therefore soon realized that even though the quantitative impact of IVF as treatment for infertility remained limited in the 1980s, there was a need for data about the safety of the technology. Indeed, published reports from single fertility clinics [1, 2] soon made it apparent that a number of important health concerns were related to the new technique, and solid data would require large samples that would optimally be obtained if national registries were established [3].

The first concern was whether children born via assisted reproductive technology (ART) had an increased risk of congenital disorders including malformations. Perhaps hitherto unseen malformations, syndromes and specific diseases would occur. This fear was evidently related to the radical and completely novel approach of in vitro handling of female gametes and embryos, and later on to oocyte donation, intracytoplasmic sperm injection (ICSI) and cryopreservation and preimplantation genetic testing.

The second concern was related to the practice of replacing several embryos, as was done in the early period of ART. This caused a huge increase in multiples, including triplets and quadruplets [3], with the inherent risks of preterm births of infants with a poor neonatal outcome and poor long-term outcome for the children.

The third concern was related to the immediate maternal risks. Evidently, the rise in multiple gestations had implications for both infant and maternal health, but additionally the introduction of aggressive gonadotropin stimulation to induce growth of multiple follicles caused an epidemic in ovarian hyperstimulation syndrome (OHSS) in the treated women. Some of these women became critically ill, and the media indeed reported on the dangers of IVF.

The fourth concern was related to long-term maternal risks. In the early 1990s, it was suggested that women exposed to repeated gonadotropin stimulation could have a long-term risk of developing severe disorders such as ovarian cancer [4]. In order to monitor such possible risks in appropriate follow-up studies, it was crucial to know the identity of treated women.

Therefore, the early development of ART surveillance was driven by safety concerns, in particular for the infants; for example, the first national recordings on ART in Sweden, Norway and Finland were based on screening and identification of pregnant women who attended antenatal care. Those who were pregnant after IVF were identified by the midwives in order to report that the newborns were conceived in vitro. Thus, registry data were based on the pregnant mothers and the infants they delivered – but no data at all were available on unsuccessful ART treatments as later reviewed by Henningsen et al. [5].

Even though the number of ART infants was very low during the 1980s, it gradually became apparent that the health of ART infants was generally good, at least among singletons. Society was thus reassured concerning safety and indeed by large single centre [6, 7] and national data [3]; Westergaard et al. [8] showed that overall there were no major health concerns with singletons born via ART.

After the early years of addressing the safety concerns, registries gradually developed to include several aspects of ART. One development was to improve the methods of data collection. Registry data were initially summary data, and still remain so from many countries, but the trend has been to obtain specific person-related data on individual cycles. This would allow more detailed analyses of outcomes, and in a number of countries identification of the couples allowed cross-linking of ART data to other health registries [9].

Overall, the main areas of focus for ART registries and the general importance of the surveillance systems that have been developed over 35 years may be summarized under three main headings: efficacy, safety and society.

General Importance of Surveillance

Efficacy

The purpose of ART treatment is the delivery of a healthy infant, and treatment efficacy remains the main determinant of any ART registry. As only a fraction of ART treatments is successful in terms of achieving live pregnancies, efficacy will involve both a numerator and a denominator, as, for instance, the traditional recording of the percentage of pregnancies per transfers, but it is clear that changes in both the numerator and the denominator will influence the percentage.

Efficacy will depend on three important issues:

1. Which numerator and denominator are used
2. How they are defined
3. How consistently and precisely the parameters are recorded in clinical practice

The Numerator and the Denominator

With efficacy reporting, the numerator may be pregnancy, but it is often defined differently. It could be a positive human chorionic gonadotropin (hCG) test, a clinical pregnancy with or without a live fetus or an ongoing live pregnancy at a certain gestational age. The numerator may also be a live birth. The latter is evidently a more appropriate end point than just pregnancies, but the drawback, and the reason why this was rarely used in the first years of ART registries, was that precise follow-up on deliveries was often not done or often not even possible – a large proportion of missing information.

Similarly, the denominator in a single stimulated ART cycle could be per initiated cycle, oocyte aspiration or embryo transfer. If cryopreserved embryos/blastocysts are used, the denominator could be either thawing or transfer. Cancellation of embryo transfer for various reasons means that the number of oocyte retrievals is a better parameter than the number of transfers to use as denominator. Additionally, some stimulated cycles are cancelled before aspiration, and thus the number of stimulated cycles begun using expensive gonadotropin stimulation is a more appropriate parameter than oocyte retrievals. The results of efficacy reporting were typically related to a single stimulated cycle but, as discussed later, the results would be highly dependent on the parameters that were put into the equation. Additionally, as discussed in later chapters, there are several reasons why the end point of an initiated cycle should be modified. The most important change has been the attempts to report cumulative birth rates after one stimulated cycle, including all births after replacement of frozen-thawed embryos or blastocysts, as detailed in Chapter 5, Reporting ART Success Rates.

Definition of Parameters Used

The second important aspect was how the parameters, such as pregnancy, were defined. Collecting national data from different countries, as, for instance, done by the European IVF Monitoring (EIM) Consortium of the European Society of Human Reproduction and Embryology (ESHRE) or by the International Committee Monitoring Assisted Reproductive Technologies (ICMART), it was apparent that there was a need to standardize the definitions. As discussed in later chapters (see Chapter 11, Global ART Surveillance: The International Committee Monitoring Assisted Reproductive Technologies (ICMART)), the work to develop and renew the definitions (see Appendix B, International Glossary on Infertility and Fertility Care) has been made by the international collaboration of ICMART and the World Health Organization (WHO), resulting in publications of updated consensus glossaries in order to harmonize the parameters that are used for reporting [10, 11, 12].

How Consistently and Precisely the Parameters Are Recorded in Clinical Practice

A third important aspect has been how consistently and accurately a parameter is recorded by the clinicians and clinics providing data to the registry. A good example is reporting of birth or live birth rates. How do you, for instance, ensure that a clinic has 100% follow-up on all pregnancies using donor oocytes, including those deliveries that may occur among foreign patients using cross-border reproductive care? In practice, data on the main efficacy parameter, which is live birth, are therefore often missing.

To summarize, even the simplest recording of efficacy per single treatment requires use of a strict definition of all recordings and complete follow-up of the end points – for instance, deliveries. In general, the lowest ratios are the most informative, such as live births per initiated cycle, and this remains the key figure reported in the annual report of national registries, as well as documented from the United States (US) [13].

Developments in Efficacy Reporting

New developments in ART include fewer embryos transferred, more embryos frozen and more use of a 'freeze-all' approach, so the most appropriate single figure for success in ART may be the total (cumulative) number of live births per initiated stimulation cycle, including those live births that resulted from cryopreserved embryos/blastocysts from that cycle. The impact of the frozen embryo replacement (FER) treatments is obviously much more important today, when the number of fresh embryos replaced is reduced and the proportion of FER cycles is increasing [14]. However, the requirements to be able to record such data on a national basis are indeed complex, as discussed in later chapters. In the annual reports, the European IVF Monitoring Consortium as part of ESHRE has for many years published an estimate of the cumulative pregnancy rate from a selected number of countries [14]. This estimate is based on the number of births/ pregnancies from all fresh cycles and all FER cycles for a specific year. As all FER treatments are the result of earlier 'fresh' cycles, this is likely to represent a good and clinically useful estimate of the cumulative efficacy of single fresh cycles. Recently, specific data from the Human Fertilisation and Embryology Authority (HFEA) in the United Kingdom (UK) have provided such cumulative birth rates after a single stimulated cycle [15]. Those registries that may be able to trace individuals over time, and when treated at different clinics, may even extend the concept of 'cumulative' birth rates to include several fresh stimulated cycles and the resulting FER cycles. Such overall cumulative efficacy data have been recorded from single clinics, and lately national registry-based datasets [15, 16].

In conclusion, registry data based on identification of individual women and men may allow extension of single cycle efficacy end points to cumulative end points after one or even several stimulated cycles. Such recordings are not currently available in summarized forms for the registry data themselves but are related to research projects using the ART registry data. These important aspects are discussed in detail in later chapters.

How Efficacy Parameters Are Used

The main reason why efficacy data are important for patients, ART professionals and society may be summarized in the following:

1. To provide patients with a reliable and realistic estimate about their chance for pregnancy or birth per cycle, and over repetitive cycles. Single public and private clinics generally provide their results, but there are indeed examples of rather selective recording of data. Selective presentation of data should be avoided. Patients can use registry data to find out their chance of birth per cycle in relation to the most important and consistent factor: female age at treatment.

2. To allow patients to know their cumulative prognosis for live birth either over time or over a number of successive cycles.

3. To allow professionals in each clinic to benchmark with national data.

4. To follow changes over time as part of the overall development in the technology and the patients exposed to these technologies.

5. To follow changes over time when introducing specific new approaches, for example, changes in efficacy with a shift from dual to single embryo transfer or a shift from slow freezing to vitrification.

6. To characterize success rates with different treatment modalities. How does standard IVF/ ICSI compare with preimplantation genetic diagnosis (PGD)/preimplantation genetic testing (PGT) for aneuploidy or oocyte donation?

Safety

In terms of safety, the treated women, professionals and society in general would like to know not only the immediate maternal complications of treatments, such as OHSS, ovarian torsion or bleeding following oocyte retrieval, but also possible long-term maternal risks of repeated ovarian stimulation. In terms of safety for the infants, there may also be immediate risks related to the newborns, such as preterm birth, stillbirth, congenital malformations or syndromes, as well as possible long-term risk of child morbidity.

Regarding the immediate risks for the treated women, such as OHSS, such data are often reported in the registries [14]. In principle, the data should thus be accurate, but there are several reasons why this may not always be the case. OHSS may occur weeks after embryo transfer in the early pregnancy, during which the woman may be admitted to another hospital. Indeed, it seems that gross underreporting may occur. For example, in the UK, the *Daily Mail* reported the official reporting system included only 16 to 60 annual cases of OHSS from 2010 to 2016. However, if data were drawn from the hospital discharge registries, 691 to 836 OHSS cases were reported. This illustrates a challenge to registries to ensure correct reporting [17].

In the early days of ART, data on outcomes of treatment included small hospital series describing infant health, but one of the strengths of national registries is their large sample size. With large datasets, it would be less likely to have coincidental findings of an apparent association. One example of this was the proposal by Dutch researchers that ART increased the risk of retinoblastomas [18]. The study from the Netherlands using expanded national data by Marees et al. [19] illustrates the value of large national data in order to assess whether specific and rare diseases are truly related to the ART technology.

In terms of immediate and long-term safety risks for both children and the mothers, registry data are today used to cross-link the parents as well as the children with other registries already available (see Chapter 9, Monitoring Long-Term Outcomes of ART: Linking ART Surveillance Data with Other Datasets). Huge datasets have been available from large countries such as the US, the UK and France, as well as combined analyses from Australia and New Zealand and the Nordic countries [20].

Another important aspect related to safety is the vigilance of ART registries in identifying possible safety issues involving new techniques, for example, the rapid introduction of ICSI, changes from slow-freezing methods to vitrification or the change from replacing cleavage-stage embryos to blastocysts. Registries thus have to develop and include recordings of new approaches. These aspects are discussed in Chapter 7, Monitoring ART Safety and Biovigilance.

Society

ART has a number of stakeholders, not only couples seeking ART as treatment, fertility clinics, ART professionals and the industry that provide drugs and equipment, but also society in general and the political systems that directly or indirectly allocate resources to ART and the regulatory authorities being responsible for health surveillance. In addition, the public in general and the media have an interest in ART data as they provide data on birth and the extent to which ART contributes to national birth rates.

Society, Ethics and Legislators. Handling of female gametes in vitro introduced a number of new treatment modalities such as egg donation, embryo donation, surrogacy and use of donor sperm in single or lesbian women. These treatments raised concerns in relation to ethics, law and regulations, as well as concerns about the psychological and physical health issues related to such techniques. Stories that appeared in the mainstream press of, for instance, postmenopausal women delivering preterm triplets after egg donation raised demands for regulation. The political system, health authorities and other regulators wanted data to assess the quantity of such treatments in order to allow/forbid certain activities.

Cost, Access to and Impact of Treatment. Australia and the EIM introduced the concept of number of treatment cycles per million inhabitants or per million women of reproductive age. These data gave useful information about to what extent ART was available and accessible in the country, and it soon became apparent that large differences existed regarding the utilization of ART, even among countries with similar wealth. In the US, marked differences were seen from state to state in the utilization of ART, as clearly shown by registry data [13]. Additionally, the EIM started a systematic comparison of the percentage of infants born after ART, and it became clear that ART had a measurable impact on the overall birth rates in many societies. In Europe, the European Parliament incorporated ART data in their *Report on the Demographic Future of Europe* from 2008, where it 'calls on the Member States to ensure the right of couples to guarantee universal access to infertility treatment and medically assisted procreation by taking steps with a view to reducing the financial and other obstacles'. This important statement was unlikely to have been presented if solid data on the impact of ART across Europe had not already been available.

Historical Development

Very early, gathering data for a better understanding of ART practice and results appeared necessary among professionals in several countries, and the registries' setup history can be described in three steps: national, world and regional, with some overlap.

General History

National Registries

Australia and France began ART data collection in 1983. In Australia [21], the first IVF pregnancy had been conceived in 1979, and the first report, based on 309 IVF pregnancies, collected retrospectively, was published in 1984, with just over 200 IVF pregnancies conceived by early 1983, followed by annual reports [3]. In France, ART professionals started a registry based on data summary sheets one year after the first French IVF birth in1982, and the data were presented at national meetings from 1982 to 1985. From January 1986, this became a cycle-based registry, with annual publications [22, 23, 24, 25].

Several other countries also began registries in the mid-1980s. In the US, the first report contained data for 1985 and 1986 [26, 27]. It was initially based on data summaries. It then became a cycle-based registry, and the Centers for Disease Control and Prevention (CDC) began ART data collection in 1995, as mandated by law (Public Law 102–493, 24 October 1992), in collaboration with the Society for Assisted Reproductive Technology (SART) [28].

In the UK, in March 1985 a Voluntary Licensing Authority (VLA) was created by the Medical Research Council and the Royal College of Obstetricians and Gynaecologists [29, 30]. In 1989, the VLA changed its name to the Interim Licensing Authority for Human In Vitro Fertilization and Embryology to better reflect its temporary status. Finally, in 1990, the Human Fertilisation and Embryology Act (HFEA) was passed by both Houses of Parliament and received Royal Assent, and the HFEA became fully operational in August 1991. The Voluntary Licensing Authority for Human In Vitro Fertilization and Embryology published a brief summary of pregnancy rates for 1985 in its Second Report in 1987. A more detailed analysis of the outcome of pregnancies for the period 1978–1987 was published later, based on a registry of children born after IVF and originally established in 1983 [31].

In Germany, in vitro fertilization groups have been voluntarily participating in a national IVF registry since 1982 and, since 1991, an annual report has been published [32, 33, 34]. By 2000, the General Directive for Assisted Reproduction, issued by the German Medical Association, had been implemented across Germany and the participation in the German IVF registry (D·I·R Registry) became compulsory for each centre. In 2009, the registry adopted its present legal form. Many countries then started national data collection, such as Belgium in 1989 [35, 36], Canada in 1999 [37], Israel [38] and Switzerland in 1992 [39].

In recent years, many other countries have either started registries or provided pooled data for international reports. Countries that have now reported their results in journals or separate reports include Belgium, Canada, the Czech Republic, Japan, Latin American countries, the Nordic countries and Taiwan.

World Registry

The idea of sharing experiences on ART at an international level appeared relatively early. Initially, data on IVF were obtained from individual IVF centres around the world and results were presented at international conferences and later published. The first concerned the cycles performed before 1984 by 65 teams reporting information on 10,028 cycles [40]. A report was then published on the cycles performed in 1985 by 55 centres on 2,432 pregnancies [41].

The first formal meeting of professionals responsible for national registries was held in Oxford in September 1990, through the initiative of P. Lancaster and J. de Mouzon, with representatives of countries in which national registries on IVF already existed or were planned. It was decided to create the International Working Group for Registers on Assisted Reproduction (IWGROAR). The main aim of this group was to collaborate on the realization of an international data collecting system.

As a preliminary step, a world report concerning the procedures performed during 1989 was established by the executive committee of the 7th World Congress on In Vitro Fertilization and Assisted Reproductive Technology in Paris (20 June – 3 July 1991) [42]. This report included information from 24 countries, 469 centres and 76,030 aspiration cycles. This was the real first world report. Due to the success of this first experience, the scientific committee for the 8th World Congress in Kyoto (12–15 September 1993) decided to repeat this experience and to create a world report on the procedures realized during 1991. Jean Cohen was charged with undertaking this report, in collaboration with IWGROAR (P. Lancaster and J. de Mouzon). For this report [43], data were obtained from:

- Established national registries (Belgium, Canada, Czechoslovakia, France, Germany, Greece, Israel, Italy, Japan, Netherlands, Singapore, Slovenia, Taiwan, UK, US), regional registries (Australia–New Zealand, Latin America [Argentina, Brazil, Chile, Colombia, Ecuador, Mexico, Panama, Paraguay and Venezuela], and the Nordic countries [Denmark, Finland, Iceland, Norway and Sweden])

- Individual centres where a national registry was not established (Austria, Egypt, India, Ireland, South Korea, Morocco, Pakistan, Poland, Portugal, Russia, Saudi Arabia, South Africa, Spain, Switzerland, Turkey)

This report was based on 13 forms with data summaries describing cycles and outcomes, age, infertility cause, ovulation induction, number of transferred embryos, multiple pregnancies and their outcomes (including gestational age) and birth defects. In total, this report included 46 countries and 760 clinics, 138,238 oocyte aspiration cycles (increase of 55%), 26,411 clinical pregnancies (increase of 70%) and 19,319 live births (increase of 90%).

IWGROAR then published biennial world reports. These reports covered treatments performed in 1993, 1995, 1996 and 1998. They were presented at world congresses on ART in Montpellier [44], Vancouver [45], San Francisco [46] and Melbourne [47], respectively. In 2001, IWGROAR changed its name to the International Committee Monitoring Assisted Reproductive Technologies (ICMART). ICMART created the world reports for cycles performed in 2000 and 2002; from 2003, these were reported annually. Since 2002, all preliminary reports were presented at the annual ESHRE meetings and all reports were published alternatively in *Human Reproduction* and *Fertility and Sterility* [48–58].

Since the first report on 1991 cycles [43] until the last on those for 2014, IWGROAR/ICMART coverage increased gradually, in terms of number of participating countries (from 46 to 77), clinics (from 760 to 2,734), cycles (from 138,238 to 1,647,777) and deliveries (from 19,319 to 311,193). The ICMART report now covers all of Europe, all of the US, Australia and New Zealand, some of Asia (India, Japan, South Korea, Taiwan) and, more recently, some centres in Africa. Data come from 4 regional registries (Europe, Latin America, Australia–New Zealand and Africa) and from national registries for other countries. For more information about ICMART, see Chapter 11, Global ART Surveillance: The International Committee Monitoring Assisted Reproductive Technologies (ICMART).

Regional Registries

The first area that organized a regional registry was Australia and New Zealand in 1985, with a report including data from Australian centres and from the first IVF unit in New Zealand [59]. It was a combined initiative of the Fertility Society of Australia and the Australian Institute of Health and Welfare National Perinatal Statistics Unit, directed by Paul Lancaster, and included all Australian and New Zealand units with annual reports [60, 61]. In 2004 it became ANZARD (the Australian and New Zealand Assisted Reproduction Database). The ANZARD collection is a collaborative effort between the National Perinatal Epidemiology and Statistics Unit (NPESU), the Fertility Society of Australia (FSA) and the fertility centres in Australia and New Zealand. ANZARD data are provided by fertility centres in Australia and New Zealand. The NPESU, previously the National Perinatal Statistics Unit, is the ANZARD data custodian for all fertility centres in Australia and New Zealand. This region has provided annual reports on ART cycles performed since 1992 (see Chapter 15, ART Surveillance in Australia and New Zealand).

The second regional registry (the Latin American Registry of Assisted Reproduction (RLA)) was organized in Latin America in 1990 as a professional initiative by several ART centres [62, 63]. The RLA is organized via the voluntary participation of individual clinics in all of Latin America. It was initially based on annual activity summaries of each participating centre, but then became a cycle-based registry with more validity controls (see Chapter 19, ART Surveillance in Latin America). It has produced annual reports from its inception, and was created in tandem with the world registry.

The European ART registry was based on the initiative of a group of professionals, but importantly was supported by ESHRE's Executive Committee and with ESHRE administrative, technical and financial support. This registry was initiated in 1999 through an invitation by ESHRE to representatives of all European ART registry representatives and, if such did not exist, to identified key persons in each country. The structure was very different from the two previous regional registries because the goal was to begin with existing national representatives and to help countries without a national registry to create one. Thus, the European IVF Monitoring (EIM) Consortium of national representatives was created, with a board. In 1999, the first report was produced on cycles performed in 1997 [64]. Since that date, the report was presented annually during the annual ESHRE meeting (June–July), and then annually in the journal *Human Reproduction* [14, 65, 66, 67, 68].

Additionally, in 2017 the EIM published the first study on trends over time [69]. For more information about the EIM Consortium, see Chapter 16, ART Surveillance in Europe.

In terms of regional registries, there has been an initiative in Africa with ANARA, supported by both ICMART and the Latin American REDLARA. The aim has been to build a regional registry for all Africa (English and French speaking), from either national registries (as in South Africa) or individual clinics. For more information, see Chapter 13, ART Surveillance in Africa.

General Evolution of Registries

The last point on the history of registries concerns their general evolution from organizational and methodological aspects. At the beginning, most of the registries were held by professional organizations, with voluntary participation and based on data summaries, with paper-based entry methods. All these aspects have changed in many countries, but not simultaneously, not in all aspects and not in all countries. However, several trends may be noted. The first registry belonging to health authorities was established in the UK (HFEA) in 1991. France had a dual level system, with a voluntary registry based on individual cycles begun in 1985, and a compulsory registry held by health authorities, based on data summaries, begun in 1992. In the last world report, among the 77 participating countries, health authorities were involved in North America (in collaboration with medical organizations), in 2 Asian countries (Japan and Taiwan), in Israel and in 19 European countries (out of 39).

Most of the registries are still voluntary. Those held by health authorities are compulsory, but this also applies to the German and the Spanish registries, even if held by a professional society. Another development is that more and more registries are now based on individual cycles, as in North America and Latin America, Australia and New Zealand, and in 17 European countries.

References

1. Wood C, Trounson A, Leeton JF, Renou PM, Walters WA, Buttery BW, et al. Clinical features of eight pregnancies resulting from in vitro fertilization and embryo transfer. *Fertil Steril.* 1982;38:22–9.

2. Diamond MP, Lavy G, Russell JB, Boyers SP, Nero F, DeCherney AH. Weight of babies conceived in vitro. *J In Vitro Fert Embryo Transf.* 1987;4:291–3.

3. Saunders DM, Lancaster P. The wider perinatal significance of the Australian in vitro fertilization data collection program. *Am J Perinatol.* 1989;6:252–7.

4. Whittemore AS, Harris R, Itnyre J. Characteristics relating to ovarian cancer risk: collaborative analysis of 12 US case-control studies. II. Invasive epithelial ovarian cancers in white women. Collaborative Ovarian Cancer Group. *Am J Epidemiol.* 1992;136:1184–203.

5. Henningsen AK, Romundstad LB, Gissler M, Nygren KG, Lidegaard O, Skjaerven R, et al. Infant and maternal health monitoring using a combined Nordic database on ART and safety. *Acta Obstet Gynecol Scand.* 2011;90:683–91.

6. Tan SL, Doyle P, Campbell S, Beral V, Rizk B, Brinsden P, et al. Obstetric outcome of in vitro fertilization pregnancies compared with normally conceived pregnancies. *Am J Obstet Gynecol.* 1992;167:778–84.

7. Bonduelle M, Legein J, Derde MP, Buysse A, Schietecatte J, Wisanto A, et al. Comparative follow-up study of 130 children born after intracytoplasmic sperm injection and 130 children born after in-vitro fertilization. *Hum Reprod.* 1995;10:3327–31.

8. Westergaard HB, Johansen AM, Erb K, Andersen AN. Danish National In-Vitro Fertilization Registry 1994 and 1995: a controlled study of births, malformations and cytogenetic findings. *Hum Reprod.* 1999;14:1896–902.

9. Andersen AN, Westergaard HB, Olsen J. The Danish in vitro fertilization (IVF) register. *Dan Med Bull.* 1999;46:357–60.

10. Zegers-Hochschild F, Nygren KG, Adamson D, de Mouzon J, Lancaster P, Mansour R, et al. The International Committee Monitoring Assisted Reproductive Technologies (ICMART) glossary on ART terminology. *Fertil Steril.* 2006;86:16–19.

11. Zegers-Hochschild F, Adamson GD, de Mouzon J, Ishihara O, Mansour R, Nygren K, et al. on behalf of ICMART and WHO. The International Committee for Monitoring Assisted Reproductive Technology (ICMART) and the World Health Organization (WHO) revised glossary on art terminology, 2009. *Hum Reprod.* 2009;24:2683–7.

12. Zegers-Hochschild F, Adamson GD, Dyer S, Racowsky C, de Mouzon J, Sokol R, et al. The International Glossary on Infertility and Fertility Care, 2017. *Hum Reprod.* 2017;32:1786–1801.

13. Sunderam S, Kissin DM, Crawford SB, Folger SG, Boulet SL, Warner L, et al. Assisted reproductive technology surveillance – United States, 2015. *MMWR Surveill Summ.* 2018;67(3):1–28.

14. European IVF-Monitoring Consortium (EIM); European Society of Human Reproduction and

Embryology (ESHRE); Calhaz-Jorge C, De Geyter C, Kupka MS, de Mouzon J, Erb K, Mocanu E, et al. Assisted reproductive technology in Europe, 2013: results generated from European registers by ESHRE. *Hum Reprod.* 2017;**32**:1957–73.

15. McLernon DJ, Maheshwari A, Lee AJ, Bhattacharya S. Cumulative live birth rates after one or more complete cycles of IVF: a population-based study of linked cycle data from 178,898 women. *Hum Reprod.* 2016;**31**:572–81.

16. Malchau SS, Henningsen AA, Loft A, Rasmussen S, Forman J, Nyboe Andersen A, et al. The long-term prognosis for live birth in couples initiating fertility treatments. *Hum Reprod.* 2017;**32**:1439–49.

17. Bentley P, Smyth S. 'Drugs made my ovaries swell to five times their usual size': Fertility clinics accused of covering up potentially fatal side effects of IVF. Daily Mail.com. 3 May 2017.

18. Moll AC, Imhof SM, Cruysberg JR, Schouten-van Meeteren AY, Boers M, van Leeuwen FE. Incidence of retinoblastoma in children born after in-vitro fertilisation. *Lancet.* 2003;**361**:309–10.

19. Marees T, Dommering CJ, Imhof SM, Kors WA, Ringens PJ, van Leeuwen FE, et al. Incidence of retinoblastoma in Dutch children conceived by IVF: an expanded study. *Hum Reprod.* 2009;**24**:3220–4.

20. Wennerholm UB, Henningsen AK, Romundstad LB, Bergh C, Pinborg A, Skjaerven R, et al. Perinatal outcomes of children born after frozen-thawed embryo transfer: a Nordic cohort study from the CoNARTaS group. *Hum Reprod.* 2013;**28**:2545–53.

21. Lancaster P. Registers of in-vitro fertilization and assisted conception. *Hum Reprod.* 1984;**11**(Suppl 4):89–109.

22. de Mouzon J. Dossier FIVETE national. Première analyse. *Horm Reprod Metab.* 1986:217–21.

23. de Mouzon J. *FIVNAT. French experience and results of a national collaborative data recording system on IVFET.* 5th World Congress on in vitro fertilization and embryo transfer. Norfolk, USA, 5–10 April 1987.

24. de Mouzon J, Bachelot A, Spira A. Establishing a national in vitro fertilization registry. Methodological problems and analysis of success rates. *Stat Med.* 1993;**12**:39–50.

25. de Mouzon J, Bachelot A, Logerot H, Spira A. French national in vitro fertilization registry FIVNAT. Analysis of 1986–1990 data. *Fertil Steril.* 1993;**59**:587–95.

26. Medical Research International, the American Fertility Society Special Interest Group. In vitro fertilization/ embryo transfer in the United States: 1985 and 1986 results from the National IVF-ET Registry. *Fertil Steril.* 1988;**49**:212–15.

27. Medical Research International, the American Fertility Society Special Interest Group. In vitro fertilization/ embryo transfer in the United States: 1987 results from the National IVF-ET Registry. *Fertil Steril.* 1989;**51**:13–19.

28. Wright VC, Schieve LA, Reynolds MA, Jeng G, Division of Reproductive Health, National Center for Chronic Disease Prevention and Health Promotion, Centers for Disease Control and Prevention (CDC). Assisted reproductive technology surveillance, United States, 2002. *MMWR Surveill Summ.* 2005;**54**:1–24.

29. McNaughton M. Regulation before the HFEA. *Hum Fertil.* 2005;**8**:61–2.

30. Nelson EL. Comparative perspectives on the regulation of assisted reproductive technologies in the United Kingdom and Canada. *Alberta Law Review.* 2006;**43**:1023–48.

31. MRC Working Party on Children Conceived by In Vitro Fertilisation. Births in Great Britain resulting from assisted conception, 1978–87. *BMJ.* 1990;**300**:1229–33.

32. Felberbaum R, Dahncke W. *DIR-Deutsches IVF Register – First Steps towards Quality Control in German ART.* ESHRE 15th annual meeting, Tours, France, 1999 (Abstract.)

33. Kupka MS, Bühler K, Dahncke W, Wendelken M, Bals-Pratsch M. Summary of the 2008 annual report of the German IVF registry. *J Reproduktionsmed Endokrinol.* 2010;**7**:34–8.

34. Bühler K, Bals-Pratsch M, Blumenauer V, Dahncke W, Felberbaum R, Fiedler K, et al. Annual 2011 – German IVF-registry. *J Reproduktionsmed Endokrinol.* 2012;**9**:453–84.

35. De Sutter P, Lejeune B, Dhont M, Leroy F, Englert Y, Van Steirteghem A. Ten years follow-up of medically assisted procreation in Belgium. *Rev Med Brux.* 2004;**25**:160–5. [In French.]

36. De Neubourg D, Bogaerts K, Wyns C, Albert A, Camus M, Candeur M, et al. The history of Belgian assisted reproduction technology cycle registration and control: a case study in reducing the incidence of multiple pregnancy. *Hum Reprod.* 2013;**28**:2709–19.

37. Gunby J, Daya S; IVF Directors Group of the Canadian Fertility and Andrology Society. Assisted reproductive technologies (ART) in Canada: 2001 results from the Canadian ART register. *Fertil Steril.* 2005;**84**:590–9.

38. Friedler S, Mashiach S, Laufer N. Births in Israel resulting from in-vitro fertilization/embryo transfer, 1982–1989: National Registry of the Israeli Association for Fertility Research. *Hum Reprod.* 1992;**7**:1159–63.

39. Van den Bergh M, Hohl MK, De Geyter Ch, Stalberg AM, Limoni C. Ten years of Swiss National IVF

Register FIVNAT-CH. Are we making progress? *Reprod Biomed Online*. 2005;**11**:632–40.

40. Seppälä M. The world collaborative report on in vitro fertilization and embryo replacement: current state of the art in January 1984. *Ann N Y Acad Sci*. 1985;**442**:558–63.

41. Cohen J, Mayaux MJ, Guihard-Moscato ML. Pregnancy outcomes after in vitro fertilization. A collaborative study on 2342 pregnancies. *Ann N Y Acad Sci*. 1988;**541**:1–6.

42. Testart J, Plachot M, Mandelbaum J, Salat-Baroux J, Frydman R, Cohen J. World collaborative report on IVF-ET and GIFT: 1989 results. *Hum Reprod*. 1992;7:362–9.

43. Cohen J., de Mouzon J., Lancaster PL. *IVF 1991 World Report*. 8th World Congress on In Vitro Fertilization and Alternate Assisted Reproduction. Kyoto, 12–15 September 1993.

44. de Mouzon J. *World Collaborative Report 1993 on IVF. Trends and Characteristics of Infertile Couples*. 15th World Congress on Fertility and Sterility. Montpellier 17–22 September 1995.

45. IWGROAR, prepared by de Mouzon J, Lancaster P. World collaborative report on in vitro fertilization. Preliminary data for 1995. *J Assist Reprod Gen*. 1997;**14**:251s–265s.

46. IWGROAR, presented by de Mouzon J, Lancaster P, Nygren K, Zegers-Hochschild F. *World Report: Preliminary Data for 1996*. 16th World Congress on Fertility and Sterility, IFFS San Francisco USA, 4–9 October 1998.

47. IWGROAR, prepared by Adamson D, Lancaster P, de Mouzon J (co-ordinator), Nygren KG (chairman) and Zegers-Hochschild F. World collaborative report on assisted reproductive technology, 1998. In DL Healy, GP Kovac, E Mclachlan, O Rodriduez-Armas (eds.), *Reproductive Medicine in the 21st Century*. London: Parthenon Publishing Group; 2001. pp.209–19.

48. ICMART, prepared by Adamson D, de Mouzon J (co-ordinator), Lancaster P, Nygren KG (chairman), Sullivan E and Zegers-Hochschild F. World collaborative report on in vitro fertilization 2000. *Fertil Steril*. 2006;**85**:1586–1622.

49. ICMART prepared by de Mouzon J, Lancaster P, Nygren KG (chairman), Sullivan E, Zegers-Hochschild F, Mansour R, Ishihara O, Adamson D. World collaborative report on assisted reproductive technology for the year 2002 activity. *Hum Reprod*. 2009;**24**:2310–20.

50. Nygren KG, Sullivan E, Zegers-Hochschild F, Mansour R, Ishihara O, Adamson D, de Mouzon J. ICMART world report on assisted reproductive technology 2003. *Fertil Steril*. 2011;**95**:2209–22.

51. Sullivan EA, Zegers-Hochschild F, Mansour R, Ishihara O, de Mouzon J, Nygren KG, Adamson GD. International Committee for Monitoring Assisted Reproductive Technologies (ICMART) world report: assisted reproductive technology 2004. *Hum Reprod*. 2013;**28**:1375–90.

52. Zegers-Hochschild F, Mansour R, Ishihara O, Adamson GD, de Mouzon J, Nygren KG, Sullivan EA. International Committee for Monitoring Assisted Reproductive Technology: world report on assisted reproductive technology, 2005. *Fertil Steril*. 2014;**101**:366–78.

53. Ishihara O, Adamson GD, Dyer S, de Mouzon J, Nygren KG, Sullivan EA, et al. International Committee for Monitoring Assisted Reproductive Technologies: world report on assisted reproductive technologies, 2007. *Fertil Steril*. 2015;**103**:402–13.

54. Dyer S, Chambers GM, de Mouzon J, Nygren KG, Zegers-Hochschild F, Mansour R, et al. International Committee for Monitoring Assisted Reproductive Technologies world report: assisted reproductive technology 2008, 2009 and 2010. *Hum Reprod*. 2016;**31**:1588–609.

55. Adamson GD, de Mouzon J, Chambers GM, Zegers-Hochschild F, Mansour R, Ishihara O, et al. International Committee for Monitoring Assisted Reproductive Technologies world report: assisted reproductive technology 2011. *Fertil Steril*. In press.

56. Adamson GD, de Mouzon J, Chambers GM, Zegers-Hochschild F, Mansour R, Ishihara O, et al. *International Committee for Monitoring Assisted Reproductive Technologies World Report: Assisted Reproductive Technology 2012*. ESHRE 32nd Annual Meeting, Helsinki (Finland), 3–6 July 2016.

57. Adamson GD, de Mouzon J, Chambers GM, Zegers-Hochschild F, Mansour R, Ishihara O, et al. *International Committee for Monitoring Assisted Reproductive Technologies World Report: Assisted Reproductive Technology 2013*. ESHRE 33rd Annual Meeting, Geneva (Switzerland), 2–5 July 2017.

58. Adamson GD, de Mouzon J, Chambers GM, Zegers-Hochschild F, Mansour R, Ishihara O, et al. *International Committee for Monitoring Assisted Reproductive Technologies World Report: Assisted Reproductive Technology 2014*. 33rd Annual Meeting, Barcelona (Spain), 1–4 July 2018.

59. Australian In Vitro Fertilization Collaborative Group. In-vitro fertilization pregnancies in Australia and New Zealand, 1979–1985. *Med J Aust*. 1988;**148**:429–36.

60. Lancaster P, Shafir E, Huang J. *Assisted Conception, Australia and New Zealand, 1992 and 1993*. Sydney: AIHW National Perinatal Statistics Unit; 1995. Assisted Conception Series No. 1.

61. Hurst T, Shafir E, Lancaster P. *Assisted Conception Australia and New-Zealand 1996*. Sydney: AIHW National Perinatal Statistics Unit; 1997. Assisted Conception Series No. 3. Available at: https://npesu .unsw.edu.au/sites/default/files/npesu/data_collection/ Assisted%20conception%20Australia%.

62. Zegers-Hochschild F, Schwarze JE, Crosby JA, de Souza MCB. Twenty years of assisted reproductive technology (ART) in Latin America. *JBRA Assist Reprod*. 2011;**15**:19–30.

63. Zegers-Hochschild F, Schwarze JE, Crosby JA, Musri C, Urbina MT. Assisted reproductive techniques in Latin America: The Latin American registry, 2014. *JBRA Assist Reprod*. 2017;**21**:164–75.

64. Nygren KG, Nyboe Andersen A; European IVF-Monitoring Programme; European Society of Human Reproduction and Embryology. Assisted reproductive technology in Europe, 1997. Results generated from European registers by ESHRE. *Hum Reprod*. 2001;**16**:384–91.

65. Nyboe Andersen A, Gianaroli L, Nygren KG; European IVF-Monitoring Programme; European Society of Human Reproduction and Embryology. Assisted reproductive technology in Europe, 2000. Results generated from European registers by ESHRE. *Hum Reprod*. 2004;**19**:490–503.

66. Nyboe Andersen A, Goossens V, Gianaroli L, Felberbaum R, de Mouzon J, Nygren KG. Assisted reproductive technology in Europe, 2003. Results generated from European registers by ESHRE. *Hum Reprod*. 2007;**22**:1513–25.

67. de Mouzon J, Goossens V, Bhattacharya S, Castilla JA, Ferraretti AP, Korsak V, et al.; European IVF-Monitoring (EIM) Consortium, for the European Society of Human Reproduction and Embryology (ESHRE). Assisted reproductive technology in Europe, 2007: results generated from European registers by ESHRE. *Hum Reprod*. 2012;**27**:954–66.

68. Kupka MS, Ferraretti AP, de Mouzon J, Erb K, D'Hooghe T, Castilla JA, et al.; European IVF-Monitoring Consortium, for the European Society of Human Reproduction and Embryology. Assisted reproductive technology in Europe, 2010: results generated from European registers by ESHRE. *Hum Reprod*. 2014;**29**:2099–113.

69. Ferraretti AP, Nygren KG, Nyboe Andersen A, de Mouzon J, Kupka M, Calhaz-Jorge C, et al.; European IVF-Monitoring Consortium (EIM), for the European Society of Human Reproduction and Embryology (ESHRE). Trends over 15 years in ART in Europe: an analysis of 6 million cycles. *Hum Reprod Open*. 2017;**2017**(2). Available at: https://doi.org/10.1093/ hropen/hox012.

Chapter

3

ART Surveillance: Who, What, When and How?

Sara Crawford, Dmitry M. Kissin and Georgina M. Chambers

The findings and conclusions in this report are those of the authors and do not necessarily represent the official position of the Centers for Disease Control and Prevention.

Introduction

According to the World Health Organization (WHO), public health surveillance is defined as "the continuous, systematic collection, analysis and interpretation of health-related data needed for the planning, implementation, and evaluation of public health practice" [1]. The United States (US) Centers for Disease Control and Prevention (CDC) uses a similar definition, adding that public health surveillance is "closely integrated with the dissemination of these data to those who need to know and linked to prevention and control" [2]. Public health surveillance serves a variety of purposes. Per CDC guidelines for evaluating public health systems, public health surveillance systems "can be used to: guide immediate action for cases of public health importance; measure the burden of a disease (or other health-related event), including changes in related factors, the identification of populations at high risk, and the identification of new or emerging health concerns; monitor trends in the burden of a disease (or other health-related event), including the detection of epidemics (outbreaks) and pandemics; guide the planning, implementation, and evaluation of programs to prevent and control disease, injury, or adverse exposure; evaluate public policy; detect changes in health practices and the effects of these changes; prioritize the allocation of health resources; describe the clinical course of disease; and provide a basis for epidemiologic research" [3].

An assisted reproductive technology (ART) public health surveillance system allows for the monitoring of treatment success, including pregnancy and live birth, and captures information that can inform practice patterns. ART surveillance systems are also used to track adverse health outcomes for the mother, such as ovarian hyperstimulation, and outcomes that increase risk for mothers and babies, such as multiple births.

While many countries recognized the importance of collecting and using ART data, ART surveillance systems and other ART data collection tools, such as registries or repositories, vary according to ownership, reporting responsibility, type of data being reported, information being reported, data quality and validation activities, public reporting of success rates, reporting requirements and data protection around the world. This chapter will explore each of these areas as they relate to ART surveillance.

ART Surveillance: Who

Owners of ART Surveillance Systems

ART surveillance systems may be owned by a governmental agency, a professional medical organization or a private entity. Sometimes, more than one organization is involved in ART surveillance. For example, in the US, both a governmental agency and a professional medical organization collect and use ART data. The CDC, a governmental public health agency [4], owns the National ART Surveillance System (NASS). This surveillance system was designed to fulfil the Fertility Clinic Success Rate and Certification Act, a law requiring the CDC to annually publish ART clinic-specific success rates [5] through the collection of data on all ART cycles from all clinics performing ART across the US, and is estimated to capture 98% of such cycles. The Society for Assisted Reproductive Technology (SART), a professional medical organization, owns an ART registry, the SART Clinical Outcomes Reporting System (SART CORS), which captures data from SART-member clinics. Approximately 81% of all reporting ART clinics in the US are SART-member clinics [6]. To avoid SART-member clinics having to report data twice (both to NASS and SART CORS), SART-member clinics typically report data to SART

CORS and then the CDC accepts data from SART on behalf of these clinics. This arrangement allows both a governmental agency and a professional medical organization to be the owners of their own ART data and to use these data according to their respective missions and goals. Of the 34 countries that reported to the European IVF Monitoring (EIM) Consortium in 2012, 15 (44%) reported to a national health authority, 16 (47%) reported to a professional medical organization and 3 (9%) reported to a private entity [7].

The choice of a national ART surveillance system owner can be determined by law, cultural or historical perspectives, availability of human and financial resources and other factors. Close collaboration between governments and professional medical organizations in operating an ART surveillance system and in using ART data (regardless of the ownership) makes an ART surveillance system stronger. It improves stability by allowing for better access to human and financial resources, thereby improving its acceptability among ART providers by considering their suggestions and concerns, and improving its usefulness for policy, research and quality assurance for the benefit of ART patients and their infants.

Entities Reporting Primary ART Data

The burden of reporting ART data primarily falls on ART clinics because, as ART providers, they are uniquely positioned to know all the details of an ART cycle. Having ART clinics report ART data is beneficial in that the source of the data is typically a medical chart and the reported data can be checked against the medical chart for a measure of accuracy such as sensitivity and specificity (i.e. data validation). Typically, the medical director of a clinic is ultimately responsible for the reporting of the data; however, other clinic personnel are sometimes responsible for the actual gathering of data and entry of the data into the reporting system. In some cases, more than one clinic is involved in a cycle (for example, if a weather event threatens to disrupt a treatment cycle that is already in progress the patient may be referred to another clinic). Data collection systems may deal with these situations differently, for example, by placing the responsibility for reporting on either the entity responsible for the embryo culture or the entity responsible for starting the cycle.

ART Surveillance: What

Type of Data Being Reported (Cycle-Level, Summary)

ART surveillance data may be reported as summary- or cycle-level data. With summary-level data, clinics report only aggregate information describing ART cycles performed and their outcomes (e.g. total number of cycles performed, total number of egg retrievals, total number of embryo transfers, total number of resulting pregnancies and live births). With cycle-level data, clinics report each cycle individually, along with characteristics of the cycle (e.g. number of oocytes retrieved or number of embryos transferred) and the cycle outcome (e.g. pregnancy or live birth). Cycle-level data could then be used to calculate summary statistics such as the total number of cycles or total number of live births. In the US, clinics report cycle-level data. In Europe, of the 34 countries that reported to the EIM Consortium in 2012, 10 (29.4%) indicated they collect cycle-level data while the remaining 24 (70.5%) indicated they collect summary-level data [7]. The reporting of aggregate data poses less of a burden to clinics, but the reporting of cycle-level data has advantages of improved data quality and usefulness.

The collection of cycle-level data allows fewer opportunities for selective reporting. In the reporting of summary-level data, clinics can make mistakes in the calculation of reported statistics or easily manipulate reported statistics, for example, altering the population of patients or cycles for which the statistics are calculated to improve cycle outcomes. Data validation can be performed to detect instances of mistaken or selective reporting, but if clinics are reporting only summary data, verification requires review of all of the medical records of procedures performed in the clinic during the reporting period, extraction of the necessary data and replication of the clinic calculations. If clinics are reporting cycle-level data, the validators can randomly select a subset of patients or cycles and compare the reported data with the data in the charts, also looking for unreported cycles, in order to make an overall assessment with regard to the accuracy of the reported data. In either case, data validation is only as good as the data reported and the medical records provided by the clinic for verification.

The collection of cycle-level data is also substantially more useful for carrying out research of ART cycles and their outcomes. Summary data are used primarily for ecological studies. Because these studies involve aggregate data, they are often unable to account for patient- or treatment-specific characteristics that may affect treatment success. However, these factors can be accounted for with cycle-level data. This allows for a better understanding of factors that influence treatment success, as well as the ability to assess and improve the quality of ART practice. More information about using ART surveillance data for clinical research can be found in Chapter 6.

Finally, the collection of cycle-level data enables linkage of ART data with other datasets such as birth and death registration data, health service data and other disease registries. If an ART surveillance system involves the collection of direct identifiers such as a unique identifying number, direct linkage can be performed between the ART surveillance data and other datasets with the same information. Otherwise, if indirect identifiers such as date of birth and residence are collected, probability-based algorithms can be used for data linkage. In the US, mother's date of birth, infant's date of birth, zip code, plurality and gravidity are used to link ART surveillance data with birth certificate and other vital records data. See Chapter 9, Monitoring Long-Term Outcomes of ART: Linking ART Surveillance Data with Other Datasets.

Information Being Reported

There is a variety of information that can be reported in an ART surveillance system, regardless of whether cycle- or summary-level data are collected. Typical elements for reporting include the source and type of gametes and/or embryos used in the ART procedure; the patient characteristics; the components of an ART cycle; the manipulations performed during the cycle; adverse patient or donor events; ART treatment outcomes; and pregnancy outcomes, if applicable. Some reporting systems may also collect medical and obstetric histories for the patients and/or donors. One of the challenges of ART surveillance is rapid changes in the field of ART that require continuous review of variables that are being collected and adding new variables to remain timely and relevant. Appendix A includes a list of variables currently collected by ART surveillance systems. The International Committee Monitoring Assisted

Reproductive Technologies (ICMART), which reports on global ART activity annually, provides an ART surveillance Tool Box to facilitate the monitoring and data collection of ART cycles and outcomes for counties and/or regions that use ART but have not yet established a surveillance system [8].

Source and Type of Gametes and Embryos

ART cycles involve the handling of oocytes or embryos for the purpose of establishing pregnancy. Depending on the type of ART cycle being conducted, the cycle may involve oocytes, sperm and/or embryos. The source of the oocytes and sperm can be the patient or partner or a donor. The source of an embryo is determined by the source of the oocytes and, therefore, can be either patient oocyte or donor oocyte. Embryos themselves can also be donated if a patient has unused embryos from an ART treatment that they wish to donate to another patient/couple. The type of oocyte, sperm or embryo used is either fresh (if never cryopreserved) or cryopreserved (if cryopreserved and thawed). The variety of options involved in an ART cycle complicates its classification (even if the state of sperm is not taken into account): fresh oocyte – fresh embryo, cryopreserved oocyte – fresh embryo, fresh oocyte – cryopreserved embryo, and cryopreserved oocyte – cryopreserved embryo.

Patient Characteristics

Typically, information about the patient undergoing treatment is collected. Common fields are demographics such as patient age and race/ethnicity, infertility diagnosis and/or the reason for undergoing ART treatment and reproductive history. If donor gametes are used, particularly donor eggs, it is also useful to collect similar information about the donor, if possible, because the characteristics of the donors play a role in the success of the treatment cycle. For example, live birth rates for women undergoing ART with their own eggs decline with patient age, while live birth rates for women undergoing ART with eggs from a young donor are fairly constant by patient age, suggesting that the age of the woman providing the oocyte plays a significant role in the success of an ART treatment [9]. In addition, collecting information about the oocyte donor or gestational carrier may help in the evaluation of the effect of ART treatment on the health of donor or carrier.

Components of an ART Cycle

The components of an ART cycle include cycle initiation, oocyte retrieval and oocyte or embryo transfer(s). Cycle initiations include cycles started with the intent to stimulate a woman's ovaries with medication to produce multiple oocytes for surgical retrieval and cycles started with the intent to allow a woman's ovaries to naturally produce an oocyte for surgical retrieval. Cycle initiations also include those started with the intent to transfer previously frozen oocytes or embryos or those started with the intent to transfer fresh oocytes or embryos retrieved from a donor. Oocyte retrievals involve the surgical removal of oocytes, while transfers involve the transfer of oocytes or embryos to a patient's uterus or fallopian tubes.

Surveillance systems may track cycles with the intent to retrieve oocytes or transfer oocytes or embryos, cycles in which a retrieval or transfer was attempted and/or cycles in which a retrieval or transfer was actually performed. It is important to capture cycle initiations, oocyte retrievals and oocyte or embryo transfers, as not all initiated cycles proceed to a retrieval. Sometimes initiated cycles are stopped prior to retrieval, i.e. cancelled, due to reasons such as illness or poor or excessive response to stimulation. In addition, sometimes cycles that proceed to oocyte retrieval do not proceed to transfer for reasons such as poor oocyte yield.

It is important to capture both the intent of the cycle and what actually happens to fully understand the success of a cycle. For example, if a cycle is initiated with the intent to retrieve oocytes and then transfer a fresh embryo but doctors end up cryopreserving all resulting embryos due to a poor response to stimulation or the risk of ovarian hyperstimulation syndrome, the 'success' of this cycle may be interpreted differently than would a cycle initiated for cryopreserving all resulting embryos.

Manipulations

Surveillance systems may track the type of gamete or embryo manipulation used during an ART cycle. These may include the use of intracytoplasmic sperm injection (ICSI), in which a single sperm is injected directly into the oocyte for fertilization; assisted hatching, in which the shell of an embryo is either thinned or punctured using chemical, mechanical or laser methods; or preimplantation genetic testing (PGT), in which oocytes or embryos undergo DNA testing to diagnose for aneuploidies, genetic defects or chromosomal abnormalities [10]. Inclusion of these and other manipulations in ART surveillance is important for evaluating their effect on ART success rates and for monitoring their safety for mothers and children.

Adverse Events

Many surveillance systems track adverse events that may arise during the course of ART treatment. One example of an adverse event is ovarian hyperstimulation syndrome (OHSS), in which a woman's body has an exaggerated response to the stimulation process, possibly leading to enlarged ovaries, a distended abdomen, nausea, vomiting or diarrhoea, fluid in the abdominal cavity or chest, breathing difficulties, changes in blood volume or viscosity and diminished kidney perfusion and function [6, 10]. Other ART-related adverse events include infection, haemorrhage, complications due to medications or anaesthetic, hospitalization and death [11]. While such events may be under-reported, their inclusion in ART surveillance can be very useful for monitoring ART safety and biovigilance (see Chapter 7 for more information).

ART Treatment Outcomes

To determine the success of ART treatment, a surveillance system needs to include information on whether each ART cycle resulted in implantation, indicated by the presence of gestational sacs or fetal hearts, and pregnancy. Pregnancy can take on a variety of definitions such as biochemical, clinical or viable, and a surveillance system may capture one or several of these definitions. For example, the NASS classifies pregnancies as either biochemical, defined as positive human chorionic gonadotropin (hCG) levels without ultrasound confirmation of a gestational sac; clinical, defined as ultrasound confirmation of a gestational sac; ectopic, defined as confirmed implantation outside the uterus; or heterotopic, defined as simultaneous clinical and ectopic pregnancies. A surveillance system may also capture information to establish that a pregnancy actually occurred (e.g. ultrasound results). Usually this outcome is evaluated by the reproductive endocrinologist before the patient, if pregnant, starts treatment with an obstetrician.

Pregnancy Outcomes

While implantation and pregnancy are intermediate measures of treatment success, patients are most interested in achieving a live birth; therefore, a surveillance system should report pregnancy outcomes. While ART providers usually do not provide prenatal care once a pregnancy has been established, follow-up with patients or prenatal providers allows for the reporting of a live birth or pregnancy loss and, possibly, other details about the pregnancy outcome such as gestational age, infant birth weight or infant gender. Obtaining this information can be challenging because of the discontinuation of care by the fertility physician and the length of time between the establishment of pregnancy and birth, but collection is important as it contributes to success rates reporting.

Data Quality and Validation

The quality of data reported to an ART surveillance system is dependent on provider evaluation of the patient (e.g. evaluation of reason for seeking treatment is variable), documentation of data in the patient ART medical chart, transcription of data from the chart to the surveillance system and access to pregnancy outcome data. A data audit can be performed to assess the quality of the submitted data. Because the auditing of data requires significant human and financial resources, few ART surveillance systems have this component. In the US, data auditing of the National ART Surveillance System (NASS) is conducted by visiting a random sample of reporting clinics and comparing the contents of the medical charts for a set of randomly selected cycles in the data reported to NASS for those cycles [6]. During this process, auditors do not quality check all data fields, but only those thought to have a greater impact on success rates. Discrepancy rates are calculated for each of the audited fields. While this methodology captures errors in transcription of the data and inconsistencies between the reported data and the definitions and guidelines provided for reporting, it has limited capacity to capture all possible issues with the quality of data. For example, if a cycle is reported to NASS with a live birth outcome, the auditing process will verify that the clinic has a notation for a live birth in the medical chart, but the validation process will not verify the live birth by other means (e.g. comparing the reported live birth with birth certificate data). However, countries that routinely link ART births with vital records data can utilize such linkage for ensuring the accuracy of a live birth in ART surveillance. In recent years, data auditing of the NASS has included variables such as patient date of birth, infertility diagnosis and reason for treatment, number of cycles reported, cycle intent, cycle cancellation, number of eggs or embryos transferred, ART treatment outcome, pregnancy outcome, number of fetal hearts on initial ultrasound and number of infants born. Discrepancy rates are typically 5% or lower, with the highest discrepancies typically found for patient diagnoses [6].

In the US, data auditing of SART CORS is conducted by SART. SART representatives visit clinics with an indicator of data problems such as a high percentage of deleted cycles, low percentage of prospectively reported cycles, high percentage of fertility preservation cycles with linked frozen embryo transfers or very high live birth rate that differs for deleted or prospectively reported cycles. Typically, about 10 clinics are visited. These clinics are educated about any reporting issues and then allowed the opportunity to correct their data. See more information about targeted auditing by SART in Chapter 18, ART Surveillance in North America.

ART Surveillance: When

Annual ART Surveillance Timeline

ART surveillance can be performed prospectively or retrospectively. In prospective reporting, some information about each ART cycle is reported around the time the ART cycle is started. For example, in the NASS, "reporting of the initial cycle intent and select patient details is required within four days of cycle initiation" [12]. The remaining information can be reported as it is attained or by a specified deadline after the cycles for a reporting period are complete. In retrospective reporting, the surveillance data are reported after the cycles are partially or fully complete. In the United Kingdom (UK), clinics are required to report prospectively to the Human Fertilisation and Embryology Authority (HFEA) within a few days after each of the key components of ART treatment: initiation of treatment, mixture of gametes, cryopreservation of oocytes or embryos, thawing of previously frozen embryos, and when treatment outcomes become known [13].

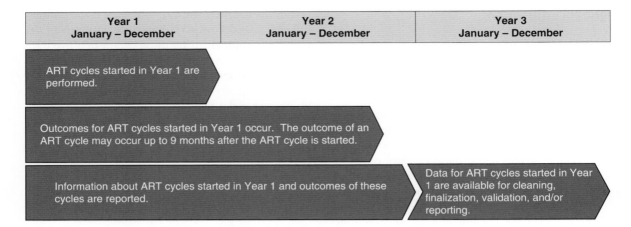

Year 1 January – December	Year 2 January – December	Year 3 January – December

ART cycles started in Year 1 are performed.

Outcomes for ART cycles started in Year 1 occur. The outcome of an ART cycle may occur up to 9 months after the ART cycle is started.

Information about ART cycles started in Year 1 and outcomes of these cycles are reported.

Data for ART cycles started in Year 1 are available for cleaning, finalization, validation, and/or reporting.

Figure 3.1 ART data reporting timeline.

Each reporting year of ART surveillance data collection spans a calendar period of approximately one year and nine months, as births resulting from ART cycles started at the end of a reporting year can occur up to nine months later. Because time must be allowed for the reporting of final cycle details and outcomes after these are complete, one could expect the reporting of one year of surveillance data to actually span a calendar period of at least two years. This is true regardless of whether data are reported prospectively or retrospectively. Additional time is then needed after reporting for data cleaning, preparation, validation and/or publication; therefore, the entire process of collecting and publishing one reporting year of ART data may span three calendar years, as shown in Figure 3.1. As some surveillance systems link oocyte retrievals and embryo transfers, and success rate calculations have moved to include the complete treatment cycle (including a retrieval of oocytes and the fresh and frozen transfer of all retrieved oocytes), success rates reporting can involve more than one year of data, thus extending this timeline further.

ART Surveillance: How

Motivation for Reporting

The reporting of ART surveillance data is dependent on the cooperation of clinics performing ART procedures, which may be affected by reporting requirements. Some countries have a voluntary reporting environment, in which there is typically a mechanism in place for the reporting of ART surveillance data, but no reporting requirement exists.

In other countries, reporting is required via some sort of mandate or law. In the US, the Fertility Clinic Success Rate and Certification Act (FCSRCA) mandates that all clinics performing ART procedures report success rates to the CDC. According to the 16th European Society of Human Reproduction and Embryology (ESHRE) report on ART, there is an association between whether reporting is required and the completeness of reporting. Among the 16 countries with voluntary reporting in 2012, only 3 had complete reporting (i.e. 100% of clinics report). Alternatively, among the 18 countries with required reporting in 2012, 15 had complete reporting [7].

ART reporting can be a burden to ART clinics with regard to both time and money. Surveillance systems, particularly those designed to handle cycle-level reporting, can be a substantial investment to create and maintain. In the US, the NASS is maintained by the CDC and reporting to the system is free for clinics. However, SART-member clinics that report data to SART CORS pay a per-cycle fee to submit data to offset the costs of data collection, an arrangement similar to the HFEA ART registry. In addition, clinics have to allocate personnel to report the data, resulting in additional time and expense. Clinics generally report data even in the face of these disincentives because of mandated reporting, resulting in more complete databases for surveillance and research.

Data Protection and Confidentiality

ART data may be considered sensitive information, particularly cycle-level information capturing patient history, ART treatment characteristics and outcomes and pregnancy outcomes. For example, in the US, data collected via the NASS do not contain direct personal identifiers such as name or social security number and are protected under an assurance of confidentiality. The assurance of confidentiality provides a formal protection for highly sensitive data and ensures that identifiable information will not be disclosed and will be used only for the purpose for which it was supplied unless individuals or institutions consent to use of the data for other purposes [14].

Attributes of an ART Surveillance System

According to the CDC guidelines for evaluating public health systems, public health surveillance systems can be assessed using the following attributes: simplicity, flexibility, data quality, acceptability, sensitivity, positive predictive value, representativeness, timeliness and stability [3]. Despite the complexities of ART, an ideal ART surveillance system has *simple* and straightforward data entry with variable definitions that are easy to understand. The system should be designed for ease of use and data extraction by the collecting body. Because ART is a rapidly changing field, an ideal system should be designed to be *flexible* and easily allow for changes to which data fields are collected, data field definitions and success rate calculations. Interoperability with electronic medical records may ease the reporting burden on clinics. In addition, the system should involve frequent review to assess the need for changes to these items.

An ideal surveillance system has high-level *data quality*. Efforts should be made to ensure that the data collected through the surveillance system are as complete and accurate as possible. Mandated reporting of cycle-level ART data facilitates the completeness of the data. Additional measures such as data validation and prospective reporting help to ensure data accuracy. The ART surveillance system should be *acceptable* to ART practitioners, who carry the main burden of reporting the data. While mandates can encourage practitioners to report despite the burden, other elements can be incorporated into the system to reduce the burden, such as having the surveillance system linked with electronic medical records, reducing the fields collected to only those necessary and making the system available at no cost. In addition, because ART can be a sensitive topic for both patients and providers, an ideal system should ensure strict

confidentiality protections to gain the trust of reporting bodies. At the same time, providing access to a clinic's own data for quality assurance purposes can demonstrate the value of ART surveillance for ART practitioners and, therefore, improve acceptability.

The ideal system should have high levels of *sensitivity*, with the ability to accurately capture all ART cycles and their outcomes. Cycle-level (instead of summary) data collection can help to prevent reporting duplications or omissions. Linking ART births with vital records can result in more accurate live birth reporting. While *positive predictive value* is typically high in ART surveillance because reporting of cycles or births that didn't occur is unlikely, strong positive predictive value can be achieved by making the tracking and reporting of live births easy and by incorporating data validation to check the accuracy of the reported live births. A population-based surveillance system will ensure *representativeness* of the data collected. Mandated reporting can ensure that all clinics are reporting their data. In Australia and New Zealand all clinics report to the regional registry as it is required by a licensing agreement [15].

An ideal system should be *timely* in collection and reporting. Because of the typical nine-month lag between ART treatment and a live birth outcome, ART data collection and reporting naturally lag behind the ART treatment procedure. However, options to improve timeliness include more frequent reporting cycles, such as quarterly reporting, or real-time reporting. Linkage to electronic health records could also expedite reporting. Finally, the reporting system should be *stable* and fully operational at all times with adequate technical support. Special care should be taken to ensure functionality during peak periods for reporting.

Conclusion

An ideal ART surveillance system provides a useful tool for evaluating treatment effectiveness and for tracking adverse outcomes and treatment and usage patterns. There is variation in ART surveillance systems around the world with regard to ownership of the system and data, the type and amount of information that is collected and when and how the ART data are collected and then reported to the public (if public reporting is conducted). In addition, attributes of ART surveillance systems can be improved to be simple, flexible, acceptable, representative, timely and stable and have high data quality and sensitivity and positive predictive values.

References

1. World Health Organization. Public health surveillance. *Health Topics*; 2018. Available at: www.who.int/topics/public_health_surveillance/en/, accessed 20 April 2018.

2. Centers for Disease Control and Prevention. CDC's vision for public health surveillance in the 21st century. MMWR Morb Mort Wkly Rep. 2012;**61**:1–40.

3. German R, Lee LM, Horan JM, Milstein R, Pertowski CA, Waller MN; Guidelines Working Group Centers for Disease Control and Prevention. Updated guidelines for evaluating public health systems: recommendations from the Guidelines Working Group. MMWR Morb Mort Wkly Rep. 2001;**50**:1–35.

4. Adashi EY, Wyden R. Public reporting of clinical outcomes of assisted reproductive technology programs: implications for other medical and surgical procedures. *JAMA*. 2011;**306**:1135–6.

5. Fertility Clinic Success Rate and Certification Act of 1992, Pub. L. No. 102-493 (1992). Available at: www.gpo.gov/fdsys/granule/STATUTE-106/STATUTE-106-Pg3146/content-detail.html.

6. Centers for Disease Control and Prevention, American Society for Reproductive Medicine, Society for Assisted Reproductive Medicine. *2015 Assisted Reproductive Technology Fertility Clinic Success Rates Report.* Atlanta, GA: US Dept of Health and Human Services; 2017. Available at: www.cdc.gov/art/reports/2015/fertility-clinic.html.

7. Calhaz-Jorge C, De Geyter C, Kupka MS, de Mouzon J, Erb K, Mocanu E, et al. Assisted reproductive technology in Europe, 2012: results generated from European registers by ESHRE. *Hum Reprod*. 2016;**31**: 1638–52.

8. Nygren KG, Zegers-Hochschild F, Adameson D, de Mouzon J, Mansour R, Ishihara O, et al. *The ICMART Tool Box for ART Data Collection.* Palo Alto, CA: International Committee Monitoring Assisted Reproductive Technologies (ICMART); 2011.

9. Centers for Disease Control and Prevention, American Society for Reproductive Medicine, Society for Assisted Reproductive Technology. *2015 Assisted Reproductive Technology National Summary Report.* Atlanta, GA: US Dept of Health and Human Services; 2017. Available at: www.cdc.gov/art/reports/2015/national-summary.html.

10. Zegers-Hoschschild R, Adamson GD, Dyer S, Racowsky C, de Mouzon J, Sokol R, et al. The International Glossary on Infertility and Fertility Care, 2017. *Fertil Steril*. 2017;**108**: 393–406.

11. Kawwass JF, Kissin DM, Kulkarni AD, Creanga AA, Session DR, Callaghan WM, et al. NASS Group. Safety of assisted reproductive technology in the United States, 2000–2011. *JAMA*. 2015;**13**(1):88–90.

12. Centers for Disease Control and Prevention, Department of Health and Human Services. Reporting of pregnancy success rates from assisted reproductive technology (ART) programs. *Federal Register*. 2015;**80** (165):51811–19.

13. Human Fertilisation and Embryology Authority. Collecting and recording information for the Human Fertilisation Embryology Authority. Ref: 0005. Version: 4. 29 October 2015. Available at: http://ifqtesting.blob.core.windows.net/umbraco-website/1551/2017-04-03-general-direction-0005-version-4-final.pdf, accessed 1 May 2018.

14. Centers for Disease Control and Prevention, Office of the Associate Director for Science. Assurances of confidentiality. Atlanta, GA: Centers for Disease Control and Prevention; 11 October 2017. Available at: www.cdc.gov/od/science/integrity/confidentiality/, accessed 1 May 2018.

15. Fitzgerald O, Paul RC, Harris K, Chambers GM. Assisted reproductive technology in Australia and New Zealand 2016. Sydney: National Perinatal Epideminology and Statistics Unit, the University of New South Wales; 2018.

Chapter

4

Future Directions for ART Surveillance and Monitoring Novel Technology

Christian De Geyter and Eli Y. Adashi

Introduction

Medical surveillance in assisted reproductive technology (ART) is defined by the continuous and systematic collection of health data needed for the analysis and interpretation of trends in medical care including their safety. Data are usually collected and scrutinized in regional or national registries. The submission of data to these registries is often made compulsory by law, but in many cases it is conducted on a voluntary basis by dedicated professional groups.

The data collected by registries differ from those resulting from randomized controlled trials (RCTs), in which selected cohorts of patients are prospectively recruited and treated under well-controlled conditions. The value of registry-based data resides in their being less biased by the strict selection criteria stipulated in elaborate research protocols, and they more clearly represent the real-life conditions of day-to-day clinical care. Another advantage of registry-based data collections is the size of the treated cohorts, far exceeding those recruited during clinical trials. Rare adverse events or complications, often missed during prospective randomized trials, may be detected through continued surveillance by professional registries.

The data collected by national or regional registries provide the information needed for surveillance. The latter requires the timely dissemination of data, including their publication in peer-reviewed journals or reports. When compared with other specialities in medicine, surveillance in ART is special because it includes data of more than one individual, i.e. both parents and the child, which are to be collected over an extended time period. As a result, surveillance in ART should therefore involve not only reproductive medicine but also obstetrics, neonatal care and, ideally, paediatrics.

Surveillance in ART has traditionally been simplified by collecting information about treatment cycles with a well-defined starting point and a well-defined end point. One single treatment cycle was defined by the initiation of controlled ovarian hyperstimulation and concluded by the result of the pregnancy test, usually approximately four weeks later. In the occurrence of a negative pregnancy test, the cycle was concluded. In the case of a positive pregnancy test, the outcome of the pregnancy was followed until the delivery of a newborn child. At the centre of such treatment trials were the collection of oocytes (oocyte pickup, OPU) and embryo transfer (ET). Individual couples were identified by numbers or codes, usually attributed at random by the treatment centre itself.

Many centres provide to their national registry aggregated data, which contain a collection of all treatment cycles carried out over a predefined time period, usually one year. The most advanced registries collect data in a prospective fashion: the initiation of a treatment is given to the registry, and by the end of the treatment the detailed information about the treatment is given six to eight weeks later in an ongoing fashion. Traditionally, data-collecting organizations and national registries analyze the incoming data of all treatment cycles over defined time intervals, usually one single year. This type of cross-sectional data acquisition and analysis requires an ultimate date of data submission, usually in the second quarter of the following year. At this point, the database may be frozen for statistical analysis and no further data can be submitted after that time. If pregnancy outcome data are collected, then a second data submission deadline is required, usually in the third quarter of the year following the treatment. For this type of data acquisition, treatments are analyzed cycle by cycle. This type of data collection and analysis has been the standard in virtually all registries, including those of the Society for Assisted Reproductive Technology (SART) and those of the European IVF Monitoring (EIM) Consortium.

Although some registries allow linkage of several subsequent treatment trials, current reporting very often fails to analyze outcome data if the treatment crosses the predefined observance period (for example, one year). In addition, if the infertile couple decides to change the treatment unit, the new institution will attribute to the couple another random code, with which it will then transmit its data to its national or supranational registry. As the codes given by both institutions are not interlinked, most registries do not allow a reliable and exact cumulative analysis of ART outcome data. Therefore, it would be preferable to have identification by codes attributable to individual patients, but this is currently not possible for privacy and other reasons in almost all registries.

Ongoing Trends in ART

Several recent developments in ART tend to make conventional cross-sectional data analysis as described above increasingly obsolete [1]. More and more, modern ART consists of sequences of short, intermediate therapeutic steps, in which the timing of the ultimate pregnancy test is deliberately delayed by a few weeks, months or even years. Fewer embryos are now being replaced per treatment cycle, preferentially one single selected embryo, and the remaining cohort of embryos may be cryopreserved for later thawing, often beyond the time limit of the annual data reporting [2]. Increasingly, all embryos are stored frozen to prevent complications such as ovarian hyperstimulation syndrome (OHSS) [3].

Other recent developments in ART extend the time interval between the initial measure and the ultimate outcome of ART to many years. Progress in oocyte vitrification results in frequent cryostorage of oocytes being carried out either in women confronted with the risk of destruction of their oocyte pool through chemotherapy or in women delaying the age of childbirth for personal reasons. In such cases, the time interval between oocyte collection and thawing may be many years. In those treatment modalities, traditional annual data collection and analysis consistently fail to link the events of oocyte collection with that of pregnancy. In addition, some of the frozen material will never be thawed or used for procreation, resulting in underestimation of treatment efficacy. This also applies to the surgical removal of ovarian tissue for later retransplantation.

Not only are the time intervals becoming more and more extended, but also space aspects have become more important in complicating ART surveillance. The more institutions that offer ART services, the higher the likelihood that stored biological material will be transported from one centre to another, sometimes across borders. Data are completely lacking concerning the sourcing, processing, transport and distribution of gametes, embryos or gonadal tissues within individual countries or across borders. These transports inherently carry many risks, such as loss of the gametes during transport, intermediate disruption of the freezing conditions, mislabelling, contamination of the receiving institution with infectious agents or commercial abuse of the transported gametes or embryos. When the biological material finally reaches the receiving institution, the many differences in the freezing and thawing protocols may render the proper handling of the frozen material difficult. The outcome of infertility treatment with transported gametes is rarely, if ever, documented in any registry.

As a result of all these developments, the strategy of conventional cross-sectional data collection systems in ART must be revisited, because they contribute not only to underreporting the outcome of therapeutic steps but also to overestimating their safety.

Surveillance in Other Fields of Medicine, or What Can We Learn from Our Colleagues?

Can we learn from other medical specialities in which single diagnostic and therapeutic steps are also distributed both in time and in space? One aspect of surveillance is vigilance, which aims at detecting serious or less serious adverse events of medical activities including the administration of drugs.

In pharmacology, the term *pharmacovigilance* denotes the collection, detection and monitoring of adverse events caused by the intake of pharmaceutical products. Information about the occurrence of adverse events may be reported both by health care professionals and patients and may be collected from postmarketing studies, literature sources, social media and the like. Although pharmacovigilance is a main duty of any drug regulatory authority, adverse event reporting is a regulatory requirement of all pharmaceutical companies. Pharmacovigilance helps to identify hazards linked to any pharmaceutical product and has become one of the most important ongoing measures of quality control in pharmacology. As such, pharmacovigilance relies on the reporting of single adverse events by prescribing physicians and medical care providers to the pharmaceutical company in charge of the suspect drug and on the transmission of each of these events by the pharmaceutical companies to the local drug regulatory authorities. A single individual case is valid only if the event can be traced to an identifiable patient by the reporting physician. Even if the identity of the patient is not transmitted to the drug regulatory authorities, traceability of the report is important to obtain additional information, for follow-up and to avoid duplicate reporting of adverse events.

Haemovigilance is another example for quality and safety assurance in clinical medicine. Vigilance in blood transfusion technology is required to identify and prevent, according to the World Health Organization (WHO), "the occurrence (or recurrence) of transfusion-related unwanted events, to increase the safety, efficacy and efficiency of blood transfusion, covering all activities of the transfusion chain from donor to recipient" (see the WHO guidelines on blood transfusion safety). Haemovigilance depends on the traceability of blood and blood products from donors to recipients and on reporting, investigation and analysis of adverse events. This requires correct identification of patients, samples and blood products through appropriate labelling. This can be achieved only by the active participation of all stakeholders in institutional quality management systems and active reporting of all incurrent adverse events associated with transfusion [4].

Other disciplines in medicine that have developed high-profile surveillance and vigilance systems include bone marrow transplantation [5].

The examples described above may be used as templates to improve surveillance in ART. In these examples, data reporting by the involved health care providers is not considered a burden but is, instead, an integral part of quality management and assurance, and all stakeholders (including the patients) are aware and involved. Full traceability is achieved through appropriate labelling. Very few of these achievements of our colleagues in other medical disciplines can be found in current surveillance in ART. In a majority of European countries, surveillance in ART by a national registry is not compulsory and (serious) adverse events are often not reported. Failure to report data leads to underreporting, and underreporting is the most significant flaw of current data management in ART. Underreporting is likely to result in underestimation of the risk of any treatment or in the overestimation of its effectiveness.

Surveillance in ART depends on accurate data collection, which requires the continuous involvement of highly motivated physicians, dedicated embryologists and other members of the various teams. This task should not be considered a burden by the caregivers but rather an opportunity to control and improve the quality of medical care to the ultimate benefit of the patients. Some registries allow benchmarking of ART practice for quality control purposes to improve clinical decision making [6]. Active participation in surveillance of ART should be communicated by the caregivers to the caretakers (e.g. the patients) and they should be made aware that surveillance in ART contributes to medical excellence.

Future Development of Surveillance in ART

The Rising Need for Cumulative Data Recording

Ever since its early beginnings, ART has been characterized by the rapid evolution of new technologies, such as intracytoplasmic sperm injection (ICSI) [7] and, more recently, vitrification for cryopreservation [8]. Historically, the introduction of many new developments in ART into routine clinical use was not based on the result of large-scale, prospective randomized studies, but resembled more a revolution-like, sudden widespread introduction of often inadequately tested new technologies. It is likely that future developments in ART will follow the same path. In contrast to the introduction of novel pharmaceutical products, which is highly regulated and under strict control, new methods in ART may become broadly implemented without much administrative control. Such a setting emphasizes the need for further improvement of surveillance in ART, as any new technology in ART may impact the health of both the mother and the offspring.

As indicated above, future developments in ART can be monitored only through the construction of prospective follow-up settings, in which the various therapeutic steps are segmented over prolonged periods of time, often in multiple institutions offering medical treatments sequentially to the same couple. Ideally, all cases treated with ART should be identified with a unique label, so that different steps of the therapeutic process can be linked. Such an identifying label can be given to the infertile individuals only in the presence of informed consent. This label should be promoted to become a standard of quality accepted worldwide.

As ART is now expanding to new areas, such as ovarian tissue collection (as in ovarian tissue banking) and oocyte freezing (as in 'social' freezing), the initial step in treatment should be to label the patient with a unique code. This label should follow the patient throughout all processes, even if she or he decides to change the caregiver or her or his country of residence. Especially in Europe, in which cross-border fertility care is common, the label should be accepted internationally [1].

The Need for Long-Term Follow-Up of Children after ART

Current surveillance of ART ends with the birth of the baby, which has often been stamped as the 'baby take home' rate. Future surveillance in ART should extend beyond the stage of the newborn child. Congenital abnormalities may become apparent much later and are well known to be greatly underreported in virtually all ART-surveillance data registries [9]. A substantial number of pregnancies in previously infertile women give rise to preterm birth, and prematurely born newborn children often suffer health problems. However, these are not recorded in the first few days after birth. Even in normally born adolescents resulting from ART, subtle differences in blood pressure and in their cardiovascular condition have been described [10, 11]. Paediatric medical societies should be involved to link surveillance in ART with a prospective long-term follow-up of children.

If data are to be linked from the first initial decision to embark on treatment not only with ongoing pregnancy but also with health data of the growing child, information must be collected by three different medical disciplines, not necessarily working closely together: (1) reproductive medicine, (2) fetomaternal medicine and obstetrics and (3) neonatology and paediatrics. This can be achieved only with the active support of national authorities, which should be aware of the need to install surveillance in ART. They should impose surveillance of all forms of ART within the frame of a common acceptance of the principles of proactive quality management and assurance.

Not only health authorities but also many other parties may be interested in good-quality and long-term ART surveillance, such as the pharmaceutical industry and health insurance companies. For data privacy purposes, only aggregated data may typically be provided by the registries to any external organization, and this requires much administrative and analytical work. Such requests are expected to become more frequent in the near future and may represent an additional source of income for high-quality registries.

Vigilance in ART

Vigilance in ART may be defined by the detection, analysis and communication of complications, errors and adverse events occurring during or after ART. Currently, some safety data in ART are recorded, such as multiple deliveries, OHSS and maternal mortality, but all are often underreported. Other severe adverse events, such as the erroneous mix-up of gametes and embryos or their unintentional loss, are not reported at all. To the general public, it seems as if these events do not happen at all or happen very rarely, and, in case of an incident, leave the afflicted individuals and the responsible caregiver(s) isolated because of an apparently unique accident. Proper reporting of all adverse events in ART will help to quantify the effect of human error in ART and may help to create a sense of objectivity through mutual trust.

The exact circumstances of severe adverse events are rarely described in detail in most registries. Vigilance consists not only of merely recording adverse events, but also of assessing underlying causes and understanding the mechanisms leading to the events. Doing so may lead to the formulation of preventive measures as part of an ongoing quality management development.

Methods for Quality Assurance in Data Management

The increasing relevance of surveillance and vigilance in ART requires quality data management. The instalment of a compulsory ART data registration through a legal framework has been demonstrated to be highly beneficial, but caregiver compliance with any imposed legal obligation needs to be controlled as well. Appropriate legislation is also important for the informed consent to be signed by every single individual undergoing ART.

Quality data management starts with continuous collection of the required information in the various institutions offering ART services and includes well-functioning data acquisition and plausibility testing by the registries, followed by professional statistical analysis of the data. Proper functioning of ART surveillance is of interest to many parties, including health authorities and health insurance companies, and an appropriate certification of the data exchange with external partners should be mandatory in all registries. The handling of aggregated data requests by external parties, such as health authorities, the pharmaceutical industry or scientists, must be formulated as standardized operating procedures (so-called SOP). The many aspects of data confidentiality should be checked on a regular basis by an appointed data protection officer, as regulations may change over time.

An external audit system by independent international experts has been shown to be effective in the Swiss ART registry in optimizing the quality of data reporting [12], as also demonstrated in an international liver transplantation registry [13]. External audits may check the completeness and accuracy of data reporting in randomly selected patient files. Repeated external audits help to motivate the teams in improving their performance, and are valuable to quantify human error in data acquisition.

Confidentiality and Protection of Privacy

Individuals suffering from infertility are potentially vulnerable, and all information resulting from the exploration of the causes of their infertility should be protected. Therefore, all activities in surveillance in ART must comply with regulations with respect to protection of privacy and confidentiality. Confidentiality is defined as the treatment of information that an individual has disclosed in a relationship of trust and with the expectation that this information will not be shared with others without agreement. All information linking the various measures of ART with pregnancy outcome and with child development can be collected after obtaining patient informed consent or through a waiver of consent. In providing their signed agreement, the infertile patients should be made aware that through this they take the responsibility of providing true anonymous data about their child to the national registry.

Following current regulations, traceability should not be organized through the names and birthdates of the treated individuals but instead by using a unique identifying code attached to each person seeking fertility treatment. As stated above, this individual identifier should follow the caretakers during the entire process of ART, pregnancy and delivery. The link between an individual code and the involved patients should reside with the treating physician and will not be passed on to the national registry. If a patient decides to change the treating institution, all data on the previous treatments and eventual biological material should be made identifiable with the code attributed at the very beginning of medical care.

References

1. De Geyter Ch, Wyns C, Mocanu E, de Mouzon J, Calhaz-Jorge C. Data collection systems in ART must follow the pace of change in clinical practice. *Hum Reprod.* 2016;**31**:2160–3.

2. Ubaldi FM, Capalbo A, Colamaria S, Ferrero S, Maggiulli R, Vajta G, et al. Reduction of multiple pregnancies in the advanced maternal age population after implementation of an elective single embryo transfer policy coupled with enhanced embryo selection: pre- and post-intervention study. *Hum Reprod.* 2015;**30**:2097–106.

3. Devroey P, Polyzos NP, Blockeel C. An OHSS-free clinic by segmentation of IVF treatment. *Hum Reprod.* 2011;**26**:2593–7.

4. WHO, National Haemovigilance System. Aide-mémoire for ministries of health. Available at: www .who.int/bloodsafety/am_National_Haemovigilance_ System.pdf?ua=1.

5. Shaw BE, Chapman J, Fechter M, Foeken L, Greinix H, Hwang W, et al. Towards a global system of vigilance and surveillance in unrelated donors of haematopoietic progenitor cells for transplantation. *Bone Marrow Transplant.* 2013;**48**:1506–9.

6. Sullivan EA, Wang YA, Norman RJ, Chambers GM, Chughtai AA, Farquhar CM. Perinatal mortality following assisted reproductive technology treatment in Australia and New Zealand, a public health approach for international reporting of perinatal mortality. *BMC Pregnancy Childbirth.* 2013;**13**:177.

7. Palermo G, Joris H, Devroey P, Van Steirteghem AC. Pregnancies after intracytoplasmic injection of single spermatozoon into an oocyte. *Lancet.* 1992;**340**:17–18.

8. Cobo A, Kuwayama M, Pérez S, Ruiz A, Pellicer A, Remohí J. Comparison of concomitant outcome achieved with fresh and cryopreserved donor oocytes vitrified by the Cryotop method. *Fertil Steril.* 2008;**89**:1657–64.

9. Boyle B, Addor MC, Arriola L, Barisic I, Bianchi F, Csáky-Szunyogh M, et al. Estimating Global Burden of

Disease due to congenital anomaly: an analysis of European data. *Arch Dis Child Fetal Neonatal Ed.* 2018;103:F22–F28.

10. Guo XY, Liu XM, Jin L, Wang TT, Ullah K, Sheng JZ, et al. Cardiovascular and metabolic profiles of offspring conceived by assisted reproductive technologies: a systematic review and meta-analysis. *Fertil Steril.* 2017;107:622–31.

11. Scherrer U, Rimoldi SF, Rexhaj E, Stuber T, Duplain H, Garcin S, et al. Systemic and pulmonary vascular dysfunction in children conceived by assisted

reproductive technologies. *Circulation.* 2012;125: 1890–6.

12. Van den Bergh M, Hohl MK, De Geyter Ch, Stalberg AM, Limoni C. Ten years of Swiss National IVF Register FIVNAT-CH. Are we making progress? *Reprod Biomed Online.* 2005;11:632–40.

13. Karam V, Gunson B, Roggen F, Grande L, Wannoff W, Janssen M, et al.; European Liver Transplant Association. Quality control of the European Liver Transplant Registry: results of audit visits to the contributing centers. *Transplantation.* 2003;75:2167–73.

Chapter

5

Reporting ART Success Rates

Georgina M. Chambers, Kevin Doody and Sara Crawford

The findings and conclusions in this report are those of the authors and do not necessarily represent the official position of the Centers for Disease Control and Prevention.

Introduction

A principal role of assisted reproductive technology (ART) registries is to report on the performance of ART in terms of treatment success. Success can be considered the attainment of a favourable or desired outcome, encapsulating the concepts of *safety, efficacy, effectiveness* and *efficiency* [1, 2]. However, operationalizing its meaning depends on the stakeholder perspective, be it patient, scientist, clinician, clinic or regulator, and the concept of success being measured. Many national ART registries were established in the 1980s primarily to monitor the safety of the rapidly evolving technology. However, the roles of the more than 90 national registries [3] and numerous jurisdictional and regional registries currently operating around the world have evolved to incorporate research, performance management, health system planning and public reporting functions. Indeed, how ART treatment success is reported to the public by individual clinics and ART registries is a widely debated topic in reproductive medicine [4, 5, 6, 7, 8, 9].

There is no single, agreed upon measure of ART success even when the stakeholder perspective is known. A recent appraisal of 142 randomized controlled trials (RCTs) of medically assisted fertility treatments identified more than 800 different computations of measures of ART outcomes [10]. The plethora of outcome measures is largely due to the complex, multilevel nature of ART treatments resulting in many possible numerators and denominators from which to choose. A 'single ART cycle' is the most traditional unit of measure and involves a series of stages, including ovarian stimulation, oocyte retrieval and embryo transfer in the case of a stimulated (fresh) cycle, and thawing/warming and embryo transfer in the case of a cryopreservation cycle. A 'complete ART cycle' accounts for all embryos resulting from an initiated stimulated cycle (or, in some cases, an oocyte retrieval) and can include a fresh embryo transfer and/or multiple

cryopreservation embryo transfer procedures [11]. Finally, taking the patient as the unit of measurement, multiple 'complete ART cycles' are possible, and indeed likely, over an entire treatment course.

Evolving laboratory and clinical practices continue to challenge how success rates from ART treatments are calculated and reported. The increasing trend of delaying embryo transfer to allow preimplantation genetic testing (PGT) of the embryos and to improve embryo–uterine synchronicity is a particular challenge, with two of the largest registries in the world, the United Kingdom (UK) Human Fertilisation and Embryology Authority (HFEA) registry and the United States (US) Society for Assisted Reproductive Technology Clinical Outcomes Reporting System (SART CORS), adopting substantially different approaches to reporting [9]. Similarly, the use of ART to support the reproductive goals of those not traditionally treated for infertility is increasing, introducing new challenges in terms of reporting measures of ART success. For example, two of the fastest growing areas of ART are the long-term cryopreservation of gametes to extend the reproductive potential of individuals for medical or non-medical ('social') reasons and the use of donated gametes and surrogacy arrangements to enable people who are not in traditional unions to have children (single, same-sex couples, transgender) [12].

The principal concern of ART treatments must be patient *safety*, reducing the risk of unnecessary harm to women and babies, and *effectiveness*, maximizing the chance of a live birth delivery in routine practice. However, many of the numerators and denominators employed to express success are often a proxy or intermediate measure of the overarching goal of ART treatments – a healthy baby.

The following sections will elaborate on these points by contextualizing the role that ART registries play in reporting ART performance outcomes, describing advantages and disadvantages of the common numerators and denominators, summarizing the challenges associated with evolving clinical practice and, finally, discussing how public reporting of ART registry data affects patient decision making.

The Role of ART Registries in Informing Stakeholders about ART Success

Greater use of health data by patients, clinicians, regulators and policy makers is a hallmark of the digital age, making the ART registry a central player in modern health care delivery. ART registries are arguably one of the most prolific clinical registries in the world, with many having been established in the early 1980s soon after the birth of the first ART baby in 1978. Indeed, the world's first national ART registry was established in 1983 in Australia and New Zealand, and recorded ART pregnancies achieved from 1979 onwards [13].

Clinical registries are generally described as standardized data collection systems which collect a defined minimum dataset from patients undergoing a particular procedure or therapy, diagnosed with a particular condition or disease or managed via a specific health care resource. Clinical registries that provide feedback for quality improvement functions are more specifically referred to as clinical *quality* registries [14, 15, 16]. Although most ART registries were initially established to monitor safety and as a source of data for epidemiological and health systems planning, they are increasingly being used for monitoring quality of care, providing feedback, benchmarking performance, reducing variation and driving best practice. The rise of performance management in the health care system since the 1990s as a way of improving quality and reducing cost has meant that the ART registry has taken on increasing quality control and public reporting functions [17].

At the level of health systems planning and governance, a number of countries use a variety of regulatory and funding mechanisms to ensure near complete ascertainment of ART treatment and outcomes data in national ART registries. Examples include the UK HFEA Act [18], the US Fertility Clinic Success Rate and Certification Act of 1992 [19] and the Australian Reproductive Technology Accreditation Committee (RTAC) Codes of Practice [20]. ART registry data are increasingly used by governments and regulators to plan and assess the impact of government policies on ART services, with decisions about public funding for ART treatment often contingent on the effectiveness of treatment based on female age and number of successive treatments [21, 22, 23].

At the clinician or provider level, ART registry data are increasingly used to assess the success rates of clinics against peers, either by public disclosure of performance ('report cards') or by feedback directly to clinics as part of clinical quality registry benchmarking. Public reporting of clinic performance is practised by the US and UK. For example, the US Act [19] stipulates that public reporting of outcomes at the clinic level is required. The challenges of publishing clinic success rates are discussed in further detail later in this chapter.

At a patient/consumer level, users of health care are increasingly turning to the Internet to inform themselves about the quality of health care providers and institutions. Approximately three-quarters of Americans searched the Internet for health-related information in 2012, and this number is likely to increase with time [24]. Consumers use public reporting to inform their decisions about selecting providers with their preferred characteristics of care, based not only on success rates but also on cost, location and the range of services provided. Consumers have come to expect transparency of health care information in line with other consumer goods and services. Indeed, new laws and market dynamics underpin and support greater provider accountability and consumer engagement in health care decision making [25]. ART registries thus have a vital role to play in informing consumers. If done well, standardized performance indicators provided by ART clinical registries are unbiased, easily understood clinical quality measures for consumers. Such publicly available performance indicators should include measures of treatment success that are meaningful to patients and encapsulate dimensions of both safety and effectiveness.

Choice of Numerators

Typically, an outcome measure includes a numerator that represents a clinical parameter of interest (e.g. live birth), and a denominator that provides the clinical context in which the outcome is measured – that is, the definition of the cohort at risk from an exposure (e.g. total number of patients or embryo transfers). Although there are many numerators that can be chosen to describe the ART outcome parameter of interest, embryo implantation, pregnancy and live birth are the most common. Measures that define a 'healthy' baby are tied to reducing harms to mothers and infants.

Implanted Embryos

Implanted embryos refer to embryos that have successfully implanted in the uterus, resulting in the formation of a gestation sac. The implantation rate is usually expressed as the number of gestational sacs observed divided by the number of embryos transferred (often expressed as a percentage and multiplied by 100) [11].

Implantation rates provide a biologically measurable outcome of reproduction and can be measured close to the time of embryo transfer, thus providing a relatively proximal, albeit intermediate, measure of treatment success. However, it is rare for ART registries to report implantation rates, and a number of researchers and clinicians have criticized the reporting of implantation rates even in the context of clinical trials [26]. Arguments centre on the presence of a 'cohort effect', wherein the implantation of one embryo predicts the implantation outcome of the remaining embryos in the cohort. An additional argument relates to the statistical problem of pooling embryos by groups of women, thereby creating a sample of interrelated observations and thus violating the independence necessary for inferential statistical testing. Furthermore, when embryo selection techniques, such as PGT, are evaluated against strategies that do not actively exclude embryos, the former usually results in a higher implantation rate because only highly selected embryos are transferred, but the overall success rates of an initiated stimulation cycle (a complete ART cycle) may actually be reduced [26, 27].

Pregnancy

Reporting pregnancy rates as a measure of ART success is common but is still an intermediate measure of treatment success from a patient's perspective, with pregnancy not guaranteeing a live birth. Furthermore, pregnancy can be variously described as being biological, clinical, viable or ongoing, all with different definitions making comparative assessment between registries, clinics, clinicians and treatment strategies problematic [10]. The reporting of pregnancy rates alone also masks safety concerns related to high multiple birth rates due to the transfer of multiple embryos.

Live (Birth) Deliveries

Live birth delivery has traditionally been used as the preferred primary outcome for ART success and is generally defined as the birth of one or more live born infants, with twins or high-order multiples (HOMs) counted as a single live birth delivery [11]. A live birth delivery provides a quantitative measure of treatment success that is clinically meaningful for patients. Furthermore, each live born child must be registered as part of national vital statistics. However, even national definitions of what constitutes a delivery, live birth and stillbirth vary based on gestational age cut-offs and birth weight, making international comparison between ART registries problematic. The International Committee Monitoring Assisted Reproductive Technologies (ICMART) glossary specifies a cut-off of gestational age of 22 weeks or birth weight of 500 grams for international comparison of ART delivery and live birthrates, and cut-offs of 22–28 weeks and 28 weeks to define late fetal loss and stillbirth, respectively [11].

Live birth delivery as a definitive measure of ART success has limitations because it may mask important safety outcomes, such as high multiple birth rates. Indeed, the focus on pregnancy or live birth rates as measures of success alone can incentivize unsafe embryo transfer practices, promoting the transfer of more than one embryo to improve pregnancy and live birth rates at the expense of a higher multiple birth rate (which increases the risk of adverse health outcomes for mother and infant).

Healthy Baby

The most significant safety challenge associated with ART treatment is the risk of multiple gestation pregnancy as a result of the transfer of more than one embryo during treatment. It is well documented that twins and HOMs pose significant health risks to both mothers and infants [28]. The ART multiple birth rate varies substantially between countries. For example, in 2015 the multiple birth rate among ART-conceived infants in the US was 35.3% compared with 4.4% in Australia and New Zealand [29, 30].

Adopting measures that provide a proxy of a healthy baby born from ART have been suggested and indeed reported using the US National ART

Surveillance System (NASS). The idea is to reduce practices that result in adverse outcomes (particularly multiple gestation) and to provide a single universal measure of ART success that combines both elements of effectiveness and safety. The most common measure is that proposed by Min and colleagues, the "birth of a healthy singleton baby at full gestation per cycle initiated" (known as birth emphasizing a successful singleton at term, BESST) [31].

The BESST outcome [31], or other similar measures [32] that shift the emphasis from pregnancy or live birth rate to a primary end point that focuses on achieving the best opportunity for a healthy baby, is intuitively attractive. However, there remains little agreement in combining both effectiveness and safety into a single measure. Effectiveness and safety are separate concepts, with effectiveness defined in terms of a *benefit* and safety defined in terms of a *risk*. The main problem with a composite measure is that it hinders the ability to capture either of these elements sufficiently, possibly resulting in misleading conclusions about the success and safety of ART treatments [32, 33].

Choice of Denominators

The selection of an appropriate denominator is important, as it provides the clinical context and captures the exposure–risk relationship. The most commonly used denominators for measuring ART success reflect the multiple stages of ART treatments.

Per Initiated Single Cycle

Measuring outcomes per initiated single cycle (stimulated or cryopreservation) based on a cross section of treatment performed over a specified time period (generally a year) is the most common measure reported by ART registries. In most ART registries, success rates per initiated single cycle are stratified by maternal age, cause of infertility and treatment modalities to provide an assessment of the probability of success based on an intention-to-treat principle (that is, the decision to commence or not to commence treatment). However, single cycle success rates do not provide any information about the chance of success with repeated treatment attempts (e.g. chance of success after a failed cycle), or the cumulative chance of ART success over the course of treatment (e.g. chance of success after several cycles). Furthermore, measuring success based on initiated single cycles does not adequately account for the

trend towards segmenting cycles wherein all oocytes or embryos from an ovarian stimulation are cryopreserved with the intention of delaying embryo transfer (segmented cycles).

Per Embryo Transfer

A common alternative to using 'initiated' single cycles as a denominator is to include only those cycles that reach embryo transfer. This approach results in higher reported success rates, particularly when intermediate numerators, such as pregnancy, are used. This is illustrated in the latest Australian and New Zealand Assisted Reproduction Database (ANZARD) report. The report shows the clinical pregnancy rate for women aged 40–44, when expressed per initiated single cycle, was 8.5%, but increased to 15.5% when expressed as clinical pregnancy per embryo transfer [29]. However, embryo transfer is often the preferred denominator because it removes some of the prognostic differences between patients, arguably providing a better measure of a clinic's performance than per initiated single cycle.

Per 'Complete Cycle'

Over the past decade, use of segmented cycles has grown steadily. Latest estimates from the ANZARD reveal that the number of cryopreservation cycles rose by 23% over the 5 years leading up to 2015 with a corresponding increase in the live delivery rate per cryopreservation cycle from 19.1% to 25.3% [29].

This shift has been driven by modern vitrification cryopreservation methods, an increasing shift towards single embryo transfer and an improved understanding of the embryo–endometrium synchrony [34]. Therefore, to capture the increasing use of cryopreservation and to provide a more holistic measure of ART treatment success that includes the contribution of all embryos resulting from one ovarian stimulation, cumulative success rates from a 'complete cycle' perspective are increasingly used for reporting ART outcomes. Using the per 'complete cycle' perspective, the numerator is the number of pregnancies or live births achieved from all embryo transfers associated with the ovarian stimulation and the denominator is the number of ovarian stimulated cycles [35, 36, 37].

This approach provides the advantage of measuring the patient's total reproductive potential from the start of the stimulation cycle and thus offers an all-inclusive success rate, which is arguably more relevant and meaningful to patients than a measure that provides a single cycle estimate. In addition, the 'complete cycle' perspective is more likely to incentivize single embryo transfer by minimizing the emphasis on pregnancy or live birth resulting from a single cycle. However, the use of this metric could potentially incentivize aggressive ovarian stimulation for the purpose of maximizing the number of embryos available for cryopreservation cycles [38].

Per Woman/Couple

Most couples undergo more than one ART treatment cycle during a course of treatment. Therefore, cumulative success rates over successive treatment cycles is a meaningful measure of success from a couple's perspective. The cumulative live birth rate per couple is defined as the overall chance of success (a live birth) from all fresh and cryopreservation cycles after a given number of cycles. A number of examples of cumulative live birth delivery rates following repeated 'complete ART cycles' derived from large registry datasets have been published [34, 35, 36, 37, 38]. Because cumulative live birth delivery rates provide the perspective of the woman/couple, a realistic representation of success following an entire course of treatment is achieved [39]. Moreover, as women are followed over multiple cycles, this measure can be used to inform patients of the average number of cycles needed to achieve a live birth delivery, as well as their chance of success over multiple ART cycles. However, measuring cumulative success rates using ART registry data requires that women can be followed longitudinally within, and increasingly across, ART clinics using a unique identifier or data-linkage methods. To facilitate the follow-up of patients across clinics, a unique reproductive code for all women undertaking ART in Europe has been proposed [5]. An extended period of time is also needed to obtain sufficient numbers of cycles to estimate accurate success rates (often three to four years of follow-up to achieve a live birth), by which time ART clinical practice techniques will have likely evolved.

Another challenge with cumulative live birth delivery rates relates to how to deal with assumptions about the likelihood of ART success for women who discontinue treatment. A common approach is to present optimal and conservative cumulative live birth rates. The conservative rate assumes that women who discontinue ART treatment would have had a zero chance of achieving a live birth delivery with continued treatment, while the optimal rate assumes that those who discontinue treatment would have had the same chance of treatment success as those who continued with treatment. The true cumulative success rate would fall somewhere between the estimates [35, 36, 37].

Aside from the measures summarized in this section, some ART registries use more novel approaches to reporting success, which are described in the following section.

Public Reporting of Clinic Success Rates in the US and UK

Unlike most other countries, the UK and the US publicly report the success rates for ART treatment cycles at both the national and clinic levels. These two countries use different approaches to reporting. In the UK, the HFEA collects the cycle-specific ART data and uses the data to publish the *Fertility Treatment: Trends and Figures* report [40]. This report contains aggregate data on the characteristics and outcomes of the reported ART cycles. The main birth rates that are published (referred to as 'headline' measures by the HFEA) include the birth rate per embryo transferred and the birth rate per treatment cycle. The birth rate per embryo transferred is calculated as the number of births divided by the number of embryos transferred. It was adopted by the HFEA because they consider it to be increasingly viewed by professionals as the best measure of clinical practice and penalizes the transfer of more embryos in a single cycle in order to achieve a live birth. However, this measure does not include the outcomes of patients who do not reach embryo transfer, thereby ignoring cycles with an early failure, such as cycles cancelled prior to retrieval (e.g. due to illness, poor reaction to stimulation) or cycles stopped after retrieval (e.g. poor oocyte yield, poor embryo quality). The HFEA also reports the birth rate per treatment cycle as a headline measure, which is calculated as the number of births divided by the number of treatment cycles started. This measure does not take into account the number of embryos transferred, but it does take into account cycles stopped prior to transfer [40].

The HFEA also publishes clinic-specific success rates on its website [41], where the clinic-specific rates are compared with the national rate. Here, the HFEA presents the birth rate per embryo transferred and the birth rate per treatment cycle. Another reported measure is the birth rate per oocyte collection. For each oocyte collection (i.e. retrieval), all transfers of those retrieved oocytes that occur within two years of the retrieval are examined for the occurrence of a birth in order to see whether that course of treatment (an oocyte retrieval followed by a series of fresh and frozen transfers of the retrieved oocytes in the effort to achieve a birth) resulted in a success. And finally, the HFEA reports multiple birth rates in order to highlight the safety issues surrounding multiple births. Website users can explore the clinic-specific success rates by time period, type of treatment (IVF or ICSI), age group and oocyte source (patient or donor).

In the US, there are two data collection systems used to collect cycle-specific ART data. The Society for Assisted Reproductive Technology Clinical Outcomes Reporting System (SART CORS) is owned and operated by SART, an ART professional society. SART collects cycle-specific data from SART-member clinics and publishes a preliminary and final report of ART success rates on its website at both national and clinic levels [42]. ART success rates reported by SART involve the assessment of cycles started with the intent to retrieve oocytes and all fresh and frozen transfers of those retrieved oocytes that occur within a year of the retrieval, focusing again on a complete treatment procedure. SART reports birth rates per primary transfer (i.e. the first transfer of the retrieved oocytes whether fresh or frozen) and birth rates per subsequent transfer (i.e. all transfers of the retrieved oocytes except for the first transfer). These rates can be explored by characteristics of the cycle such as embryo state (fresh or frozen), ICSI use, PGT use, elective single embryo transfer use, embryo stage (cleavage or blastocyst), level of stimulation and patient diagnosis. Similar to the birth rate per oocyte collection in the UK, SART also reports the cumulative live birth rate, or the number of births occurring from any transfer of retrieved oocytes divided by the number of cycles started with the intent to retrieve oocytes. Finally, SART reports the live birth rate per patient among patients new to an infertility clinic starting their first retrieval of their own eggs. In addition to live birth rates, SART reports singleton, twin and triplet or higher-order birth rates as well as term, preterm and very preterm birth rates. Success rates are reported by patient age group where appropriate.

The Centers for Disease Control and Prevention (CDC) collects ART cycle-specific data from all clinics performing ART in the US. It publicly reports clinic-specific and national ART treatment success rates both in published reports (the *ART Fertility Clinic Success Rates Report* and the *ART National Summary Report*) as well as on the CDC website [43, 44, 45]. Current reporting at national and clinic levels focuses on single event success rates, such as live births per cycle started, live births per retrieval or live births per transfer. Success rates are presented separately for cycles using fresh embryos from nondonor eggs, cycles using frozen embryos from nondonor eggs and cycles using donor eggs, and are presented by female age where appropriate. Success rates can be explored by patient diagnosis and, in some cases, embryo stage and the number of embryos transferred. In addition to live births, measures of success also include pregnancies, twin live births, singleton live births, and full-term, normal birth weight, singleton live births. Similar to SART, future success rates reporting will explore the outcomes of all transfers of oocytes from a single retrieval, with a focus on live birth rates and singleton live birth rates per cycle started with the intent to retrieve oocytes, per cycle involving the actual retrieval of oocytes and per cycle involving the transfer of oocytes or embryos. Future reporting of success rates will also include live birth rates for patients new to ART.

Challenges of Public Reporting of Clinic Success Rates

Public reporting of clinic-specific ART success rates is designed to improve quality and patient decision making by making clinic performance transparent. However, the public reporting of clinic-specific ART success rates has the potential for both positive and negative consequences. Public reporting of ART success rates allows for better transparency of outcomes and more informed consumers. In the US, clinics performing ART are required to report their ART cycle and outcome data to the CDC as a result of the Fertility Clinic Success Rate and Certification Act, a law that was initially passed because of concerns about the quality and comparability of ART success rates data [19]. Requiring the standard collection of cycle-level data and standard reporting of ART success rates across clinics provides information for potential ART patients to inform decision making with regard to treatment. However, ART success rates may have unintended consequences, such as selective reporting or service shifts. Either clinics may choose not to report data for patients with poor ART cycle outcomes, or clinics may limit services to only those associated with high success rates. In the US, consumers of these publicly available clinic-specific success rates are cautioned that comparisons across clinics may not be meaningful because of differences in patient populations (e.g. some clinics may treat a greater proportion of poor prognosis patients) and differences in ART treatment practices (e.g. some clinics may choose to transfer fewer embryos per attempt at pregnancy in order to lower the chances of patients having a multiple birth).

However, because consumers (and clinics) can still use these data to compare clinics, this can result in potentially negative effects on clinical care as well as reporting quality. For example, with regard to clinical care, clinics may deny care to poor prognosis patients because their chance of success is typically lower. Clinics may also use more aggressive stimulation protocols, even though these are riskier to the patient, in order to generate a better oocyte yield, or clinics may transfer more embryos at a time in order to improve the chance of pregnancy and live birth from a single cycle, thereby creating a greater risk of multiple gestation pregnancy. With regard to data quality, clinics may not report failed cycles (i.e. cycles not proceeding to retrieval or transfer). Such negative consequences occur because the process of measurement itself can alter the behaviour of clinics and clinicians. As such, any public reporting of clinic success rates should be designed to minimize and detect such unintended consequences to the greatest extent possible [17].

While the effects of public reporting of ART data on clinician or patient behaviour have not been studied, a systematic review studying the effects of the public reporting of surgical outcomes found that the most commonly studied effect was the impact on patient selection. The majority of studies found surgeons were more likely to avoid taking higher risk patients after the public reporting was instituted [46]. Both presenting and providing feedback to clinics on performance indicators that account for differences in the case-mix of the patients treated by clinicians are challenging. When patient registries are used to produce public 'report cards', it is imperative that additional measures be put in place. Prospective reporting requirements can decrease the chance that cycles cancelled prior to egg retrieval or transfer are unreported. External data review and selective on-site validation via inspection of medical and laboratory records are encouraged to identify systematic reporting errors that might mislead the public. Data quality remediation protocols may be established to handle significant data collection errors when identified. However, on balance, reporting feedback to clinicians and publishing 'report cards' based on clinical quality registries have been shown to be effective in improving professional practice [16, 47].

Prediction Models/Patient Calculators

The public reporting of clinic-specific success cannot be used to predict success for individual patients. Although publicly reported success rates are stratified by age, a variety of other factors are known to contribute to prognosis. These factors include (but are not limited to) diagnosis or reason for ART, body mass index, ethnicity, ovarian reserve, prior successful pregnancy and the number and details of prior failed IVF cycles. Creating filters by these prognostic factors for clinic-specific success rates would likely be inappropriate, as the number of patients within an average individual clinic dataset that would have similar characteristics to a prospective patient could be too few to generate a reliable estimate of success. The development of robust patient predictor tools is necessary to overcome this limitation. These predictor tools are appropriately built using the full registry dataset rather than subsets derived from individual clinics. SART has constructed one such predictor tool and has made it available to patients online since 2014 [48, 49]. This first generation of the SART patient predictor tool is limited in that it does not take into account frozen embryo transfers and, therefore, is not indicative of the total reproductive potential related to a cycle started with the intention of egg retrieval (SART's current primary success metric). Furthermore, the first treatment cycle may not succeed. Many patients embarking on IVF will undergo several complete cycles – each involving a fresh embryo transfer potentially followed by one or more frozen embryo transfers in order to achieve a live birth. Investigators from the University of Aberdeen have developed a novel calculator based on the HFEA registry designed to predict the cumulative chances of a live birth per patient through six completed cycles (each cycle includes all fresh and frozen embryo transfers following one ovarian stimulation) [50, 51]. Additionally, this predictor tool has a second tool to estimate success after the characteristics of a first attempt are known. The addition of first cycle details (number of eggs retrieved, embryos transferred and cryopreserved) improves the accuracy of the estimate. SART plans to model a second-generation predictor tool to incorporate these concepts. These calculators will continue to be refined over time to include very specific predictors that have only been collected in more recent years (e.g. anti-Müllerian hormone level). Because the practice of ART continues to evolve over time and success rates may change, it is ideal that these predictor tools use data from recent years that collect details of new techniques.

Patient predictor tools can help shape patients' expectations, allowing them to plan their treatments more efficiently and to prepare emotionally and financially for a full course of treatment. However, they are not without limitation and may not be reliable in a different context from the setting for which they were developed [52].

Concluding Remarks

The increasing complexity of ART treatments for an expanding list of indications, together with a recognition of the importance of patient-centred outcomes, makes ART registries a central resource for informing stakeholders about the performance of ART from an international, jurisdiction, clinic and patient perspective. As approaches to ART treatments become more varied, so do the options for reporting ART treatment success. The multipart nature of ART treatments gives rise to a multitude of possible measures of outcomes. Which of these are the most appropriate and important depends on the stakeholder perspective and the purpose of the measure.

ART registries are being used as a source for measuring ART performance, particularly for reporting at a clinic level, and to inform patients about their individual chances of success through web-based prediction tools. While a number of countries have laws and/or licensing arrangements that mandate clinics report treatment and outcomes to central ART registries, the US and UK also report the performance of individual clinics publicly. Although undocumented, there is concern that this type of reporting may lead to unintended incentives to increase success rates at the expense of treatment safety (i.e. transferring more embryos at once, leading to multiple pregnancies), as well as selective reporting or limiting access to poor prognosis patients.

While health data transparency generally leads to better decision making and clinical performance, ART registry reports and individualized patient predictors may be designed to present information in a format that minimizes negative consequences, such as incentivizing multiple embryo transfer to maximize pregnancy rates. Modern ART registries link all patient treatments and outcomes so that elective single embryo transfer is not penalized in a cumulative success metric. Furthermore, reporting that emphasizes a complete ART cycle per stimulation cycle or live births per 'first transfer' or per 'subsequent transfer' (regardless of whether from a fresh or cryopreserved embryo) provides a more holistic and patient-centred reflection of ART treatment.

We believe that the future of ART registry reporting will likely evolve to include a number of reporting platforms and tools to meet individual stakeholder needs, such as the patient predictor tools discussed above. Public reports will likely become more interactive with user-driven menus rather than large static reports, and while public reports should not be used by patients to predict their own likelihood of success, they will continue to be critical for policy making and research, particularly when linked with other data collections. Well-designed and validated patient predictor tools for counselling patients about their individual chances of ART success will become more common and a central tool used to assist clinicians in counselling patients about treatment choices.

In conclusion, the ubiquitous expectation of timely, accurate and accessible health data will continue to make ART registries the most important source of performance measures of ART treatment. Governments and fertility organizations maintaining ART registries are encouraged to keep pace with ART clinical practice and stakeholder, particularly patient, expectations.

References

1. Haynes B. Can it work? Does it work? Is it worth it?: the testing of healthcare interventions is evolving. *BMJ.* 1999;**319**(7211):652–3.

2. Runciman W, Hibbert P, Thomson R, Van Der Schaaf T, Sherman H, Lewalle P. Towards an International Classification for Patient Safety: key concepts and terms. *Int J Qual Health Care.* 2009;**21** (1):18–26.

3. Dyer S, Chambers GM, de Mouzon J, Nygren KG, Zegers-Hochschild F, Mansour R, et al. International Committee for Monitoring Assisted Reproductive

Technologies world report: assisted reproductive technology 2008, 2009 and 2010. *Hum Reprod.* 2016;**31**(7):1588–609.

4. Abdalla HI, Bhattacharya S, Khalaf Y. Is meaningful reporting of national IVF outcome data possible? *Hum Reprod.* 2010;**25**(1):9–13.

5. De Geyter C, Wyns C, Mocanu E, de Mouzon J, Calhaz-Jorge C. Data collection systems in ART must follow the pace of change in clinical practice. *Hum Reprod.* 2016;**31**(10):2160–3.

6. Doody KJ. Public reporting of assisted reproductive technology cycle outcomes is not simple. *Fertil Steril.* 2016;**105**(4):893–4.

7. Heijnen EMEW, Macklon NS, Fauser BCJM. What is the most relevant standard of success in assisted reproduction? The next step to improving outcomes of IVF: consider the whole treatment. *Hum Reprod.* 2004;**19**(9):1936–8.

8. Schieve LA, Reynolds MA. What is the most relevant standard of success in assisted reproduction? Challenges in measuring and reporting success rates for assisted reproductive technology treatments: what is optimal? *Hum Reprod.* 2004;**19**(4):778–82.

9. Wilkinson J, Roberts SA, Vail A. Developments in IVF warrant the adoption of new performance indicators for ART clinics, but do not justify the abandonment of patient-centred measures. *Hum Reprod.* 2017;**32**(6):1155–9.

10. Wilkinson J, Roberts SA, Showell M, Brison DR, A. V. No common denominator: a review of outcome measures in IVF RCTs. *Hum Reprod.* 2016;**31**:2714–22.

11. Zegers-Hochschild F, Adamson GD, Dyer S, Racowsky C, de Mouzon J, Sokol R, et al. The International Glossary on Infertility and Fertility Care, 2017. *Fertil Steril.* 2017;**108**(3):393–406.

12. Inhorn MC. The egg freezing revolution? Gender, technology, and fertility preservation in the twenty-first century. In *Emerging Trends in the Social and Behavioral Sciences.* New York: John Wiley & Sons, Inc.; 2015.

13. Australian In-Vitro Fertilization Collaborative Group. In-vitro fertilization pregnancies in Australia and New Zealand, 1979–1985. *Med J Aust.* 1988;**148**(9):429–36.

14. Australian Commission on Safety and Quality in Health Care. *Logical Design: Australian Clinical Quality Registries.* Sydney: ACSQHC; 2012. Available at: www.safetyandquality.gov.au/wp-content/uploads/2012/03/Logical-Design-for-CQR_v1.0_FINAL-DRAFT_March-2012_1.58MB.pdf, accessed March 2018.

15. Hoque D, Kumari V, Hoque M, Ruseckaite R, Romero L, Evans S. Impact of clinical registries on quality of patient care and clinical outcomes:

a systematic review. *PLoS ONE.* 2017;**12**(9):e0183667. Available at: https://doi.org/10.1371/journal.pone.

16. van der Veer SN, de Keizer NF, Ravelli ACJ, Tenkink S, Jager KJ. Improving quality of care. A systematic review on how medical registries provide information feedback to health care providers. *Int J Med Inform.* 2010;**79**(5):305–23.

17. Bird SM. Performance indicators: good, bad, and ugly. *J R Stat Soc: Ser A (Stat Soc).* 2005;**168**(1):1–27.

18. Human Fertilisation and Embryology Act 1990 (UK). Available at: www.legislation.gov.uk/ukpga/1990/37/contents, accessed March 2018.

19. Fertility Clinic Success Rate and Certification Act of 1992, Pub. L. No. 102–493 (1992).

20. Reproductive Technology Accreditation Committee (RTAC) of the Fertility Society of Australia (FSA). Codes of Practice. Revised 2005. Available at: www.fertilitysociety.com.au/rtac/, accessed December 2014.

21. Australian Government Department of Health; Assisted Reproductive Technologies Review Committee. *Report of the Independent Review of Assisted Reproductive Technologies.* Canberra: Australian Government Department of Health; last updated 2007. Available at: www.health.gov.au/internet/main/publishing.nsf/Content/ART-Report, accessed March 2018.

22. National Collaborating Centre for Women's and Children's Health. *Fertility: Assessment and Treatment for People with Fertility Problems.* London: Royal College of Obstetricians and Gynaecologists; 2013.

23. Vaidya A, Stafinski T, Nardelli A, Motan T, Menon D. Assisted reproductive technologies in Alberta: an economic analysis to inform policy decision-making. *J Obstet Gynaecol Can.* 2015;**37**(12):1122–30.

24. Fox S. *The Social Life of Health Information.* Washington, DC: Pew Research Center; 15 January 2014. Available at: www.pewresearch.org/fact-tank/2014/01/15/the-social-life-of-health-information/.

25. Findlay SD. Consumers' interest in provider ratings grows, and improved report cards and other steps could accelerate their use. *Health Aff.* 2016;**35**(4):688–96.

26. Griesinger G. Beware of the 'implantation rate'! Why the outcome parameter 'implantation rate' should be abandoned from infertility research. *Hum Reprod.* 2016;**31**(2):249–51.

27. Romanski P, Goldman R, Farland L, Srouji S, Racowsky C. Impact of quality of the entire embryo cohort on implantation potential of the transferred blastocyst. *Fertil Steril.* 2017;**108**(3):e341.

28. Kissin DM, Kulkarni AD, Mneimneh A, Warner L, Boulet SL, Crawford S, et al. Embryo transfer practices and multiple births resulting from assisted

reproductive technology: an opportunity for prevention. *Fertil Steril.* 2015;**103**(4):954–61.

29. Fitzgerald O, Harris K, Paul RC, Chambers GM. *Assisted Reproductive Technology in Australia and New Zealand 2015.* Sydney: National Perinatal Epidemiology and Statistics Unit, the University of New South Wales Sydney; 2017.

30. Sunderam S, Kissin D, Crawford S, Folger S, Boulet S, Warner L, et al. Assisted reproductive technology surveillance – United States, 2015. *MMWR Surveill Summ.* 2018;**67**(SS-3):1–28.

31. Min JK, Breheny SA, MacLachlan V, Healy DL. What is the most relevant standard of success in assisted reproduction? The singleton, term gestation, live birth rate per cycle initiated: the BESST endpoint for assisted reproduction. *Hum Reprod.* 2004;**19**(1):3–7.

32. Braakhekke M, Kamphuis EI, Mol F, Norman RJ, Bhattacharya S, van der Veen F, et al. Effectiveness and safety as outcome measures in reproductive medicine. *Hum Reprod.* 2015;**30**(10):2249–51.

33. Land JA, Evers JLH. What is the most relevant standard of success in assisted reproduction? Defining outcome in ART: a Gordian knot of safety, efficacy and quality. *Hum Reprod.* 2004;**19**(5):1046–8.

34. Wong KM, Mastenbroek S, Repping S. Cryopreservation of human embryos and its contribution to in vitro fertilization success rates. *Fertil Steril.* 2014;**102**(1):19–26.

35. Chambers GM, Paul R, Harris K, Fitzgerald O, Boothroyd CV, Rombauts L, et al. Assisted reproductive technology in Australia and New Zealand: cumulative live birth rates as measures of success. *Med J Aust.* 2017;**207**(3):114–18.

36. McLernon DJ, Maheshwari A, Lee AJ, Bhattacharya S. Cumulative live birth rates after one or more complete cycles of IVF: a population-based study of linked cycle data from 178,898 women. *Hum Reprod.* 2016;**31**(3):572–81.

37. Smith AC, Tilling K, Nelson SM, Lawlor DA. Live-birth rate associated with repeat in vitro fertilization treatment cycles. *JAMA.* 2015;**314**(24):2654–62.

38. Doody KJ. Cryopreservation and delayed embryo transfer-assisted reproductive technology registry and reporting implications. *Fertil Steril.* 2014;**102**(1):27–31.

39. Maheshwari A, McLernon D, Bhattacharya S. Cumulative live birth rate: time for a consensus? *Hum Reprod.* 2015;**30**(12):2703–7.

40. Human Fertilisation and Embryology Authority. *Fertility Treatment 2014–2016: Trends and Figures.* London: HFEA; 2018. Available at: www.hfea.gov.uk/media/2563/hfea-fertility-trends-and-figures-2017-v2.pdf, accessed April 2018.

41. Human Fertilisation and Embryology Authority. Welcome to the HFEA. Available at: www.hfea.gov.uk/, accessed April 2018.

42. Society for Assisted Reproductive Technology. Find a clinic. Available at: www.sart.org/clinic-pages/find-a-clinic/, accessed April 2018.

43. Centers for Disease Control and Prevention (CDC). ART success rates. Available at: www.cdc.gov/art/artdata/index.html, accessed April 2018.

44. Centers for Disease Control and Prevention, American Society for Reproductive Medicine, Society for Assisted Reproductive Technology. *2015 Assisted Reproductive Technology Fertility Clinic Success Rates Report.* Atlanta, GA: US Dept of Health and Human Services; 2017.

45. Centers for Disease Control and Prevention, American Society for Reproductive Medicine, Society for Assisted Reproductive Technology. *2015 Assisted Reproductive Technology National Summary Report.* Atlanta, GA: US Dept of Health and Human Services; 2017.

46. Behrendt K, Groene O. Mechanisms and effects of public reporting of surgeon outcomes: a systematic review of the literature. *Health Policy.* 2016;**120**(10):1151–61.

47. Campanella P, Vukovic V, Parente P, Sulejmani A, Ricciardi W, Specchia ML. The impact of public reporting on clinical outcomes: a systematic review and meta-analysis. *BMC Health Serv Res.* 2016;**16**(1):296.

48. Luke B, Brown MB, Wantman E, Stern JE, Baker VL, Gibbons W, et al. A prediction model for live birth after assisted reproductive technology. *Fertil Steril.* 2014;**102**:744–52.

49. Society for Assisted Reproductive Technology. What are my chances with ART? Available at: www.sartcorsonline.com/predictor/patient, accessed April 2018.

50. McLernon DJ, Steyerberg EW, Te Velde ER, Lee AJ. Predicting the chances of live birth after one or more complete cycles of in vitro fertilization: population based study of linked cycle data from 113,873 women. *BMJ.* 2016;**355**:i5735.

51. University of Aberdeen. Outcome prediction in subfertility. Available at: https://w3.abdn.ac.uk/clsm/opis, accessed April 2018.

52. Steyerberg EW, Vickers AJ, Cook NR, Gerds T, Gonen M, Obuchowski N, et al. Assessing the performance of prediction models: a framework for some traditional and novel measures. *Epidemiology.* 2010;**21**(1):128–38. doi:10.1097/EDE.0b013e3181c30fb2.

Chapter

6

Using ART Surveillance Data in Clinical Research

Valerie L. Baker, Sheree L. Boulet and Anja Bisgaard Pinborg

The findings and conclusions in this report are those of the authors and do not necessarily represent the official position of the Centers for Disease Control and Prevention.

Introduction

Assisted reproductive technology (ART) surveillance databases have developed in multiple parts of the world. In the United States (US), the Fertility Clinic Success Rate and Certification Act of 1992 requires each ART program to report pregnancy success rates annually through the Centers for Disease Control and Prevention (CDC) [1]. The National ART Surveillance System (NASS) is the CDC's web-based reporting system for the collection of ART data [2]. Most clinics in the US report data to the professional group called the Society for Assisted Reproductive Technology (SART) [3], which then submits the data to the CDC on behalf of the clinic; other clinics report their data directly to the CDC. Both the CDC and SART publish annual reports describing success rates for ART clinics [2, 3]. In Europe, the European IVF Monitoring (EIM) Consortium [4] collects data from participating countries and publishes regular reports with ART success rates. The Latin American Registry of Assisted Reproduction collects and reports data from institutions in 15 countries [5]. There have also been world reports using aggregate data submitted by participating countries to the International Committee Monitoring Assisted Reproductive Technologies (ICMART) [6].

Although ART surveillance databases are not necessarily designed for research purposes, they can be used for research aimed at improving the effectiveness and safety of ART [7]. Research using surveillance data ultimately benefits patients and can inform clinical practice and additional surveillance needs. For example, if research suggests that a certain factor increases risk for an adverse outcome, surveillance systems can be modified to collect additional or more targeted data about that factor. Many ART surveillance databases include large numbers of ART treatment cycles. This large sample size can facilitate precise estimation of the relationships between patient or treatment factors and outcomes of success such as

live birth rate, as well as permit detection of rare outcomes. Surveillance databases are also useful for studying trends over time, such as utilization of elective single embryo transfer [8]. However, ART surveillance systems may lack detail that is available when data are collected specifically with the intent of research. Surveillance data allow the researcher to assess associations between patient characteristics or specific treatment parameters and outcomes but cannot prove causation and may detect relationships with statistical but not clinical significance. Despite limitations, many clinically important research questions have been addressed using ART surveillance databases, particularly databases with cycle-level and patient-level data, which take into account important factors that influence effectiveness and safety. This chapter will describe the use of ART surveillance data to study ART effectiveness and safety and will outline the benefits and limitations of using ART surveillance data for research.

Using ART Surveillance Data to Study ART Effectiveness

ART surveillance data can be used to study the effectiveness of various ART methods. More than 100 manuscripts have been published using the SART Clinical Outcomes Reporting System (SART CORS) alone, with a comprehensive review of effectiveness studies beyond the scope of this chapter. Measures of ART effectiveness include rates of embryo implantation, clinical pregnancy, miscarriage and, most important, live birth. Patient factors predictive of live birth have been examined such as race/ethnicity [9, 10], body mass index [11], ovarian reserve [12] and female age [13]. The effectiveness of various ART methods (exposures) has been examined, such as intracytoplasmic sperm injection (ICSI) [14, 15], gestational carrier [16], donor vs. autologous cycles, fresh vs. frozen cycles [17], cleavage vs. blastocyst stage of embryo development, assisted hatching [18], gonadotropin dose [19], preimplantation genetic screening [20] and number of embryos transferred [21]. Markers of response to treatment such as embryology morphology [22] and number of oocytes retrieved [23, 24] have also been shown to be predictive of live birth rate. Although it is difficult to prove [1], findings reported in these manuscripts have likely influenced patient care.

To best understand the efficacy of in vitro fertilization (IVF) for an individual patient, it is important to link all cycles for the same patient [25, 26]. Cumulative live birth rates are a very important aspect of assessment of ART efficacy, particularly in the light of freeze-all (also known as freeze-only) strategies [27]. In the US, since 2014 in SART CORS it is possible to report embryo transfers in which eggs from more than one retrieval are utilized [3]. In the past, the success rate of a fresh IVF cycle in which all embryos were frozen was counted as zero. It is also now possible in SART CORS to report success rates taking into account the fact that the first (primary) embryo transfer may be a frozen and not a fresh embryo transfer. Starting with the 2016 reporting year, this type of linkage will be possible with data collected by the CDC. In addition, for greatest accuracy and transparency regarding success rates, it is important to report all initiated cycles [28]. In SART CORS, previously 'hidden cycles' are now reported [29], such as those that employed preimplantation genetic testing with no euploid embryo.

Based on the Danish IVF registry, which was initiated in 1994 and has included intrauterine insemination (IUI) cycles since 2007, cumulative live birth rates after finished treatment courses in the same women have been reported [30]. Hence, a long-term prognosis can be provided to the individual couple when initiating fertility. Similarly, cumulative live birth rates including risks of ovarian hyperstimulation syndrome (OHSS) and thromboembolic diseases have been published based on the Swedish Quality Registry (Q-IVF) [31].

Using ART Surveillance Data to Study ART Safety

Worldwide, more than 5 million children have been born after ART [32]. Approximately 1.7% of the US birth cohort and 2–6% of the European birth cohorts are conceived by ART [4, 33]. Since the first IVF child, Louise Brown, was born in 1978, the world has observed a tremendous increase in the number of ART cycles performed. However, new and advanced techniques such as ICSI, assisted hatching, oocyte and embryo freezing and preimplantation genetic testing have been implemented with limited safety assessments prior to use.

ART surveillance data can be used to study ART safety. The mandatory recording of all ART cycles in IVF registries since 1982 in Sweden and the early 1990s in the other Nordic countries has made short- and long-term follow-up of the children possible [34]. In the Nordic countries, all citizens have a unique personal identification number (PIN), which is provided immediately after birth and enables linking of a specific ART cycle to the mother and, via the medical birth registries, the maternal PIN can be paired to the child. The national health registries can provide data on diagnoses and drug prescription, and data can be merged to the ART mother and child safety databases [34]. The following national registries are available for follow-up in most Nordic countries: birth, hospital and outpatient, drug prescription, cancer, causes of death, diabetes and socio-economic registries. Further linkage to national clinical quality databases can provide additional data on specific diseases such as childhood diabetes and epilepsy.

An important factor affecting the safety of IVF is the increased risk of multiple pregnancy and associated risks of adverse perinatal outcomes such as preterm birth. In the beginning of the IVF era, many embryos were transferred, resulting in multiple birth rates of approximately 30%, with almost half of the ART children born as twins or high-order gestations [35]. ART success rates reports from the ICMART [6], US reports from SART and the CDC [2] and the EIM [4] are some of the sources that have included multiple birth rates. In addition to reporting the number of ART cycles performed, these reports have, over the years, emphasized the need for a reduction in the multiple births attributable to ART. National societies have recommended and encouraged single embryo transfers. Based on ART surveillance data and recommendations from professional societies, preterm birth rates associated with multiple gestation considerably diminished after single embryo transfer recommendations were introduced [36]. In those countries with the steepest increase in the proportion of single embryo transfers, the most pronounced decline in preterm birth rates after ART has been observed [37].

In addition to the increased risk of multiple birth, there are many other safety outcomes that can be monitored using ART surveillance data, including OHSS [30, 38], maternal complications [39] and other infant morbidity and mortality [37]. In the United Kingdom (UK), national ART surveillance data have shown that in singleton pregnancies the risk of preterm birth and low birth weight is higher, with a very high number of oocytes in fresh IVF cycles encouraging milder ovarian stimulation regimens [40]. In addition, cycles with freezing and thawing of embryos result in lower preterm birth and low birth weight rates; however, frozen embryo transfers are more likely to be associated with large-for-gestational-age babies [41, 42].

In some countries, surveillance data also include information on other techniques, such as blastocyst transfer. The Swedish Q-IVF registry has included blastocyst transfer as a parameter after the registry was initiated in 2007. Based on the Swedish surveillance data, the registry demonstrated no increased risk of birth defects related to blastocyst transfer; however, risks of perinatal mortality and perinatal complications were higher [43]. These serve as examples of the valuable information we can gain by adapting ART surveillance for specified ART procedures to the surveillance data at an early stage of the implementation.

To surveille ART safety there are two primary requirements. The first is a database with inclusion of all ART cycles performed with specific cycle data on the number of embryos transferred, fresh or frozen embryo transfer, freezing method, donor vs. autologous gametes, culture length, culture media and type of drugs used. Key variables should include the female identification number and data regarding female and male age, parity, previous number and type of ART cycles and so on. The second requirement is that information in the database includes data on additional birth and reproductive outcomes including multiple birth, birth weight, gestational age at delivery, monozygotic twinning, OHSS, ectopic pregnancy, infection, miscarriage and fetal death, thromboembolism and female death. When these two requirements are met, researchers are able to assess risks of adverse outcomes associated with specific exposures, such as the number of oocytes retrieved [30].

To surveille long-term morbidity and mortality in children conceived by ART, coupling of the mother and child, by a personal identification code, such as PINs in Nordic countries, is very helpful.

Identification of individuals without PINs by specific obstetric parameters can also be used for linking to a specific ART treatment, as was done with ART and childhood cancers in the UK [44]. National biobanks with cord blood and placental tissue samples do not yet exist but would provide opportunities to examine epigenetic alterations in children born after specific ART methods. Longer-term impacts of interest, such as possible increased cardiometabolic risks in ART children, can be evaluated on a long-term basis only by following the children for subsequent cardiovascular events and deaths (see Chapter 9, Monitoring Long-Term Outcomes of ART: Linking ART Surveillance Data with Other Datasets, for further discussion of this important topic).

All of this requires large databanks and extended knowledge concerning data harmonizing and storage. It requires organizational bodies with the expertise to handle and monitor these kinds of data. In smaller countries, cross-border coupling of safety data can be an opportunity. The Committee of Nordic Assisted Reproductive Technology and Safety (CoNARTaS) was established in 2008 with the aim of surveillance of perinatal outcomes in ART children by using a matched cohort design with data from the medical birth registries up to 2007 in each country [34]. The current research focus is to explore short- and long-term health for children born after ART and for their mothers, compared with the background population of naturally conceived children and their mothers, respectively. Long-term outcomes include metabolic diseases, hormonal and pubertal disturbances, cardiovascular disease, diabetes, cancer and mental health. However, registration practices in the Nordic medical birth registries vary tremendously between the countries, i.e. gestational age can be coded in days or weeks and nulliparity can be coded as either 0 or 1. Hence, data should be harmonized and all variables coded similarly before merging the data.

One challenge in conducting research regarding safety is identifying an appropriate comparison group. Couples undergoing ART may have underlying medical conditions, which increase their risk of pregnancy complications and long-term adverse outcomes irrespective of whether they had undergone ART. Comparison with the general population may lead to an overestimation of the risk for complications associated with ART. A subfertile comparison group can be advantageous [45], but couples requiring ART may still have more serious co-morbidities than sub-fertile couples able to conceive without ART. It is important for researchers to control for potential confounders to the greatest extent possible to maximize the accuracy of conclusions regarding the safety of ART. However, information about potentially important confounders may be missing. Sibling studies are another way of overcoming biases in the selection of a control group. By including only mothers who gave birth to both an IVF and a naturally conceived child, many maternal factors may be stable when also adjusted for birth order and maternal age. This approach has been used in Nordic cohort studies, but requires that siblings can be identified in the surveillance datasets, which may not be possible in other datasets [46, 47].

ART surveillance data can provide important information on ART practices and corresponding associations with maternal and infant health outcomes. However, assessment of safety is limited in some ART surveillance systems due to challenges in collecting information on outcomes that are rare (e.g. OHSS) or distal from exposure (e.g. birth defects). Underreporting of adverse outcome measures is a problem for many public health surveillance systems [48], particularly where surveillance databases are not readily linked to other databases for assessment of longer-term outcomes such as risk of cancer. However, studies using ART surveillance databases have already led to significant improvements in ART safety, such as the reduction in the risk of multiple pregnancies and related complications such as pre-term birth [37]. Further refinements and linkage to other databases will provide information to support the continued improvement of ART safety.

Advantages, Disadvantages and Potential Solutions in Using ART Surveillance Data for Clinical Research

The use of ART surveillance data for clinical research is advantageous for a number of reasons (Table 6.1). First, outside of individual treatment centres or programs, the type of detailed information collected in ART surveillance systems is unlikely to be available from other sources, making the data a valuable resource for answering clinical questions. Next, surveillance data are often collected at the national level or across multiple sites, allowing sufficient sample size for studying rare outcomes such as monozygotic

twinning, ectopic pregnancy or OHSS. In turn, because the data are collected across different populations, research findings are more representative of the ART population at large than single centre studies. Finally, if the surveillance system regularly and systematically validates the reported data via medical record review, accuracy of the data fields is likely to be high.

There are also several limitations to consider when using ART surveillance data for research purposes (see Table 6.1). Because the intent of ART surveillance is to monitor the safety and efficacy of the procedures, not to conduct research, information on relevant outcomes or confounders may not be collected. In some cases, proxy measures can be used (i.e. the number of embryos cryopreserved as surrogate indicator of embryo quality) [49]. However, the potential for residual confounding remains an important consideration. Notably, demographic characteristics such as maternal education, income and race/ethnicity are rarely collected in routine ART surveillance and, if collected, may be poorly reported. In the US, race/ethnicity, a factor associated with birth outcomes, is missing in approximately one-third of ART surveillance data [50]. When using multivariate regression models, listwise deletion of cases with missing data has been shown to bias estimates of effect when the data are not missing completely at random [51, 52]. Imputation methods can be used to replace missing values [46]; multiple imputation approaches are generally preferred over single imputation because standard errors are more likely to be correctly estimated [50, 52, 53].

In addition, incomplete collection of cycle-level data may occur if clinics fail to report all cycles or selectively exclude cycles with suboptimal outcomes. Prospective reporting can reduce the likelihood of incomplete or selective reporting but may be difficult to implement and enforce. Furthermore, errors in data entry can affect the validity of the reported fields and contribute spurious research findings. The use of clear definitions for data fields, appropriate training for staff responsible for data entry and data validation to identify systematic discrepancies can improve data quality. To maintain accuracy of data entry, the amount of data collected should be limited to the most important fields and be within scope of what a clinic can practically do. See Chapter 3, ART Surveillance: Who, What, When and How?, for more information. In the US, SART and the CDC

Table 6.1 Using ART surveillance data for research: advantages, limitations and potential ways to address the limitations

Advantages
Multisite, national and multinational data are representative of populations. Large sample size allows research questions with important outcomes such as live birth rate and enables the study of rare outcomes.
Data are generally high quality (when data fields are regularly validated).
Cycle-level data collection facilitates evaluation of treatment procedures and corresponding outcome.

Limitations	Potential solutions
Large sample size can lead to statistically significant findings that may not be clinically important.	• Lower *p*-value thresholds • Rely on interpretation of point estimates and confidence intervals • Use Bayesian methods or false discovery rate approach • Abandon significance testing • Use caution when interpreting effect estimates within a certain range
Information on important confounders (e.g. race and ethnicity) may not be collected or may be missing for a large proportion of cycles.	• When confounder variables are missing for some but not all cycles, use imputation methods to replace missing information
Data are correlated for women undergoing more than one cycle of treatment and for patients who are treated in the same clinic.	• Use generalized estimating equations or hierarchical regression • Calculate cumulative success rates for a single patient over multiple cycles
There is confounding by indication.	• Use multivariable regression models, stratified analyses or propensity scores • Consider biological pathways
There is incomplete or selective reporting of ART cycles.	• Prospective reporting • Limit data collection to fields that are essential to minimize reporting burden on clinics
Errors occur in data entry.	• Clearly define data fields • Regularly train staff on data entry • Validate reported information using medical records

have engaged in discussions that led to the addition of new fields, modification of others and deletion of fields with limited value [3]. Finally, because data from ART surveillance systems cannot be fully compiled until information on all resultant births in a given time period is collected, the data are typically one to two years old before they can be analyzed.

Although the large sample size of surveillance data facilitates the examination of rare outcomes, the increased precision can lead to statistically significant findings for associations with small effect sizes that are clinically irrelevant. In addition, increased precision is not necessarily indicative of improved validity, as residual confounding or selection bias can still influence estimates from large observational studies [54]. A number of methods have been proposed to address the issue of statistical significance, including lowering *p*-value thresholds [55], abandoning statistical significance altogether [56], relying on interpretation of point estimates and confidence intervals [57] or using Bayesian methods or other inferential approaches such as false discovery rates [58]. To reduce the likelihood of reporting spurious

associations in observational epidemiology, it has also been suggested that effect sizes within certain ranges (odd ratios between 0.33 and 3 or relative risks between 0.5 and 2) are potentially biased and should be interpreted with caution [54].

An important source of bias in observational studies is confounding by indication, which refers to situations in which the indication for a certain treatment is also associated with the outcome [59]. For example, confounding by indication may occur when comparing clinical outcomes for cycles using cleavage versus blastocyst stage embryos. If patients with poorer quality oocytes are more likely to transfer cleavage stage embryos, live birth rates may appear lower in the cleavage stage group. The methodological approach to addressing confounding by indication is the same as confounding in general – use of multivariable regression models, stratified analyses or propensity scores [59, 60]. However, even when these methods are applied correctly, residual confounding can still bias results when information on a critical confounder is not captured in the surveillance system or when investigators lack understanding of the underlying biological mechanisms for the outcomes under investigation. In addition, when propensity score methods are used, biased estimates can still result if the models used to generate the scores are mis-specified [61].

Lastly, when collected at the cycle level, data for patients undergoing more than one treatment are not independent. Likewise, outcomes for a particular clinic are also likely correlated because of clinic practice patterns, patient selection or use of a common laboratory. If these correlations are ignored during data analysis, variance estimates can be biased, leading to inaccurate interpretation of effect estimates [62]. One method of accounting for cycle-level correlation is to limit the analysis to one cycle for a particular patient. This may not be ideal, as it reduces sample size and fails to account for within-subject variability [62]. Other methods for addressing correlation include use of generalized estimating equations (GEEs) or hierarchical regression, also known as multilevel modelling. In general, GEE approaches are appropriate when there is an interest in comparing responses averaged over a population, while hierarchical models are used to compare changes in an individual's response [63, 64]. Another strategy for addressing cycle-level correlation involves linking multiple cycles for a single patient and estimating cumulative outcomes, such as live birth rate per patient [25]. However, this approach does not account for correlation of outcomes within clinics and requires certain assumptions about women who do not return for treatment, which should be explicitly stated in publications of analytic results.

Providing Access to Data

Registries can be useful for research only if individuals with research expertise have access to the ART surveillance data. In the US, SART has developed an online research portal, which can be used by any SART member to request a dataset from SART CORS [3]. SART's Research Committee must review and approve each dataset request, with guidance provided to researchers who are initially less familiar with SART CORS. A SART member interested in conducting research using SART CORS must provide the SART Research Committee with a description of the research question, specific fields that they want to be included in the dataset and documentation of Institutional Review Board approval for the project. Only de-identified datasets are provided, which do not include patient name or any other protected

health information. Linked datasets can now be generated, so that the researcher can conduct analyses including multiple fresh and frozen cycles linked for each patient. This allows the researcher to examine cumulative outcomes, such as cumulative live birth rate at the patient level, rather than conducting analyses only at the cycle level. Dates (other than year) are not provided, but SART will calculate elapsed time variables (e.g. days of ovarian stimulation, or time between oocyte retrieval and embryo transfers) if needed for a particular research question. Although clinic-specific pregnancy rates are publicly available, patient- and cycle-level data are provided to researchers only in the aggregate for all practices in the US or by geographic region. Data are released to researchers in a way that allows analysis of details about each cycle and each patient, but the researcher is not given information that identifies specific clinics. Thus, SART protects the confidentiality of each patient and each clinic, while still providing access to data with a level of detail that permits the researcher to address clinically important research questions. Since 2006, SART has partnered with an epidemiologist who uses SART CORS to study ART outcomes and obtains funding from the National Institutes of Health [3] for linkages of SART CORS to other databases to examine longer-term outcomes. See Chapter 9, Monitoring Long-Term Outcomes of ART: Linking ART Surveillance Data with Other Datasets, for more information on these linked databases

Likewise, the CDC provides several options for accessing data from the NASS. In addition to the annual publication of the *Fertility Clinic Success Rates Report* and the *National Summary Report*, the CDC provides access to a spreadsheet containing treatment and outcome data for all reporting clinics in the US each year. For researchers interested in examining cycle-level data, the CDC's Research Data Center can be used to access de-identified NASS datasets from 2004 and later. This secure environment allows researchers with approved proposals to conduct analyses while assuring that confidentiality of the data is protected. All research projects require a proposal, which is reviewed by subject matter experts for scientific merit, appropriate methodology and overlap with other projects.

The access to data varies between the Nordic countries. In Finland, IVF data are registered in the medical birth register and there is no specific IVF registry, while in Sweden, Norway and Denmark specific IVF registries exist but the level of details in the registrations differs. Access to data from the health care registries for research purposes is through the national boards of health, and research projects should be approved by the national data protection authorities. In Norway and Sweden, approval from the scientific ethics committee is required. Moreover, the research institutions have to pay the national authorities for access to data.

Conclusions

Surveillance data are important for assessing ART effectiveness and safety. Although efforts to obtain aggregate data from clinics throughout the world are to be applauded as a great start, cycle-level data and patient-level data allow the most detailed analyses and are ultimately of most value to patients. In using these data for research, it is important to recognize not only the strengths but also the limitations of surveillance data. Appropriate analytic strategies should be employed to address the limitations whenever possible. ART surveillance data should be available to interested and responsible researchers. Continued efforts to expand ART surveillance to countries throughout the world will benefit the diverse population of women and men who are attempting to build their families using ART.

References

1. Adashi EY, Wyden R. Public reporting of clinical outcomes of assisted reproductive technology programs: implications for other medical and surgical procedures. *JAMA*. 2011;**306**:1135–6.

2. Centers for Disease Control and Prevention, American Society for Reproductive Medicine, Society for Assisted Reproductive Technology. *2015 Assisted Reproductive Technology Fertility Clinic Success Rates Report*. Atlanta, GA: US Dept of Health and Human Services; 2017.

3. Toner JP, Coddington CC, Doody K, Van Voorhis B, Seifer DB, Ball GD, et al. Society for Assisted Reproductive Technology and assisted reproductive technology in the United States: a 2016 update. *Fertil Steril*. 2016;**106**:541–6.

4. Calhaz-Jorge C, De Geyter C, Kupka MS, de Mouzon J, Erb K, Mocanu E, et al.; European IVF-Monitoring Consortium (EIM); European Society of Human Reproduction and Embryology (ESHRE). Assisted reproductive technology in Europe, 2013: results generated from European registers by ESHRE. *Hum Reprod*. 2017;**32**:1957–73.

5. Zegers-Hochschild F, Schwarze JE, Crosby JA, Musri C, Urbina MT. Assisted reproductive techniques in Latin America: the Latin American Registry, 2014. *JBRA Assist Reprod*. 2017;**21**:164–75.

6. Dyer S, Chambers GM, de Mouzon J, Nygren KG, Zegers-Hochschild F, Mansour R, et al. International Committee for Monitoring Assisted Reproductive Technologies world report: assisted reproductive technology 2008, 2009 and 2010. *Hum Reprod*. 2016;**31**: 1588–609.

7. Kissin DM, Jamieson DJ, Barfield WD. Monitoring health outcomes of assisted reproductive technology. *N Engl J Med*. 2014;**371**:91–3.

8. Styer AK, Luke B, Vitek W, Christianson MS, Baker VL, Christy AY, et al. Factors associated with the use of elective single-embryo transfer and pregnancy outcomes in the United States, 2004–2012. *Fertil Steril*. 2016;**106**:80–9.

9. Baker VL, Luke B, Brown MB, Alvero R, Frattarelli JL, Usadi R, et al. Multivariate analysis of factors affecting probability of pregnancy and live birth with in vitro fertilization: an analysis of the Society for Assisted Reproductive Technology Clinic Outcomes Reporting System. *Fertil Steril*. 2010;**94**:1410–16.

10. Luke B, Brown MB, Stern JE, Missmer SA, Fujimoto VY, Leach R. Racial and ethnic disparities in assisted reproductive technology pregnancy and live birth rates within body mass index categories. *Fertil Steril*. 2011;**95**:1661–6.

11. Luke B, Brown MB, Stern JE, Missmer SA, Fujimoto VY, Leach R, et al. Female obesity adversely affects assisted reproductive technology (ART) pregnancy and live birth rates. *Hum Reprod*. 2011;**26**: 245–52.

12. Seifer DB, Tal O, Wantman E, Edul P, Baker VL. Prognostic indicators of assisted reproduction technology outcomes of cycles with ultralow serum antimüllerian hormone: a multivariate analysis of over 5,000 autologous cycles from the Society for Assisted Reproductive Technology Clinic Outcome Reporting System database for 2012–2013. *Fertil Steril*. 2016;**105**: 385–93.e3.

13. Yeh JS, Steward RG, Dude AM, Shah AA, Goldfarb JM, Muasher SJ. Pregnancy outcomes decline in recipients over age 44: an analysis of 27,959 fresh donor oocyte in vitro fertilization cycles from the Society for Assisted Reproductive Technology. *Fertil Steril*. 2014;**101**:1331–6.

14. Nangia AK, Luke B, Smith JF, Mak W, Stern JE; SART Writing Group. National study of factors influencing assisted reproductive technology outcomes with male factor infertility. *Fertil Steril*. 2011;**96**:609–14.

15. Grimstad FW, Nangia AK, Luke B, Stern JE, Mak W. Use of ICSI in IVF cycles in women with tubal ligation

does not improve pregnancy or live birth rates. *Hum Reprod*. 2016;**31**:2750–5.

16. Murugappan G, Farland LV, Missmer SA, Correia KF, Anchan RM, Ginsburg ES. Gestational carrier in assisted reproductive technology. *Fertil Steril*. 2018;**109**:420–8.

17. Maheshwari A, Raja EA, Bhattacharya S. Obstetric and perinatal outcomes after either fresh or thawed frozen embryo transfer: an analysis of 112,432 singleton pregnancies recorded in the Human Fertilisation and Embryology Authority anonymized dataset. *Fertil Steril*. 2016;**106**:1703–8.

18. Kissin DM, Kawwass JF, Monsour M, Boulet SL, Session DR, Jamieson DJ; National ART Surveillance System (NASS) Group. Assisted hatching: trends and pregnancy outcomes, United States, 2000–2010. *Fertil Steril*. 2014;**102**:795–801.

19. Baker VL, Brown MB, Luke B, Smith GW, Ireland JJ. Gonadotropin dose is negatively correlated with live birth rate: analysis of more than 650,000 assisted reproductive technology cycles. *Fertil Steril*. 2015;**104**:1145–52.e1-5.

20. Barad DH, Darmon SK, Kushnir VA, Albertini DF, Gleicher N. Impact of preimplantation genetic screening on donor oocyte-recipient cycles in the United States. *Am J Obstet Gynecol*. 2017;**217**:576.e1–576.e8.

21. Kissin DM, Kulkarni AD, Kushnir VA, Jamieson DJ; National ART Surveillance System Group. Number of embryos transferred after in vitro fertilization and good perinatal outcome. *Obstet Gynecol*. 2014;**123**(2 Pt 1):239–47.

22. Racowsky C, Stern JE, Gibbons WE, Behr B, Pomeroy KO, Biggers JD. National collection of embryo morphology data into Society for Assisted Reproductive Technology Clinic Outcomes Reporting System: associations among day 3 cell number, fragmentation and blastomere asymmetry, and live birth rate. *Fertil Steril*. 2011;**95**:1985–9.

23. Baker VL, Brown MB, Luke B, Conrad KP. Association of number of retrieved oocytes with live birth rate and birth weight: an analysis of 231,815 cycles of in vitro fertilization. *Fertil Steril*. 2015;**103**:931–8.e2.

24. Steward RG, Lan L, Shah AA, Yeh JS, Price TM, Goldfarb JM, et al. Oocyte number as a predictor for ovarian hyperstimulation syndrome and live birth: an analysis of 256,381 in vitro fertilization cycles. *Fertil Steril*. 2014;**101**:967–73.

25. Luke B, Brown MB, Wantman E, Lederman A, Gibbons W, Schattman GL, et al. Cumulative birth rates with linked assisted reproductive technology cycles. *N Engl J Med*. 2012;**366**:2483–91.

26. Stern JE, Brown MB, Luke B, Wantman E, Lederman A, Hornstein MD, et al. Cycle 1 as predictor of assisted reproductive technology treatment outcome over multiple cycles: an analysis of linked cycles from the Society for Assisted Reproductive Technology Clinic Outcomes Reporting System online database. *Fertil Steril*. 2011;**95**:600–5.

27. Roque M. Freeze-all policy: is it time for that? *J Assist Reprod Gen*et. 2015;**32**(2):171–6.

28. Kushnir VA, Vidali A, Barad DH, Gleicher N. The status of public reporting of clinical outcomes in assisted reproductive technology. *Fertil Steril*. 2013;**100**:736–41.

29. Doody KJ. Public reporting of ART cycle outcome data is not simple. *Fertil Steril*. 2016;**105**:893–4.

30. Malchau SS, Henningsen AA, Loft A, Rasmussen S, Forman J, Nyboe Andersen A, et al. The long-term prognosis for live birth in couples initiating fertility treatments. *Hum Reprod*. 2017;**32**:1439–49.

31. Magnusson Å, Källen K, Thurin-Kjellberg A, Bergh C. The number of oocytes retrieved during IVF: a balance between efficacy and safety. *Hum Reprod*. 2018;**33**:58–64.

32. Adamson GD, Tabangin M, Macaluso M, de Mouzon J. The number of babies born globally after treatment with the assisted reproductive technologies (ART). *Fertil Steril*. 2013;**100**:S42.

33. Sunderam S, Kissin DM, Crawford SB, Folger SG, Boulet SL, Warner L, et al. Assisted Reproductive Technology Surveillance – United States, 2015. *MMWR Surveill Summ*. 2018;**67**:1–28.

34. Henningsen AK, Romundstad LB, Gissler M, Nygren KG, Lidegaard O, Skjaerven R, et al. Infant and maternal health monitoring using a combined Nordic database on ART and safety. *Acta Obstst Gynecol Scand*. 2011;**90**:683–91.

35. Pinborg A. IVF/ICSI twin pregnancies: risks and prevention. *Hum Reprod Update*. 2005;**11**:575–93.

36. Practice Committee of the American Society for Reproductive Medicine, Practice Committee of the Society for Assisted Reproductive Technology. Guidance on the limits to the number of embryos to transfer: a committee opinion. *Fertil Steril*. 2017;**107**:901–3.

37. Henningsen AA, Gissler M, Skjaerven R, Bergh C, Tiitinen A, Romundstad LB, et al. Trends in perinatal health after assisted reproduction: a Nordic study from the CoNARTaS group. *Hum Reprod*. 2015;**30**:710–16.

38. Luke B, Brown MB, Morbeck DE, Hudson SB, Coddington CC 3rd, Stern JE. Factors associated with ovarian hyperstimulation syndrome (OHSS) and its effect on assisted reproductive technology (ART) treatment and outcome. *Fertil Steril*. 2010;**94**:1399–404.

39. Kawwass JF, Kissin DM, Kulkarni AD, Creanga AA, Session DR, Callaghan WM, et al. National ART Surveillance System (NASS) Group. Safety of assisted

reproductive technology in the United States, 2000–2011. *JAMA*. 2015;**313**:88–90.

40. Sunkara SK, La Marca A, Seed PT, Khalaf Y. Increased risk of preterm birth and low birthweight with very high number of oocytes following IVF: an analysis of 65,868 singleton live birth outcomes. *Hum Reprod*. 2015;**30**:1473–80.

41. Wennerholm UB, Henningsen AK, Romundstad LB, Bergh C, Pinborg A, Skjaerven R, et al. Perinatal outcomes of children born after frozen-thawed embryo transfer: a Nordic cohort study from the CoNARTaS group. *Hum Reprod*. 2013;**28**:2545–53.

42. Luke B, Brown MB, Wantman E, Stern JE, Toner JP, Coddington CC 3rd. Increased risk of large-for-gestational age birthweight in singleton siblings conceived with in vitro fertilization in frozen versus fresh cycles. *J Assist Reprod Genet*. 2017;**34**:191–200.

43. Ginström Ernstad E, Bergh C, Khatibi A, Källén KB, Westlander G, Nilsson S, et al. Neonatal and maternal outcome after blastocyst transfer: a population-based registry study. *Am J Obstet Gynecol*. 2016;**214**:378.e1-378.e10.

44. Williams CL, Bunch KJ, Stiller CA, Murphy MF, Botting BJ, Wallace WH, et al. Cancer risk among children born after assisted conception. *N Engl J Med*. 2013;**369**:1819–27.

45. Declercq E, Luke B, Belanoff C, Cabral H, Diop H, Gopal D, et al. Perinatal outcomes associated with assisted reproductive technology: the Massachusetts Outcomes Study of Assisted Reproductive Technologies (MOSART). *Fertil Steril*. 2015;**103**:888–95.

46. Romundstad LB, Romundstad PR, Sunde A, von Düring V, Skjaerven R, Gunnell D, et al. Effects of technology or maternal factors on perinatal outcome after assisted fertilisation: a population-based cohort study. *Lancet*. 2008;**372**:737–43.

47. Pinborg A, Henningsen AA, Loft A, Malchau SS, Forman J, Andersen AN. Large baby syndrome in singletons born after frozen embryo transfer (FET): is it due to maternal factors or the cryotechnique? *Hum Reprod*. 2014;**29**:618–27.

48. Deneux-Tharaux C, Berg C, Bouvier-Colle MH, Gissler M, Harper M, Nannini A, et al. Underreporting of pregnancy-related mortality in the United States and Europe. *Obstet Gynecol*. 2005;**106**:684–92.

49. Stern JE, Lieberman ES, Macaluso M, Racowsky C. Is cryopreservation of embryos a legitimate surrogate marker of embryo quality in studies of assisted reproductive technology conducted using national databases? *Fertil Steril*. 2012;**97**:890–3.

50. Wellons MF, Fujimoto VY, Baker VL, Barrington DS, Broomfield D, Catherino WH, et al. Race matters:

a systematic review of racial/ethnic disparity in Society for Assisted Reproductive Technology reported outcomes. *Fertil Steril*. 2012;**98**:406–9.

51. Donders AR, van der Heijden GJ, Stijnen T, Moons KG. Review: a gentle introduction to imputation of missing values. *J Clin Epidemiol*. 2006;**59**:1087–91.

52. Perkins NJ, Cole SR, Harel O, Tchetgen Tchetgen EJ, Sun B, Mitchell EM, et al. Principled approaches to missing data in epidemiologic studies. *Am J Epidemiol*. 2018;**187**:568–75.

53. Harel O, Mitchell EM, Perkins NJ, Cole SR, Tchetgen Tchetgen EJ, Sun B, et al. Multiple imputation for incomplete data in epidemiologic studies. *Am J Epidemiol*. 2018;**187**:576–84.

54. Grimes DA, Schulz KF. False alarms and pseudo-epidemics: the limitations of observational epidemiology. *Obstet Gynecol*. 2012;**120**:920–7.

55. Ioannidis JPA. The proposal to lower *P* value thresholds to .005. *JAMA*. 2018;**319**:1429–30.

56. Leek J, McShane BB, Gelman A, Colquhoun D, Nuijten MB, Goodman SN. Five ways to fix statistics. *Nature*. 2017;**551**:557–9.

57. Savitz DA. Commentary: reconciling theory and practice: what is to be done with *p* values? *Epidemiology*. 2013;**24**:212–14.

58. Wasserstein RL, Lazar NA. The ASA's statement on *p*-values: context, process, and purpose. *Am Stat*. 2016;**70**:129–33.

59. Kyriacou DN, Lewis RJ. Confounding by indication in clinical research. *JAMA*. 2016;**316**:1818–19.

60. Psaty BM, Koepsell TD, Lin D, Weiss NS, Siscovick DS, Rosendaal FR, et al. Assessment and control for confounding by indication in observational studies. *J Am Geriatr Soc*. 1999;**47**:749–54.

61. Austin PC. An introduction to propensity score methods for reducing the effects of confounding in observational studies. *Multivariate Behav Res*. 2011;**46**:399–424.

62. Cannon MJ, Warner L, Taddei JA, Kleinbaum DG. What can go wrong when you assume that correlated data are independent: an illustration from the evaluation of a childhood health intervention in Brazil. *Stat Med*. 2001;**20**:1461–7.

63. Hu FB, Goldberg J, Hedeker D, Flay BR, Pentz MA. Comparison of population-averaged and subject-specific approaches for analyzing repeated binary outcomes. *Am J Epidemiol*. 1998;**147**:694–703.

64. Hubbard AE, Ahern J, Fleischer NL, Van der Laan M, Lippman SA, Jewell N, et al. To GEE or not to GEE: comparing population average and mixed models for estimating the associations between neighborhood risk factors and health. *Epidemiology*. 2010;**21**:467–74.

Chapter

7

Monitoring ART Safety and Biovigilance

Luca Gianaroli, Anna Pia Ferraretti and Borut Kovačič

Introduction

Collecting data regarding assisted reproductive technology (ART) worldwide is of the utmost usefulness to ensure safety and quality of treatments provided, to detect potential problems and to implement practices aimed at reducing risks and improving outcomes. Today, registries have been set up in most countries. Regulations and guidelines for the monitoring of all clinical and laboratory aspects of ART have been issued based on data collected thus far. Currently available evidence should be the basis for a further improvement of medical and laboratory practices.

Monitoring ART Safety[*]

Safety of medical treatments implies the absence of all their side effects on patients, including both short- and long-term effects. With reference to ART, subjects involved are prospective parents (especially mothers) and their children, as well as donors of gametes and gestational carriers.

Since the early application of in vitro fertilization (IVF), operators have agreed on the importance of monitoring these new techniques in order to build and maintain trust in them. National data collections were first set up in Germany (1982), Australia (1983), France (1986) and the United Kingdom (1990). In North America, the Society for Assisted

---

[*] Data reported in this section were extracted from annual reports of the following registries: (1) Reports from Europe (European IVF Monitoring (EIM) Consortium) are available at: www.eshre.eu/Data-collection-and-research/Consortia/EIM/Publications.aspx; (2) reports from the United States (US) are available at: www.cdc.gov/art/reports/archive.html; (3) reports from Australia and New Zealand are available at: https://npesu.unsw.edu.au/data-collection/australian-new-zealand-assisted-reproduction-database-anzard; (4) International Committee Monitoring Assisted Reproductive Technologies (ICMART) reports are available at: www.icmartivf.org/icmart-publications.html.

Reproductive Technology (SART) began to publish annual reports in 1988 [1] and, by an Act of Congress, in 1992 the task was assumed by the Centers for Disease Control and Prevention (CDC) [2]. Other regional data collections have been implemented in Australia and New Zealand since 1984 and in Latin America since 1997 [3, 4]. In Europe, an IVF monitoring program was organized by the European Society of Human Reproduction and Embryology (ESHRE) in 1997, collecting data from already existing registries and from countries without a national monitoring system on a voluntary basis [5]. All these national and regional data collection systems are aimed at generating and publishing annual reports. Data collection methods, validation systems and data dissemination strategies have presented many differences among countries. In spite of this, since 1997 all people involved and/or interested in ART (inside and outside the ART professional community) can make use of systematic reports from the United States (US), Australia and Europe. More recently, some national and regional data collections have been initiated in Asia and Africa. In addition, since 1989 world reports have been presented during the World Congresses on IVF, and since 2000 they have been published systematically by the International Committee Monitoring Assisted Reproductive Technologies (ICMART) in scientific journals. Forty years after the birth of the first IVF baby, it is possible to state that the goal of monitoring ART in an effective way was achieved in an efficient manner that very few other fields of medicine can claim. ART reports provide information to patients, to health professionals, to health authorities and to the general public, not only on availability and efficacy but also on safety.

The majority of reports focus on multiple pregnancies, which are considered the most frequent and severe complication of IVF, but some of them present data on other side effects, such as ovarian hyperstimulation syndrome (OHSS) and egg retrieval complications.

Thanks to the availability of data from a long period of monitoring, we are today able to evaluate trends regarding several aspects of ART safety and suggest different policies to adopt in order to improve ART practice.

In this section, an update on the most relevant aspects of ART safety from a clinical point of view is presented.

Multiple Pregnancies

From 1980 to 1995, the incidence of multiple pregnancies grew dramatically as a result of increasingly aggressive ovarian stimulation protocols and the common practice of transferring multiple embryos in order to improve success rates. Women undergoing IVF faced a 20-fold increased risk of twins and a 400-fold increased risk of high-order pregnancies. In 1996, regional reports available at that time and collected globally by ICMART registered an incidence of twins of 30% and of triplets or higher-order pregnancies of 6%: 50% of all children born from IVF were twins or triplets. Certainly, multiple pregnancies are associated with greater risks of morbidity and mortality for both mothers and fetuses compared with singleton pregnancies [6]. Because of the dramatically high frequency of this iatrogenic adverse effect of ART (for which the ART professional community felt partly responsible), policies aimed at reducing the number of embryos transferred started to be adopted. In 2001, the WHO recommended that "no more than two embryos should be transferred per cycle" and that "elective single embryo transfer (eSET) should be encouraged" in patients with a good prognosis [7].

Methods adopted to address this problem varied among countries: in some countries, the number of embryos to be transferred has been regulated by law, in others, by professional guidelines. In 2007, according to International Federation of Fertility Societies (IFFS) surveillance, 46% (26/54) of countries had regulations on this issue, but the majority of them limited the number of embryos to three and, in some countries, transfer of more than three embryos was permitted in specific cases. Only five countries (Denmark, Israel, Norway, New Zealand and the UK) limited by law the number of embryos to two, and some countries (e.g. Japan and some northern European countries) introduced eSET into their practice (which has been compulsory by law in Belgium since 2004) [8]. Despite these different approaches, the years that followed registered a decline in the multiple birth rate (MBR) worldwide [9]. Ten years later, the proportion of countries with regulations on this subject had increased to 55% (41/74, 14 enforced by law and 27 by professional organizations or guidelines). In most cases, the number of embryos was reduced to two and eSET was more frequently adopted. However, several countries have not yet addressed this problem [10].

Opposition against the reduction of the number of embryos to be transferred has always been motivated by the fear that it would cause a decrease in pregnancy rates. The need to find a balance between safety and the willingness to maximize chances of pregnancy has been approached in different ways. A clear example of this difference can be provided by the comparison of data from Australia, North America and Europe regarding policies on the number of embryos transferred between 1997 and 2015 (Fig. 7.1).

Australia was one of the first countries in the world to reduce the number of embryos to be transferred. In 1997, in the majority of cycles, only 2 embryos were transferred, and since 2006, single embryo transfer (SET) became predominant (86% in 2015). Transfers with ≥3 embryos were less than 1%.

In North America, the number of embryos per transfer is recommended by guidelines issued by the American Society for Reproductive Medicine (ASRM). The first guidelines were published in 2000 and subsequently modified several times, with the last update occurring in 2017 and including criteria for eSET [11]. Beginning in 2000, the number of embryos transferred has been reported in the ASRM annual registry. The proportion of transfers with ≥3 embryos, which were still the majority in 2003 (56%), decreased slowly, and in the last report, published in 2015, it was 15%.

Data from Europe should be interpreted with caution because they represent an average from several countries (more than 30 in the past 10 European IVF Monitoring (EIM) Consortium reports) with different embryo transfer policies and regulations, as clearly documented in annual reports. However, a clear trend towards transferring fewer embryos was observed: dual embryo transfer has been the most frequently used strategy since 2000 and, since 2006, transfer of ≥3 embryos has shown a constant decline. At the same time, SET registered a slow but constant increase, thanks to some northern European countries (Finland, Norway, Sweden, Belgium and Denmark), which have been pioneers in eSET for years.

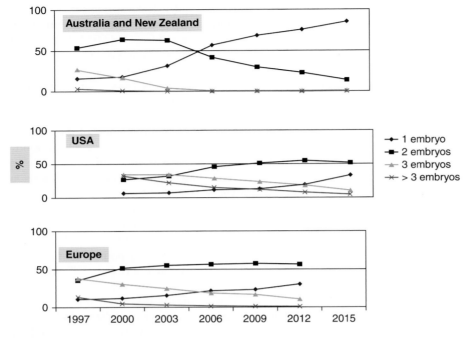

Figure 7.1 Distribution of embryo transfers per number of embryos transferred.

Sources: This figure was created using annual reports from the following registries:
Reports from Europe (EIM) are available at: www.eshre.eu/Data-collection-and-research/Consortia/EIM/Publications.aspx.
Reports from the US are available at: www.cdc.gov/art/reports/archive.html.
Reports from Australia and New Zealand are available at: https://npesu.unsw.edu.au/data-collection/australian-new-zealand-assisted-repro
duction-database-anzard.

Different policies adopted in these three continents have had a variable impact on multiple birth rates (Fig. 7.2): in Australia triplets (or more) have constituted less than 1% of births since 2000 (0.1% in 2015) and twin pregnancies declined from 19% in 1997 to 4.3% in 2015. In the US, triplets (or more) constituted less than 1% in the last reports and twin pregnancies still account for more than 20%. In Europe, triplets or more have constituted less than 1% since 2006 (0.5% in 2012) and twin pregnancies have constituted less than 20% since 2009, although they were still at 17.5% in 2012.

Globally, despite substantial regional differences, ICMART reports recorded a decline in multiple delivery rates, which according to the most recent data available is 20.4% for twins and 1.1% for triplets. Following World Health Organization (WHO) recommendations, a global trend towards the transfer of two embryos in the majority of cycles seems to have been achieved, as well as the reduction of high-order births. Thanks to data collections and reports, it has been shown that transfer of more than two embryos does

not substantially improve pregnancy rate but instead causes multiple pregnancies [9]. At this stage, the next goal should be to reduce the twin delivery rate, which is still considered too high. To achieve this, it is necessary to further improve eSET policies. To evaluate the efficacy of eSET without compromising final outcomes, some important factors should be taken into account: evaluation of the outcome as cumulative (single) delivery rate per egg retrieval, quality of laboratory procedures in terms of embryo culture to blastocyst stage, embryo selection and, very important, cryopreservation techniques. Costs should also be taken into consideration, including both direct treatment costs and indirect social costs for multiple deliveries. A number of studies have indicated that the cost patients pay for ART treatment is associated with the number of embryos transferred [12].

Elective SET was first evaluated in a randomized controlled trial (RCT) in 1999 [13]. Since 2000, as previously described, eSET was introduced by means of national laws or professional guidelines and leadership in Australia and New Zealand, in some northern

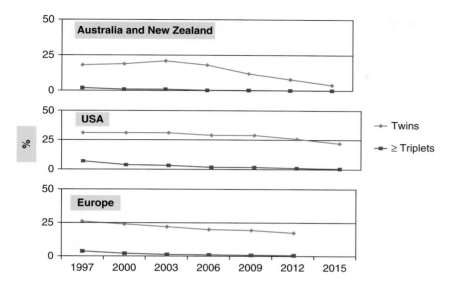

Figure 7.2 Distribution of twins and triplets between 1997 and 2015.

Sources: This figure was created using annual reports from the following registries:

Reports from Europe (EIM) are available at: www.eshre.eu/Data-collection-and-research/Consortia/EIM/Publications.aspx.

Reports from the US are available at: www.cdc.gov/art/reports/archive.html.

Reports from Australia and New Zealand are available at: https://npesu.unsw.edu.au/data-collection/australian-new-zealand-assisted-reproduction-database-anzard.

European countries (Belgium, Sweden, Denmark and Finland) and subsequently in Japan, where eSET represented 80% of all transfers performed in 2015.

In order to produce evidence on this topic, several RCTs and observational studies have been published and were subsequently reviewed in 2013 by the National Institute for Health and Care Excellence (NICE) [14]. The conclusion of the review was that evidence in favour of eSET was defective because of the poor quality of RCT studies and because of the different criteria used to compare eSET with double embryo transfer (DET). Furthermore, large RCTs using similar criteria, taking into account all clinical benefits and carefully selected arms of eSET compared with DET, are needed. In spite of this, observational evidence from large collected datasets and multicentre comparative studies was considered sufficient to reconfirm and expand recommendations for eSET [14].

The birth of a single baby should be the goal of ART, primarily for children and patients but also for society, as adverse medical outcomes associated with multiple pregnancies significantly increase health care costs [15]. "Regardless of the approach taken to valuing ART treatment, the implied or explicit monetary value of providing ART treatment far exceeds the cost per child conceived, suggesting that ART treatment is indeed good value for money – particularly if ART children are born as singletons" [16].

Ovarian Hyperstimulation Syndrome (OHSS) and Other Complications

The number of OHSS cases requiring hospitalization is reported on a yearly basis in Europe and Australia. Over the years, their incidence has shown a clear decline in both contexts (in Europe, from 1.2% in 1999 to 0.4% in 2013; in Australia, from 2.4% in 1999 to 0.6% in 2015). The cause of this decline could be related to the availability of better predictive markers of excessive response and of better preventive measures [17]. The absolute number in Europe was 32,829 OHSS cases out of more than 6.5 million cycles. Despite its low incidence, but because of its severity for each individual patient, further efforts should be made towards achieving "an OHSS-free clinic" [18].

Other complications of ART may include haemorrhages, infections and even maternal deaths. Out of 5,115,835 egg retrievals performed in Europe between 1997 and 2013, a total of 8,564 bleedings (0.16%) and 1,528 infections (0.03%) requiring surgical or medical interventions were reported. Incidence has remained the same throughout the years. The number of ART-associated maternal deaths reported in Europe during the same time period was 25 [5]. These figures, however, might be an underestimation, because in the US, between 2000 and 2011, out of 1,135,206 autologous cycles, 18 stimulation-related deaths and 40 maternal deaths prior to infant birth were reported. With reference to donor cycles, out of 112,254 cycles, there were no donor deaths reported, while 13 maternal deaths prior to infant birth were reported among oocyte recipients [19].

Obstetric and Perinatal Outcomes

Speculations about potential differences between ART pregnancies (including maternal and neonatal risks) and spontaneous pregnancies have been the subject of discussion for professionals and scientific societies since the early days of IVF. Thanks to the constant monitoring of this issue (annual reports from the ART registries and systematic reviews), several data on this subject are currently available. Some of them are based on a high level of evidence, while for others further evidence is required.

For many years [6], no doubts existed regarding the increased risks related to multiple pregnancies induced by ART both for fetuses (preterm and very preterm deliveries account for more than a 4-fold increase of perinatal mortality for twins and a 6-fold increase for triplets) and for mothers (a 2-fold increase of OHSS for twins and a 6-fold increase for higher order, a 3- to 7-fold increase of pregnancy-induced complications, a 4- to 10-fold increase of perinatal morbidity and mortality) compared with singletons. At the same time, some data show that singleton pregnancies by fresh transfers are at higher risk of 'small for gestational age' and preterm delivery and low birth weight compared with spontaneous pregnancies [20], and these findings have been confirmed [21]. On the other hand, some recent data [22, 23, 24] suggest that frozen pregnancies have a lower risk of preterm delivery and low birth weight compared with fresh pregnancies, and a higher rate of 'large for gestational age' compared with spontaneous pregnancies. A recent review and meta-analysis comparing egg donation pregnancies and IVF and spontaneous conceptions showed increased risk of hypertensive disorders, pre-eclampsia, postpartum haemorrhage, caesarean section, preterm birth, low birth weight versus IVF and spontaneous pregnancies, while there was no difference in the incidence of 'small for gestational age' and gestational

diabetes mellitus [25]. Other data analyzing blastocysts transfer versus earlier cleavage stages among singleton pregnancies [26, 27, 28] suggest a higher incidence of monozygotic twinning, of preterm or very preterm delivery and of placenta anomalies in blastocyst conceptions. A recent review of 124,215 ART and 6,054,729 non-ART singleton pregnancies found increased risk of placental anomalies (placenta praevia, placental abruption, morbidly adherent placenta and cord insertion anomalies) following ART [29]. These defects may also be responsible for higher rates of maternal and fetal morbidity and mortality in singleton pregnancies. ART pregnancies are different from spontaneous conceptions not only for the higher incidence of multiplicity but also for other risk factors also present in singletons. Research into the mechanisms that cause these conditions is required.

General consensus is that monitoring the health of babies and mothers and offering parental counselling prior to fertility treatment are crucial.

Biovigilance in Europe

This section describes biovigilance governance and procedures in the field of reproductive medicine that are currently in place in the European Union (EU). Despite the rapid development of reproductive medicine over the past 30 years, the ART success rate is still below 50% per cycle. Since the very early days, these techniques, which are now routinely used, were developed by clinicians and scientists through an approach based on diligent recording and analysis of as many parameters as possible to track their impact on ART procedures' success rates, especially in case of deviations from standards. At first, monitoring in IVF was aimed at verifying the efficiency of novelties (scientific approach), monitoring clinical results (clinical approach) and, at a later stage, at keeping the system under constantly controlled conditions (safety and quality approach) and at following up on the health of children conceived with ART (epidemiological approach) [30]. In principle, the basis for this is an optimally set up and effective monitoring system.

At present, almost every European IVF centre manages one or more databases of patients, intrauterine insemination (IUI) cycles, fresh IVF/ICSI cycles or thawing cycles. These databases contain information about recovered oocytes, fertilized oocytes, embryos and their fate after completion of in vitro cultivation and embryo transfer [31]. Each IVF centre should also maintain a diligently managed written or electronic supervision system for cryopreservation of gametes, reproductive tissues and embryos; identify and locate frozen biological materials; and keep records on the expiration of the storage period, which may be institutionally or legally restricted. Ideally, information on cryo cycles should be linked to information on fresh cycles from which biological material was obtained. By doing so, it is possible to monitor the cumulative success rate of treatments after one stimulated IVF cycle, including thawed embryo transfer outcomes.

Most EU member states have established their own national ART registries. By collecting data from them, the ESHRE EIM program monitors most of the medically assisted reproduction (MAR) cycles performed in Europe [5]. On its website, it also advises what key parameters national ART registries should contain. In collaboration with the European Commission's Directorate for Health and Food Safety (DG SANTE), it is appealing to national registries to introduce online 'cycle-by-cycle' registration of all MAR cycles, which would provide much better control over the quality of treatments in comparison with summary registries.

With the introduction of the European Union Tissue and Cells Directive (EUTCD), monitoring of factors that could in any way affect quality and safety of cells, tissues and embryos intended for infertility treatment has become a legal obligation for treatment providers in European Union member states [32, 33]. Their constant supervision is called *vigilance* and is defined as the state of constant watchfulness for potential dangers or threats. In ART laboratories, this could be defined as *medical biotechnology vigilance* and it applies to all activities aimed at detecting, assessing, understanding and preventing adverse events or reactions related to laboratory equipment, embryo culture environment, products or treatments that could have a harmful effect on biological material used in infertility treatment or that could negatively affect the health of patients or that of children conceived from ART.

Biomedical technology vigilance includes the following categories:

1. Technical vigilance
2. Pharmacovigilance
3. Medical devices vigilance
4. Bio/Histovigilance

An effective surveillance in an ART laboratory requires the following:

1. Constant monitoring of physico-chemical parameters of the equipment for in vitro culture of cells, by means of the quality management system.
2. Postmarket surveillance of medical devices that come in contact with human reproductive tissues, cells and embryos.
3. In vitro post-treatment surveillance (monitoring of gamete and/or embryo survival and/or development).
4. In vivo post-treatment surveillance (follow-up of treated patients, follow-up of offspring).

The main goal of monitoring systems in ART laboratories is to measure effectiveness and quality of the system and to identify factors that could result in complications during an infertility treatment. All actions related to identification of any weaknesses in the system with the aim of preventing complications are defined as *risk management*, which is one of the main components of the quality management system [34].

The quality management system focuses on preventing errors and maintaining consistent safety standards related to tissues and cells released for clinical application. If for any reason the system deviates from expected functioning, such a deviation represents an *incident*. Incidents are procedural errors of various severity levels depending on their different consequences for patients, their gametes, reproductive tissues or embryos and, consequently, for offspring.

Incidents are categorized as follows:

1. Near-miss events: occurrences that would probably have become an adverse incident but were identified and prevented.
2. Adverse events: unexpected occurrences that are procedural failures and might lead to harm in a patient or to a loss of any irreplaceable autologous reproductive tissues, cells or embryos.
   2.1. Serious adverse events are those that may be associated with collection, processing, storage or distribution of reproductive tissues, gametes or embryos intended for human application and which might lead to the transmission of a communicable disease, death or life-threatening, disabling or incapacitating conditions, or might result in prolonged hospitalization or illness; this also includes events in which gametes or embryos were misidentified or mixed up.

3. Adverse reactions: unintended adverse responses that have occurred, causing harm to a donor, a recipient or a child born through ART procedures.

　3.1. Serious adverse reactions include a communicable disease, in the donor or in the recipient associated with gamete collection or application of reproductive tissues, cells and embryos that is fatal, life-threatening, disabling or incapacitating or which results in, or prolongs, hospitalization or morbidity.

An adverse event may or may not cause an adverse reaction. Directive 2006/86/EC requires that all serious adverse events or reactions be reported to competent authorities (CAs). However, legislation in some countries requires that non-serious events or reactions should also be reported to the CA. In any case, all incidents that happen or might happen must be critically analyzed and assessed to ensure appropriate investigation as well as corrective and preventive actions.

In the framework of the European Union-funded projects Vigilance and Surveillance of Substances of Human Origin (SOHO V&S) and the European Union Standards and Training for the Inspection of Tissue Establishments (EUSTITE) Project, specific guidance was designed for reporting, evaluating and managing serious adverse reactions (SARs) and serious adverse events (SAEs) [35, 36, 37]. In fact, these tools can be applied to all incidents and near-miss events, not only to those considered serious. The EUSTITE tool helps to evaluate on a scale from 0 (or 1) to 4:

1. Imputability (for adverse reactions only): to evaluate whether the adverse reaction was caused during medical treatment for gamete collection or after use of gametes/embryos
2. Severity (for adverse reactions only)
3. Possibility of recurrence (for adverse reactions and events)
4. Consequences: impact of adverse events or reactions on individuals, ART service provision, availability of reproductive cells/embryos

Notification Criteria

According to the EUTCD, SAEs and SARs must be reported to CAs. The reporting criteria scoring system was set up for easier assessment of incident or reaction severity. The criteria for reporting of adverse events or reactions are based on consequences and on probability of recurrence. This scoring system helps to make decisions on whether to report the adverse event or reaction to the CA.

If the reporting criteria scores are 0–3, the ART centre usually manages the incident according to quality management principles by introducing corrective and preventive actions and by paying special attention to risk factors that caused the incident itself.

In case the reporting criteria scores are 4–6, the ART centre must interact with the CA, which may request an inspection.

For all adverse events and reactions with a notification criteria score of 7–20, the CA must be informed immediately. It will most probably designate representatives to participate in corrective and preventive action plans.

Since the recording of incidents and unwanted occurrences is an important part of the quality management system within the ART centre, it is essential to conduct an overview of incidents, carry out critical analyses and indicate corrective and preventive measures [38]. Incidents management is primarily aimed at improving the system. For this reason, it is essential that quality managers, clinical directors, laboratory heads and CAs do not immediately implement punitive measures. Incidents with high scores must be treated in an educational way.

It is recommended that the list of incidents be included in the existing IVF cycle monitoring system or in a separate database. According to SOHO V&S, such a database should contain at least the following information:

- Type of incident
- Description of the incident
- Type of vigilance into which the event falls
- Tissues and cells involved
- Number of patients involved
- Time that elapsed between the incident and its detection
- Process during which the incident occurred
- Imputability grade
- Severity grade
- Possibility of recurrence
- Notification
- Consequences
- Corrective and preventive actions
- Estimated occurrence

However, the majority of existing IVF registries do not contain any of the suggested information.

Most incidents should be reported to the CAs either as immediate notifications or as a list of adverse occurrences in an annual report. All incidents, adverse events and reactions in which biological and medical products of human origin are involved can be directly registered in the Notify Library, a global vigilance and surveillance database for medical products of human origin (www.notifylibrary.org/). The Notify Library is of interest to all stakeholders in ART. Under the heading 'Reproductive Cells', the electronic register provides an overview of reported incidents, including their more detailed description and related assessments, which define the severity and consequences of an adverse event or reaction.

By scrolling through the register, one can quickly establish the most common incidents that ART clinics report (Table 7.1).

Equipment

An IVF laboratory is categorized as a high-tech laboratory and it contains complex equipment that must operate flawlessly. The most sensitive pieces of equipment are undoubtedly incubators for embryo culture. In modern incubators, continuous monitoring of key physical and chemical parameters is featured in the incubator itself. These parameters include temperature, gas concentration and, consequently, culture media pH, which can change to critical levels, either because of a malfunction of the incubator or human error. Deviations of these parameters from the physiological level may affect oocyte and embryo vitality (technical vigilance).

Culture Media

Common errors in the process of embryo culture can also arise from culture media (medical device vigilance). Quality of media categorized as medical devices is currently checked at several levels. In accordance with the EUTCD, each medium quality certificate must be checked in each IVF laboratory [39]. Interestingly, a protein supplement, such as human serum albumin, may be added to the medium at a later stage. This, however, completely changes its chemical characteristics (pH, osmolality, concentration of media components), which means that a quality certificate issued for a medium no longer applies after albumin addition. It has also been found

Table 7.1 The Notify Library's list of adverse occurrences related to human reproductive cells, tissues and embryos (www.notifylibrary.org/)

ID	Sperm
91	Spinal Muscular Atrophy transmission by donor sperm
974	Salpingitis after intrauterine insemination
1105	Mix-up of sperm, partner
1113	Sperm of deceased partner mistakenly destroyed
1153	Sperm processing error
982	Fraud with sperm
1925	Loss of donor sperm belonging to 250 patients

ID	Oocyte
482	Acquired haemophilia
695	ABO Haemolytic Disease of the Newborn (HDN)
832	Ovarian abscess after oocytes retrieval
834	Ovarian hyperstimulation syndrome (OHSS) requiring intensive care
987	Transportation device with follicle fluid too hot
988	Oocyte placed in a dish with oocytes of another patient
958	Oocytes lost in the pipette
964	Loss of oocytes
970	Loss of oocytes
972	In vitro fertilisation cycle lost
973	Oocytes lost after cleaning
980	All oocytes of 1 cycle lost
988	Oocyte placed in a dish with oocytes of another patient
1377	*Wuchereria bancrofti* (parasite) in follicular fluid
1596	Haemorrhage requiring transfusion within 12 weeks of ART cycle initiation
1642	Infection within 12 weeks of ART cycle initiation

ID	Embryo
959	Fungal infection in embryo culture
961	Embryo for fertility preservation lost
969	Embryos of two couples lost
971	Mix-up of embryos
977	Genetically abnormal embryo (Huntington's disease) was transferred after preimplantation diagnosis
978	Mix-up of embryos
979	Cryopreservation error of embryos
981	Embryotoxic oil
983	Wrong cryopreservation program used
984	Embryotoxic dishes used
986	Technical fault of the freezer

Table 7.1 (cont.)

ID	
989	Loss of preimplantation embryos
1111	Embryo selection error
1124	Microbial contamination in dishes of 5 couples
1116	Loss of embryos of 5 couples
1117	Loss of embryos of 2 couples
1119	Bacterial infection after embryo transfer
1121	Loss of embryos of 12 couples due to an incorrect mix of cryopreservation medium
1679	Misdiagnosis, Preimplantation Genetic Diagnosis (PGD)
1680	Intrauterine Transfer of Mosaic Aneuploid Blastocysts results in birth of healthy babies
1926	Embryos of seven patients did not progress as expected and were not suitable for embryo transfer
ID	**Ovarian tissue**
1115	Incorrect cryopreservation run of ovarian tissue for maternity preservation
ID	**Combined**
92	Spinal Muscular Atrophy transmission by donor sperm and oocyte

that concentrations of salts, proteins, energy substrates, growth factors and hormones in culture media change significantly from the moment of delivery until the moment of use, and during incubation at 37 °C. Moreover, it was observed that in commercial culture media it is possible to find cell-free DNA and RNA, most likely derived from human serum albumin. These findings demonstrate that occasional deviations from optimal embryo morphology and morphokinetics and drops in clinical results of IVF may be due to nonoptimal media or to their contamination with unknown embryotoxic components that are probably derived from human protein preparations, such as human serum albumin [40].

It is very difficult to estimate the impact of suboptimal culture conditions, atmosphere, temperature or culture media on cells, embryos and, consequently, on children born. It is also known that, in suboptimal conditions, embryo development can be apparently normal. In addition, human embryo metabolism can partially adapt to nonphysiological conditions. The negative impact of suboptimal cultivation conditions on embryonic development can, therefore, manifest itself at a later developmental stage. Implantation rate may decrease, and the proportion of miscarriages may increase [41].

The impact may, however, be observed later, e.g. as a change in the birthweight of newborns conceived through ART [42]. For this reason, the imputability level is not assessable in most of these situations.

Nevertheless, medium inadequacy may also be identified. It is recommended that pH values and osmolality of media are independently measured with appropriate apparatuses [38]. Because of commercial interests, culture media manufacturers have been concealing the concentration of components, a practice that is opposed by those who work in the field of reproductive medicine [40]. However, attempts are being made to independently measure media composition and check the values of quality parameters printed on accompanying certificates [43].

In case the tracking of media serial numbers shows and confirms that there was a significant deviation in laboratory IVF results during the period of application of a specific batch, it is imperative that this occurrence is registered with the CA. Medical devices also include most of the laboratory consumables. Withdrawal of specific batches of ICSI pipettes, vitrification straws, denudation pipettes and embryo transfer catheters has occurred in the past. A toxic batch of Petri dishes was also detected and registered (see Table 7.1).

If the incident involves medical devices or biological materials identified as causing agents of an SAE or SAR, the CA may decide to initiate a product recall procedure and to trigger a rapid alert between tissue establishments (TEs) and CAs at national and/or EU/EEA levels via the rapid alert system for human tissues and cells (RATC).

Cryotank Failure

A technical-vigilance event with severe consequences for patients is the accidental thawing of stored biological samples in cryotanks, caused by cryotank failure, failure of the automatic liquid nitrogen filling system or human error. Effective alarm systems are therefore of utmost importance for cryobanks [38]. The constant presence of a backup container with liquid nitrogen, which can be used to move frozen samples in the event of failure of a cryo-storage tank, is also recommended.

Processing of Semen Samples, Oocytes and Embryos

Special attention should be paid to errors during semen sample processing, as these can cause SARs, such as oocyte contamination during sperm–oocyte co-culture in conventional IVF procedures and the subsequent cancellation of embryo transfer. An error in semen processing leading to the destruction of a sample is often solved by repeating semen collection, unless it is the only sample available (frozen sperm or testicular tissue from cancer patients and patients with azoospermia).

The Notify Library's biovigilance list includes several cases of loss or destruction of gametes and embryos. These adverse events occur primarily during processing, human error during cell and embryo pipetting being the most common cause. Destroyed oocytes may also be the result of poor-quality or inadequately matured oocytes. Oocytes can be destroyed during oocyte pickup, denudation, ICSI, pipetting, culture, vitrification and warming. Damage to only a few oocytes out of all of the oocytes from one patient is usually not registered as an adverse event, even though a part of the biological material intended for treatment is destroyed. The proportion of failed cells at individual stages of processing is recorded in the quality management system and presented with key performance indicators (KPIs) [44]. Destruction or loss of all cells leading to cancellation of the IVF cycle is considered an SAE.

Contamination

Fungi or bacteria contamination of culture dishes mainly derives from biological material itself, but culture media may be contaminated during preparation in the laboratory because of improper handling or inadequate hygiene standards. It is difficult for culture infections to arise from the surrounding air if culture media handling and culture dish preparation are performed in laminar flow hoods. Additionally, culture media are protected from air contamination by a layer of paraffin oil.

Semen mainly contains bacterial flora. Even if semen is adequately laboratory-washed and antibiotics are added to the media, bacterial colonies and fungi can also proliferate in culture dishes. Each biological material contamination is an SAE, requiring corrective actions for prevention of contamination of other samples. Corrective actions include incubator sterilization and laboratory decontamination. In the latter case, aggressive disinfecting agents should not be used to avoid affecting other gametes and embryos in the laboratory at the time of decontamination.

Transferring embryos from contaminated media may cause health problems for the recipient.

Mix-Up and Genetic Defects

One SAE that can cause an SAR is the mix-up of gametes or embryos. To avoid or minimize this risk, a plan of corrective actions must be prepared. The severity of an adverse event depends on the stage in which the error is detected: during gamete processing, insemination, embryo manipulation, embryo transfer or, later, after the birth of the child.

SARs arising from laboratory work also include births of affected children following use of donor gametes carrying genetic diseases. In this case, it is necessary to immediately recall other samples that may be available at all tissue establishments. Birth of an affected child following misdiagnosis in preimplantation genetic testing (PGT) is also a common SAR (see Table 7.1).

Conclusions

In conclusion, it is worth noting that most EUTCD and CA inspections certainly raised the safety and quality levels of working procedures in individual laboratories. This probably explains why most SAEs and SARs in the Notify Library relate to laboratory work on reproductive cells and tissues. However, the annual histovigilance reports of the Human Fertility and Embryology Authority, a report from the joint registry of MAR cycles and adverse occurrences, show that out of the 465 incidents reported in 2014, 212 were clinical, 114 were laboratory errors and 102 were administrative errors [45]. This suggests that adverse events are underreported in voluntary registers. Greater attention should therefore be given to all aspects of ART procedures and to their outcomes both in the short and in the long term.

Given that registration of cycles in national and ESHRE registries has already become well established, it would make sense to adapt these registries accordingly to monitor biovigilance as well. Compulsory registering of individual IVF cycles, including data on drugs used, ovarian stimulation protocols, types of culture media, incubation conditions (types of incubators, gas concentrations), perinatal data and, possibly, information on the subsequent development of children conceived by MAR, would significantly contribute to the establishment of an effective biovigilance governance. To use the existing ART registries for timely reporting of adverse events, such registries should have all IVF cycles registered online, from the start of patient preparation for IVF. Competent authorities could have direct access to the data. In such a system, a delay of reporting as a result of the need to wait until treatment outcomes are available would not influence the need for immediate reporting of adverse events or reactions with any impact on the processed biological material or treated patients.

References

1. Medical Research International. The American Fertility Society Special Interest Group. In vitro fertilization/embryo transfer in the United States: 1985 and 1986 results from the National IVF/ET Registry. *Fertil Steril*. 1988;**42**:212–15.

2. Fertility Clinic Success Rate and Certification Act of 1992. Public Law No. 102–493, 24 October 1992.

3. National Perinatal Statistics Unit and Fertility Society of Australia. *In Vitro Fertilization Pregnancies, Australia, 1980–1983*. Sydney: National Perinatal Statistics Unit; 1984.

4. Zegers-Hochschild F, Galdames IV. *Registro Latinoamericano de Reproduccion Asistida 1997*. RED Latinoamericana de Reproduccion Asistida; 1997.

5. Ferraretti AP, Nygren K, Nyboe Andersen A, de Mouzon J, Kupka M, Calhaz-Jorge C, et al., The European IVF-Monitoring Consortium (EIM), for the European Society of Human Reproduction and Embryology (ESHRE). Trends over 15 years in ART in Europe: an analysis of 6 million cycles. *Hum Reprod Open*. 2017;**2017**(2): hox012.

6. The ESHRE CAPRI Workshop Group. Multiple gestation pregnancy. *Hum Reprod*. 2000;**15**:1856–64.

7. Vayena E, Rowe PJ, Griffin PD (eds.). *Current Practices and Controversies in Assisted Reproduction*. Geneva: World Health Organization; 2002.

8. Jones HW Jr, Cohen J. IFFS Surveillance 2007. *Fertil Steril*. 2007;**87**(Suppl 1):S3–S67.

9. Templeton A, Morris JK. Reducing the risk of multiple births by transfer of two embryos after in vitro fertilization. *N Engl J Med*. 1998;**339**(9):573–7.

10. IFFS. IFFS surveillance 2016. *Global Reproductive Health*. 2016;**1**(e1):1–143.

11. Practice Committee of the American Society for Reproductive Medicine. Guidance on the limits to the number of embryos to transfer: a committee opinion. *Fertil Steril*. 2017;**107**(4):901–3.

12. Chambers GM, Hoang VP, Sullivan EA, Chapman MG, Ishihara O, Zegers-Hochschild F, et al. The impact of patient costs on access to assisted reproductive technologies and embryo transfer practices: an international analysis. *Fertil Steril*. 2014;**101**(1):191–8.

13. Gerris J, De Neubourg D, Mangelschots K, Van Royen E, Van de Meersche M, Valkenburg M. Prevention of twin pregnancy after in-vitro fertilization or intracytoplasmic sperm injection based on strict embryo criteria: a prospective randomized clinical trial. *Hum Reprod*. 1999;**14**(10): 2581–7.

14. National Institute for Health and Care Excellence (NICE). *Fertility. Assessment and Treatment for People with Fertility Problems*. NICE Clinical Guideline 156. London: NICE; February 2013.

15. Lemos EV, Zhang D, Van Voorhis BJ, Hu XH. Healthcare expenses associated with multiple vs singleton pregnancies in the United States. *Am J Obstet Gynecol*. 2013;**209**(6):586.e1–586.e11.

16. Chambers GM, Adamson GD, Eijkemans MJ. Acceptable cost for the patient and society. *Fertil Steril*. 2013;**100**(2):319–27.

17. Broer SL, Dolleman M, Oopmer BC, Fauser BC, Mol BW, Broekmans FJ. AMH and AFC as predictors of excessive response in controlled ovarian hyperstimulation: a metanalysis. *Hum Reprod Update*. 2011;**17**:46–54.

18. Devroey P, Polyzos NP, Blockeel C. An OHSS-free clinic by segmentation of IVF treatment. *Hum Reprod*. 2011;**26**:2593–7.

19. Kawwass JF, Kissin DM, Kulkarni AD, Creanga AA, Session DR, Callaghan WM, et al., for the National ART Surveillance System (NASS) Group. Safety of assisted reproductive technology in the United States, 2000–2011. *JAMA*. 2015;**313**(1):88–90.

20. Koudstaal J, Braat DDM, Bruinse HW, Naaktgeboren N, Vermeiden JPW, Visser GHA. Obstetric outcome of singleton pregnancies after IVF: a matched control study in four Dutch university hospitals. *Hum Reprod*. 2000;**15**(8):1819–25.

21. Pinborg A, Wennerholm UB, Romundstad LB, Loft A, Aittomaki K, Söderström-Anttila V, et al. Why do singletons conceived after assisted reproduction technology have adverse perinatal outcome? Systematic review and meta-analysis. *Hum Reprod Update*. 2013;**19**(2):87–104.

22. Wennerholm UB, Henninsen AK, Romunstadt LB, Bergh C, Pinborg A, Skjaerven R, et al. Perinatal outcome of children born after frozen-thawed embryo transfer: a Nordic cohort study from the CoNARTaS group. *Hum Reprod*. 2013;**28**(9):2545–53.

23. Ishihara O, Araki R, Kuwahara A, Itakura A, Saito H, Adamson GD. Impact of frozen-thawed single-blastocyst transfer on maternal and neonatal outcome: an analysis of 277,042 single-embryo transfer cycles from 2008 to 2010 in Japan. *Fertil Steril.* 2014;**101**:128–33.

24. Wong KM, van Wely M, Mol F, Repping S, Mastenbroek S. Fresh versus frozen embryo transfer in assisted reproduction. *Cochrane Database Syst Rev.* 2017;**2017**(3):CD 011184.

25. Storgaard M, Loft A, Bergh C, Wenerholm UB, Söderström-Anttila V, Romundstad LB, et al. Obstetric and neonatal complications in pregnancies conceived after oocyte donation: a systematic review and metanalysis. *BJOG.* 2017;**124**(4):561–72.

26. Mateizel I, Santos-Ribeiro S, Done E, Van Landuyt L, Van de Velde H, Tournaye H, et al. Do ARTs affect the incidence of monozygotic twinning? *Hum Reprod.* 2016;**31**(11):2435–41.

27. Ginstrom Ernstad E, Bergh C, Khatibi A, Kallen KB, Westlander G, Nilsson S, et al. Neonatal and maternal outcome after blastocyst transfer: a population-based registry study. *Am J Obstet Gynecol.* 2016;**214**(3):378. e1–378.e10.

28. Dar S, Lazer T, Shah PS, Librach CL. Neonatal outcomes among singleton births after blastocyst versus cleavage stage embryo transfer: a systematic review and metanalysis. *Hum Reprod Update.* 2014;**20** (3):439–48.

29. Vermey B, Buchanan A, Chambers GM, Kolibianakis EM, Bosdou J, Chapman MG, et al. Are singleton pregnancies after assisted reproduction technology (ART) associated with a higher risk of placental anomalies as compared to non-ART singleton pregnancies? A systematic review and meta-analysis. *BJOG* (forthcoming). Available at: https://doi.org/10.1111/1471-0528.15227.

30. Cohen J, Trounson A, Dawson K, Jones H, Hazekamp J, Nygren K, Hamberger L. The early days of IVF outside the UK. *Hum Reprod Update.* 2005;**11**: 439–59.

31. Levkov L, Tomas C. Laboratory information and document management systems. In AC Varghese, P Sjöblom, K Jayaprakasan (eds.), *A Practical Guide to Setting Up an IVF Lab, Embryo Culture Systems and Running the Unit.* New Delhi: Jaypee Brothers Medical Publishers; 2013. pp.195–212.

32. European Commission. 32006L0017: Commission Directive 2006/17/EC of 8 February 2006 implementing Directive 2004/23/EC of the European Parliament and of the Council as regards certain technical requirements for the donation, procurement and testing of human tissues and cells (Text with EEA relevance). Official Journal of the European Union. 2006:162–74.

33. European Commission. 32006L0086: Commission Directive 2006/86/EC of 24 October 2006 implementing Directive 2004/23/EC of the European Parliament and of the Council as regards traceability requirements, notification of serious adverse reactions and events and certain technical requirements for the coding, processing, preservation, storage and distribution of human tissues and cells (Text with EEA relevance). Official Journal of the European Union. 2006:32–50.

34. Mortimer D, Mortimer ST. *Quality and Risk Management in the IVF Laboratory.* Cambridge: Cambridge University Press; 2005.

35. SOHO V&S. *Guidance on Vigilance and Surveillance in Assisted Reproductive Technologies in the European Union. (Work Package 5, Deliverable 5).* Available at: www.tripnet.nl/wp-content/uploads/2017/07/Deliverable-5-Vigilance-in-ART.pdf, accessed 24 April 2018.

36. Fehily D, Sullivan S, Noel L, Harkin D. Improving vigilance and surveillance for tissues and cells in the European Union: EUSTITE, SOHO V&S and Project Notify. *Organs Tiss Cells.* 2012;**15** (2):85–95.

37. EUSTITE Project. *Vigilance and Surveillance of Tissues and Cells in the European Union. Final Recommendations, June 2012.* Strasbourg: Council of Europe; 2012.

38. De los Santos MJ, Apter S, Coticchio G, Debrock S, Lundin K, Plancha CE, et al. Revised guidelines for good practice in IVF laboratories (2015). *Hum Reprod.* 2016;**31**(4):685–6.

39. Council of Europe. *Guide to the Quality and Safety of Tissues and Cells for Human Application*, 3rd edn. Strasbourg: Council of Europe; 2018.

40. Sunde A, Brison D, Dumoulin J, Harper J, Lundin K, Magli MC, et al. Time to take human embryo culture seriously. *Hum Reprod.* 2016;**31**(10):2174–82.

41. Gardner DK, Kelley RL. Impact of the IVF laboratory environment on human preimplantation embryo phenotype. *J Dev Orig Health Dis.* 2017;**8**(4): 418–35.

42. Kleijkers SH, Mantikou E, Slappendel E, Consten D, van Ecten-Arends J, Wetzels AM, et al. Influence of embryo culture medium (G5 and HTF) on pregnancy and perinatal outcome after IVF: a multicenter RCT. *Hum Reprod.* 2016;**31**(10):2210–30.

43. Chronopoulou E, Harper JC. IVF culture media: past, present and future. *Hum Reprod Update.* 2015;**21** (1):39–55.

44. ESHRE SIG Embryology, Alpha Scientists in Reproductive Medicine. The Vienna Consensus: report of an expert meeting on the development of art laboratory performance indicators. *Hum Reprod Open*. 2017;**12**(2):1–17.

45. HFEA. *Adverse Incidents in Fertility Clinics: Lessons to Learn. January–December 2014*. London: HFEA; 2015. Available at: https://ifqlive.blob.core.windows.net/umbraco-website/1146/incidents_report_2014_designed_-_web_final.pdf.

Chapter

8

Quality Assurance of ART Practice: Using Data to Improve Clinical Care

Kevin Doody, Carlos Calhaz-Jorge and Jesper Smeenk

Introduction

Assisted reproductive technology (ART) registries are constructed for a variety of reasons. Broadly, ART registries focus on the improvement of ART practice. While this can be done using ART registry data for research and policy purposes, quality assurance is one of the most effective ways to achieve this goal. In this chapter, we describe how ART registries can be used for quality assurance using specific examples from two registries: the Society for Assisted Reproductive Technology (SART) Clinical Outcomes Reporting System (CORS) in the United States (US) and the Human Fertilisation and Embryology Authority (HFEA) Registry in the United Kingdom (UK).

The Society for Assisted Reproductive Technology and its registry were created in 1985 to monitor safety and efficacy of what at the time was a relatively new procedure/health service [1]. The SART registry was used for an additional purpose following the passage in 1992 of a law requiring the Centers for Disease Control and Prevention (CDC) to annually publish clinic-specific success rates for all US-based ART programs [2]. The publication of these success rates was aimed at protecting the consumers of these fertility services by requiring clinics to be transparent regarding their success/failure rates. These success rates were initially calculated using the SART registry; however, in 2004 the CDC constructed a parallel, but distinct, registry – the National ART Surveillance System (NASS). In the UK, the HFEA, an executive, non-departmental, public body of the Department of Health, was established in 1991 to regulate the ART field, including keeping a database of every IVF treatment carried out since that date and a database relating to all cycles and use of donated gametes (egg and sperm). Other ART registries have been constructed so that countries can better understand the types and numbers of ART cycles that are being performed within their borders. This information

can be helpful for the development of health care policy. No matter what the intent of the creation of these registries, they are also very valuable for research. This is especially true if cycle-specific data are collected rather than aggregate clinic data.

It is important to understand what is meant by quality, both currently and in a historical context, beginning with a description of commonly applied terminology and definitions. Important concepts include quality, quality control (QC), quality assurance (QA), quality management (QM) and quality improvement (QI). These words and phrases are 'business' terms used to describe important characteristics of services and products.

In general, a *quality* product or service is defined as one that meets the needs of the marketplace. In the special case of ART, the marketplace is largely shaped by the consumers of ART services (e.g. infertile patients, patients requesting fertility preservation or reduction in risk of genetic disease of offspring). The needs of ART consumers are not likely to be static. As new ART procedures are developed and evaluated, the perception of quality may change. ART quality management programs should be designed to take this into account.

Quality control is the most basic level of attempting to provide quality products or services. QC involves the identification of problems and defects. For an ART practice, QC will involve serial, ongoing measurements of performance of machines, instruments and personnel that are necessary for the provision of good ART care.

Quality assurance developed from the realization that quality could be improved by looking 'further up the line'. QA emphasizes planning. It is aimed at preventing non-conformities/defects. For an ART program, QA would typically involve construction of a set of procedures to prevent issues that would be identified by QC. As an example, QC might involve the daily measurement of incubator temperature,

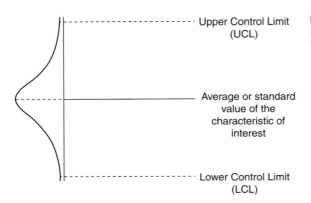

Figure 8.1 Basic form of a control chart. Reprinted from Ryan TP, *Statistical Methods for Quality Improvement.* New York: John Wiley & Sons; 2011.

while QA would further aim to prevent or quickly resolve incubator malfunction or failure through preventive maintenance, replacement with age, alarm strategies and availability of backup equipment.

Quality management recognizes that efforts should extend beyond just QA and QC to a systems approach. Quality management depends on looking at management systems and quality in the broadest of contexts. In the US, for example, the College of American Pathologists accredits reproductive laboratories and requires documentation of an active quality management program. More recently, emphasis has extended beyond quality management towards *quality improvement*. This concept recognizes that we can always do better to meet the needs of our customers/patients. An ART program should have a QM/QI program that includes both laboratory and clinic processes.

The following sections will elaborate on these points by describing the evolution of QM in industry. The rise of medical and patient registries to provide data for quality management will be reviewed. More specifically, the role that ART registries can play in quality control as well as broader continuous quality improvement for ART programs from both a laboratory and clinical perspective will be discussed.

History of QA in Industry

The desire to improve the quality of produced goods has been present since the earliest human civilizations. In the distant past, the responsibility to ensure quality was borne by the individual artisan or craftsperson. The Industrial Revolution changed this. Large numbers of people were brought together to create one product, and a supervisor was charged with the

responsibility of ensuring quality. At the beginning of the twentieth century, the mass manufacture of complex products led to the need to develop standardized design and component manufacturing processes. Henry Ford achieved great success in the automotive industry through the recognition of the benefit of inspectors. He employed inspectors in each department to cover all operations at frequent intervals to prevent faulty operations that might result in the manufacture of large numbers of bad parts. This earliest form of quality control involving inspection was innovative but was not informed by a statistical approach, which had not yet been developed.

Walter A. Shewhart (1891–1967), as the originator of the statistical process control, was instrumental in the development of the modern concept of quality control [3]. Shewhart came up with the idea of the control chart in 1924 while working at Bell Telephone Laboratories. A control chart is a time sequence plot (x-axis) with 'decision lines' added (Fig. 8.1). These decision lines are used to try to determine whether a process is in control. Ideally, it is preferred to detect such a situation as soon as possible. On the other hand, there is a desire to minimize 'false alarms'. The use of statistics allows a balance to be struck. Control charts remain at the heart of quality management programs.

William Edwards Deming (1900–1993) was a prominent statistician and is frequently cited as one of the pioneers of quality management [4]. He was greatly inspired by Shewhart. While Shewhart focused on manufacturing, Deming extended this concept of monitoring and controlling variance to management and business processes. He is frequently credited with helping the Japanese progress from having poor quality products prior to 1950 to later being able to manufacture products of superior quality. The concept of 'Plan-Do-Check (or Study)-Act' is referred to as 'Deming's Wheel', although he referred to it as the 'Shewhart Cycle'. This idea is the basis for all contemporary QM/continuous QI programs [5].

Several quality management/quality improvement programs have gained traction over the past few decades [6]. Quality management programs are always 'internal' to the business, but QA audits or inspections can be performed by internal or by external mechanisms. 'Peer review' is one of the common external QA mechanisms in medicine. In industry, ISO 9000 is a family of standards published by the International Organization for Standardization (ISO). ISO 9001 deals with the requirements that must be fulfilled, including the need for external review of compliance by third-party certification bodies. ISO focuses on processes and procedures rather than individual employees [7]. Other quality management programs such as Total Quality Management and Six Sigma are applied internally and differ somewhat in structure. In general, however, all these programs strive to improve quality by defining and designing processes followed by measuring, analyzing and reducing variance.

QA in Medicine through the Use of Data Collection and Patient Registries

Quality assurance in medicine is a rather 'new' topic, related to the availability of data and consequently adequate registries. In the 1960s, we talked about improving the quality of care primarily in terms of increasing access and lowering costs; in the 1970s, peer review was supposed to improve the quality of care. From the 1980s, quality assurance became the main driver in improving quality of care.

For a long time, quality could not be convincingly counted or measured: monitoring of and improvement in quality were generally left to individual professionals to ensure high-quality medical care. Hospitals routinely only monitored poor outcomes locally, such as deaths or infections, to identify ways to improve the quality of care. An example is the Health Care Financing Administration's (now the Centers for Medicare & Medicaid Services) program for measuring and publishing hospital mortality rates among Medicare patients in the US. After many years of publishing such statistics, the agency came to the conclusion that without a better method to adjust for the severity of illness, the data were too inaccurate to be useful, and the program was abandoned.

Data used in quality assessment are obtained from diverse sources, such as clinical records maintained by health care professionals, survey data collected for quality-assessment purposes and direct observations of the physician–patient encounter. Quality measurement and improvement have also been strongly affected by progress in information systems, computer technology and communication techniques. Along with these technological advances, the field of quality assurance developed from a local initiative before the 1960s, via regional networks in the 1960s–1970s to nationwide and even worldwide systems from the 1990s onwards. Traditionally, cancer registries have been frontrunners in this respect.

The health care systems are increasingly challenged to maintain a high quality of care while facing increasing demands and scarce resources. Comprehensive, yet confidential, health information should be available to any stakeholder in the health system in a standardized manner. If information is lacking or not well-organized, important quality characteristics, including continuity of care, safety and patient-centredness, become compromised and continuing quality improvements are impeded. To ensure the transparent monitoring of health care quality, comprehensive, standardized and understandable health information needs to be in place.

The World Health Organization (WHO) has developed three reference classifications – the International Classification of Diseases (ICD; currently in its 11th revision), the International Classification of Functioning, Disability and Health (ICF; first released in 2001) and the International Classification of Health Interventions (ICHI; under development, version 2 released in 2014) – each of which can serve as a standard language for defining aspects of health and health care–related information [8]. Their respective coding systems serve as examples that aim to ensure consistency and comparability of health and related information.

As a consequence of the implementation of information and communications systems, health care organizations are collecting clinical and administrative data on a large scale. Many nations use these 'Big Data' to support improvements in health outcomes, drug safety, health surveillance and care delivery processes. Electronic health care data are often considered to be of sufficient quality to enable this, but the reality is that many electronic health data sources are of suboptimal quality and unfit for particular uses.

What Can We Learn from Others on Surveillance Data?

Oncology

Cancer registries have always been an example to others, since much pioneering with respect to quality assurance was done within the field of oncology. As an example, within the Netherlands, guidelines were formed to improve the quality of care based on experiences and involvement in setting up patient registries in oncology. Being one of the first structured registries in the Netherlands, these experiences were incorporated elsewhere. As the monitoring and evaluation of patient care is often the primary goal (the Why), it is important to align the objectives of the registry and agree on a clear and functional governance structure with all stakeholders (the Who). There is often a trade-off between reliability, validity and specificity of data elements and feasibility of data collection (the What). Patient privacy should be carefully protected and address (inter-) national and local regulations. Patient registries can reveal unique safety information, but it can be challenging to comply with pharmacovigilance guidelines (the How) [9].

Haemovigilance

In 2002, the European Community adopted the Directive 2002/98/EC with legally binding requirements for the quality and safety of blood and blood components, including haemovigilance systems. A good example is the Serious Hazards of Transfusion (SHOT) scheme in the UK, being an independent, professionally led haemovigilance system focused on learning from adverse events.

In the US, the Massachusetts Department of Public Health's registry is a paper-based method of reporting to a web-based system. This standardized, actionable dataset can facilitate interfacility comparisons, benchmarking and opportunities for improvement of haemovigilance and patient safety. Users adhere to specified data entry guidelines, resulting in data that are comparable and standardized. Keys to successful adoption of this reporting method include

strong partnerships with local experts and epidemiologists and the engagement of regulatory bodies.

Although reporting of haemovigilance data offers several major advantages over the paper-based system, there are limitations to the data collected. As with any surveillance system that relies on interpretation of case definitions for reporting, it is possible that, despite established guidelines and clearly outlined definitions, some variation in interpretation can be seen. Furthermore, the data are often self-reported and are not yet externally validated. Evaluations suggest that, although inconsistent interpretation of case definitions and underreporting occur, these can be minimized by simplifying case definitions and enhancing education for those reporting the data [10, 11].

Organ Transplantation

Quality strategy is increasingly affecting transplantation practice, as exemplified by quality assessment and performance improvement (QAPI) regulations for pretransplantation and posttransplantation care. Transplantation providers consider not just patient comorbidities, donor quality and business constraints but also regulatory mandates when deciding how to care for transplantation candidates and recipients. The heavily regulated system of care and remuneration for transplantation involves extensive QAPI processes and outcome requirements, and assessment of lifelong, risk-adjusted data from the national, audited, publicly reported electronic registry. Transplantation is a model-integrated delivery system, with payment bundling and accountability for equitable access to high quality, efficient, cost-sensitive and multidisciplinary care. However, transplantation QAPI requires expensive resources, and this needs to be weighed against the benefits [12].

Rare Diseases

Registries on rare diseases are considered crucial to develop clinical research, to facilitate the planning of appropriate clinical trials and to improve patient care and health care planning. With the growing number of rare disease registries being established, there is a need to develop a quality validation process to evaluate the quality of each registry. A clear description of the registry is the first step when assessing data quality or the registry evaluation system. Determining the quality of data is possible through data assessment against several dimensions: completeness and validity; coherence and comparability; accessibility; usefulness; timeliness; prevention of duplicate records. Many other factors may influence the quality of a registry: e.g. development of a standardized case report form and security/safety controls of informatics infrastructure [13].

Ophthalmology

The purpose of the IRIS° (Intelligent Research in Sight) registry is to support and promote continued improvement of care. By adhering to the principles of the registry (local experts' ownership of all patient data, data protection safeguards, strict protection of individual patient-identifiable data and non-burdensome data entry), this registry has become the largest clinical registry within a short period of time. The development of electronic health records and innovative data extraction methods has obviously enabled this success, as manual data entry had been a major barrier for participation in the registry. The professionals are in the lead regarding the registry (American Academy of Ophthalmology) and no external influence or funding is accepted (industry or federal); moreover, no fees are paid for participation. The IRIS registry has proved that it can empower practitioners to improve their practice and, furthermore, that it can become a success rapidly if the barriers for participation are being met effectively [14]. It should be noted that a major contributor to its success was the fact that this software facilitates the reporting of the large number of quality measures that are required to obtain optimal reimbursement for patient care from the federal government (Medicare).

The Centers for Disease Control and Prevention (CDC) developed criteria for evaluation of public health surveillance systems. The guidelines address the need for (1) the integration of surveillance and health information systems, (2) the establishment of data standards, (3) the electronic exchange of health data and (4) changes in the objectives of public health surveillance to facilitate the response of public health to emerging health threats (e.g. new diseases) [15].

Quality Assurance of ART Practice: Using Data to Improve Clinical Care

Assisted reproductive technology (ART), defined as "all interventions that include the in vitro handling of

both human oocytes and sperm or of embryos for the purpose of reproduction" [16], includes a complex of clinical and laboratorial interventions that are applied to patients with much more diversified characteristics. Its complexity requires the existence of a QA system to control and monitor all possible steps and quickly identify deviations from the defined parameters.

Quality indicators are the pillars upon which this system can be built. The most commonly used are the performance indicators (PIs), which are measurable parameters that evaluate domains of a specific activity. They are necessary for systematically monitoring and evaluating either individual procedures or the achievement of global objectives. Any PI must be objective and reliable, and relevant qualifiers, confounders and end points should be identified. Key performance indicators (KPIs) are PIs deemed essential for evaluating a technique or process, establishing minimum standards for proficiency, monitoring ongoing performance, benchmarking and quality improvement. The definition of acceptable and optimal values for KPIs is essential to make them the anchor of drift identification and the driver for improvement. Considering the overwhelming amount of literature in the field of ART, published studies about PI are practically nonexistent.

In general, in ART we may envisage outcome and process indicators.

Outcome Metrics

In spite of a clear, desirable final outcome of the treatment – a healthy baby with normal developmental potential and lifespan – the complexity of the process has led to the use of many intermediate indicators to describe the success of these techniques. Pregnancy rate and live birth rate are the most routinely used, considering either started cycle or oocyte retrieval or embryo transfer as the denominator. Over the past years, cumulative rates per started cycle (including results of fresh and all frozen transfers of embryos obtained from a single ovarian stimulation and aspiration) have started to become the correct way to value an ART treatment (see Chapter 5, Reporting ART Success Rates).

Multiple pregnancy is one outcome indicator that deserves some consideration, as it must be considered part of the wider approach to QA. This consequence of ART is dependent on a balance of decisions made by clinicians and patients. The number of embryos transferred is paramount, but other variables must be

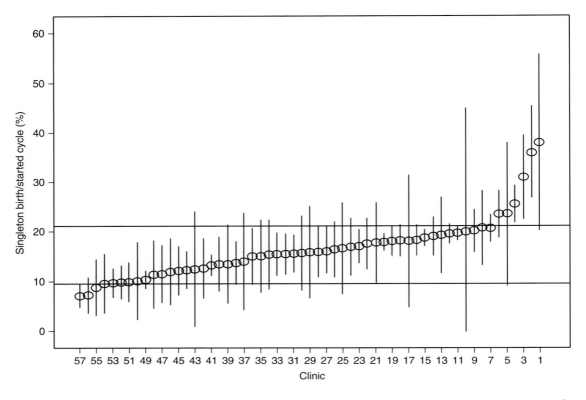

Figure 8.2 League table of singleton birth rate per started cycle. Reprinted from Castilla JA et al. Defining poor and optimum performance in an IVF programme. *Hum Reprod.* 2008;23(1):85–90.

taken into account. For instance, in Europe, for several years there has been a clear trend to a lower number of transferred embryos [17]. Nevertheless, the proportion of multiple pregnancies remains as high as 18%, which may mean that either better embryos are being transferred or the number of transfers of blastocysts is increasing, or both. In some countries, the elective single embryo transfer (eSET) in all patients younger than 35 years is mandatory. In others, there is no legal rule, but strong recommendations to take a similar approach are followed by the whole ART community. Naturally, those countries have a very low rate of multiples. However, the impact of public funding as a major factor in decision making in this context must be recognized. In fact, the implementation of principles underlying QA are here shaped by the broader reality.

Those global indicators of success of ART are somewhat late indicators and do not allow quick identification of the origin of clinical or laboratory issues. However, they may be very useful as a benchmarking tool to compare clinics and determine when a clinic is

performing less well than comparators. Several modalities can be used for that purpose [18].

One modality that seems to be appropriate is the league table, which shows/compares the performance of different ART centres considering defined outcomes. Figure 8.2 shows singleton birth rate and 95% confidence interval (CI) per started cycle for 57 clinics using data from the IVF/ICSI Register of the Spanish Fertility Society. Top and bottom horizontal lines are the 50th percentile of the lower and upper 95% CI. However, this is a very sensitive and disputed field considering the numerous potential confounder variables and the evolution of the clinical/scientific policies in individual centres [19].

This 'external QA/peer review' enables identification of outliers with regard to success (low live birth rates) and complications (high multifetal gestation rates). SART has a process to contact outliers, provide external review and recommendations and ultimately to terminate membership if the clinic is unable to remediate. In European countries, many different systems are in place regarding identification of ART performance by individual clinics depending on the national registry system. In European Union member states, periodical inspections are mandatory. Outliers and other issues are identified during those inspections, and appropriate corrective action, according to national legislation, is taken.

Process Metrics

In the clinical setting, in addition to the outcome indicators referred to above, efforts have been focused mainly on defining individualized strategies that optimize ovarian response to stimulation using prognosis according to relevant clinical variables (e.g. female age, duration of infertility, previous ovarian surgery, body mass index) and accepted so-called ovarian reserve markers (antral follicle count (AFC), follicle stimulating hormone (FSH), anti-Müllerian hormone (AMH)) to determine type and/or dosage of medication. Although this clinical approach makes sense, suggested practical alternatives to calculate initial dose of drugs have never been widely used. As a consequence, there are no reliable data on their effectiveness. Moreover, recently published randomized controlled trials (RCTs) have even questioned the benefits of this practice when based on AFC [20, 21, 22].

As stated before, a PI must be reliable. In the clinical setting, the confounders related to the individual characteristics of patients submitted to ART create difficulties not easy to overcome. To define and apply stratification of patients requires considering so many variables that only centres with an extremely high volume of activity will be able to accumulate sufficiently robust clinical information on which to base their QA system.

Although PI use has a long tradition in general medical laboratories, most indicators in ART do not have their scientific soundness and usefulness supported by any evidence [23]. A recent and detailed consensus paper resulting from the work of experts of the ESHRE Special Interest Group of Embryology and Alpha Scientists in Reproductive Medicine [24] has tried to fill this gap in the ART field. It proposes 19 indicators, 12 KPIs, 5 PIs and 2 reference indicators (Table 8.1), the latter referring to procedures prior to any action in the lab. For all of them, 'competency' and 'benchmark' values are proposed based on a search of the literature and on surveys sent to ART laboratory directors and clinical embryologists.

Table 8.1 Quality indicators for ART laboratories

Reference indicators	Proportion of oocytes recovered (stimulated cycles)
	Proportion of MII oocytes at ICSI
Performance indicators	Sperm motility postpreparation (for IVF and IUI)
	IVF polyspermy rate
	1PN rate (IVF)
	1PN rate (ICSI)
	Good blastocyst development rate
Key performance indicators	ICSI damage rate
	ICSI normal fertilization rate
	IVF normal fertilization rate
	Failed fertilization rate (IVF)
	Cleavage rate
	Day 2 embryo development rate
	Day 3 embryo development rate
	Blastocyst development rate
	Successful biopsy rate
	Blastocyst cryosurvival rate
	Implantation rate (cleavage stage)
	Implantation rate (blastocyst stage)

1PN, single-pronucleate; ICSI, intracytoplasmic sperm injection; IUI, intrauterine insemination; IVF, in vitro fertilization; MII, metaphase II

In spite of recognizing the need to define key performance indicators and use them to establish benchmarks, the ESHRE experts and Alpha scientists made no comment regarding the application of statistical process control for the purpose of prompt identification when these processes are 'out of control'. In 1950, S. Levey and E.R. Jennings suggested the use of graphs similar to Shewhart's control chart for the purpose of monitoring quality control data in clinical laboratories [25]. Levey-Jennings charts like the one in Figure 8.3 have traditionally been used to determine whether the instruments and testing processes are performing properly.

Statistical analyses, such as the application of Westgard rules, are employed to determine whether the results from the control samples are within range so that patient test samples can be reported [26].

More recently, this type of control charting has been used for the purpose of QA in assisted reproductive technology programs.

These performance graphs do not use controls, but rather assess performance in the treated patient population. Variance can occur because of patient factors or program (clinical + laboratory) variance. Some examples are shown in Figures 8.4–8.7.

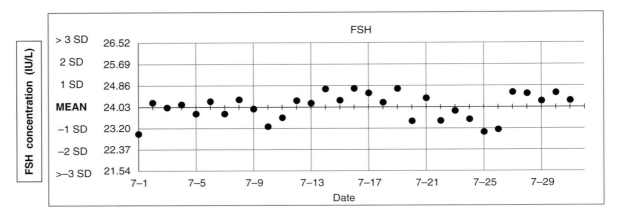

Figure 8.3 A typical Levey-Jennings chart. The same control sample is run each day.

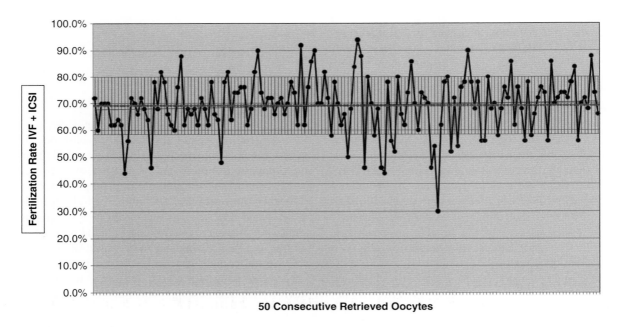

Figure 8.4 Fertilization control chart: each dot represents 50 consecutive retrieved oocytes exposed to sperm by either conventional insemination or ICSI. (Doody KJ, unpublished data). A colour version of this figure is provided in the plate section.

It is important to recognize that each dot/data point in Figures 8.4–8.6 is calculated by grouping a fixed number of consecutively retrieved eggs or fertilized eggs together. In this way, each dot is of equal 'weight' or importance. In Figures 8.4 and 8.5, this means that eggs from multiple retrievals will frequently be combined to form one data point. It is

important to handle this properly. For example, if two retrievals combined produce 40 eggs and the next retrieval produces 20, only 10 of the eggs from the third retrieval should go into the first data point. The remaining 10 will go towards the next data point. If 14 of the eggs from the third retrieval were to fertilize normally, 7 of the fertilized eggs should be

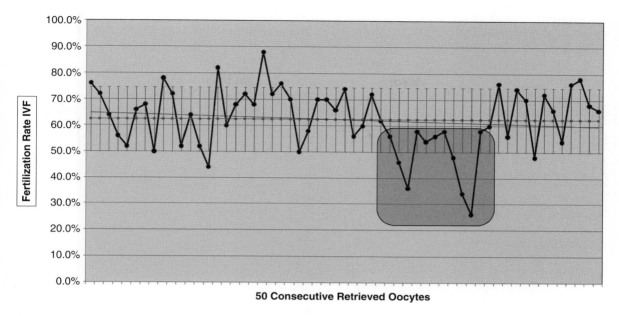

Figure 8.5 Fertilization control chart: each dot represents 50 consecutive retrieved oocytes exposed to sperm by conventional insemination with identified performance issue. (Doody KJ, unpublished data) A colour version of the figure is provided in the plate section.

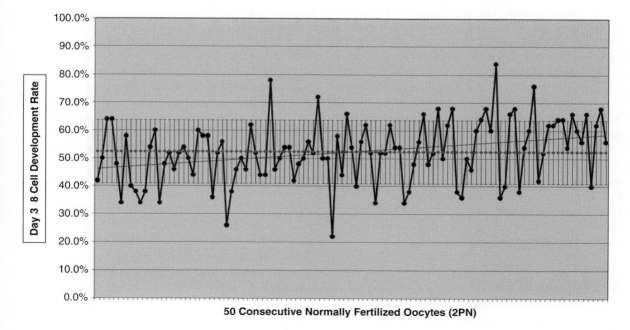

Figure 8.6 Early embryo development control chart: number of 8 cell embryos per 50 consecutive normally fertilized eggs (two-pronuclear (2PN) zygotes). (Doody KJ, unpublished data) A colour version of the figure is provided in the plate section.

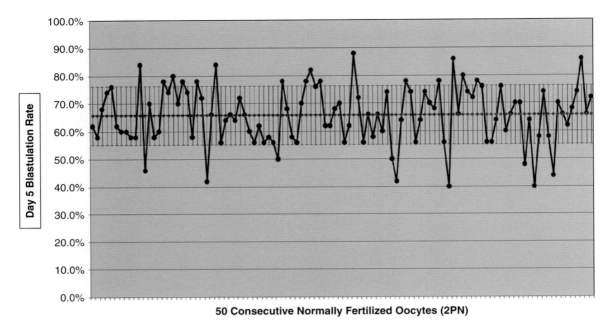

Figure 8.7 Performance graph demonstrating performance with early and late embryo culture: blastulation rate per 50 consecutive fertilized oocytes. (Doody KJ, unpublished data) A colour version of the figure is provided in the plate section.

apportioned into each of the two consecutive data points. It would be wrong to apportion 10 to the first point and only 4 to the next.

Construction of control charts using cycle-specific data can be performed internally for clinic QM/QI programs. Graphs are easily constructed to identify differences in performance of individual physicians and embryologists. SART is in the process of constructing 'QA dashboards' using similar graphs for SART-member clinics in the US. As a registry, these same data can be used for external quality assurance programs. Individual clinic performance can be compared with the aggregate of reporting clinics for benchmarking and for identification of outlier performance. Collection of data fields such as laboratory product (media, protein source, oil overlay and other contact material), manufacturer and lot number can assist in the troubleshooting of performance issues.

Concluding Remarks

The provision of ART services involves complex clinical and laboratory processes. It is well understood that the quality of care experienced by individual patients can vary. Quality management/quality improvement programs are used in a wide range of

businesses (manufacturing, service providers etc.). Health care businesses including ART programs are similarly well served by the application of these concepts.

Internal QM/QI efforts require data to determine when laboratory and clinical processes are not well controlled. Birth rates (stratified by age) are widely tracked because the delivery of a baby is a main reason that patients undergo ART treatments. These success rates are useful for benchmarking purposes (comparing with aggregate/national rates). A major limitation, however, is that this information cannot be used to track current or recent performance. It is also frequently difficult to determine the cause of low success rates. For this reason, programs should define key performance indicators for all relevant processes that can be tracked. Analysis of these indicators on an infrequent basis (e.g. quarterly) or in a table-type format is also not optimal. Shewhart-type control charts should be used to detect and resolve problems quickly.

It is likely that existing and new ART registries will evolve to collect a full set of process metrics (key performance indicators). Standardized collection using EMR software with registry interface will facilitate this data collection. Construction of 'real time'

QA dashboards will likely lead to large improvements in both internal and external QA mechanisms and translate directly to an improved quality of ART care.

References

1. In vitro fertilization/embryo transfer in the United States: 1985 and 1986 results from the National IVF/ET Registry. Medical Research International. The American Fertility Society Special Interest Group. *Fertil Steril.* 1988;**49**(2):212–15.

2. Fertility Clinic Success Rate and Certification Act of 1992, Pub. L. No. 102–493 (1992).

3. Shewhart WA. *Economic Control of Quality of Manufactured Product.* New York: D. Van Nostrand Company; 1931.

4. Deming WE. *Quality, Productivity, and Competitive Position.* Cambridge, MA: Massachusetts Institute of Technology, Center for Engineering Study; 1982.

5. Walton M. *The Deming Management Method.* London: Perigee/Penguin; 1986.

6. Ryan TP. *Statistical Methods for Quality Improvement.* New York: John Wiley & Sons; 2011.

7. Bhat S. *Business Process Improvement for Manufacturing and Service Industry.* Taos, NM: Paradigm Publications; 2015.

8. Dorjba D, Cieza A, Gmünder H, Scheel-Sailer A, Stucki G, Üstün B, et al. Strengthening quality of care through standardized reporting based on the World Health Organization's reference classifications. *Int J Qual Health Care.* 2016;**28**(5):626–33.

9. de Groot S, van der Linden N, Franken MG, Blommestein HM, Leeneman B, van Rooijen E, et al. Balancing the optimal and the feasible: a practical guide for setting up patient registries for the collection of real-world data for health care decision making based on Dutch experiences. *Value Health.* 2017;**20**(4): 627–36.

10. Cumming M, Osinski A, O'Hearn L, Waksmonski P, Herman M, Gordon D, et al. Hemovigilance in Massachusetts and the adoption of statewide hospital blood bank reporting using the National Healthcare Safety Network. *Transfusion.* 2017;**57**(2):478–83.

11. Stainsby D, Jones H, Asher D, Atterbury C, Boncinelli A, Brant L, et al.; SHOT Steering Group. Serious hazards of transfusion: a decade of hemovigilance in the UK. *Transfus Med Rev.* 2006;**20** (4):273–82.

12. Reich DJ. Quality assessment and performance improvement in transplantation: hype or hope? *Curr Opin Organ Transplant.* 2013;**18**(2):216–21.

13. Kodra Y, Posada de la Paz M, Coi A, Santoro M, Bianchi F, Ahmed F, et al. Data quality in rare diseases registries. *Adv Exp Med Biol.* 2017;**1031**:149–64.

14. Parke Ii DW, Lum F, Rich WL. The IRIS° Registry: purpose and perspectives. *Ophthalmology.* 2017;**114**: 1–6.

15. German RR, Lee LM, Horan JM, Milstein RL, Pertowski CA, Waller MN; Guidelines Working Group Centers for Disease Control and Prevention (CDC). Updated guidelines for evaluating public health surveillance systems: recommendations from the Guidelines Working Group. *MMWR Recomm Rep.* 2001;**50**(RR-13):1–15.

16. Zegers-Hochschild F, Adamson GD, Dyer S, Racowsky C, de Mouzon J, Sokol R, et al. The International Glossary on Infertility and Fertility Care, 2017. *Hum Reprod.* 2017;**32**(9):1786–801. doi:10.1093/humrep/dex234.

17. Calhaz-Jorge C, De Geyter C, Kupka MS, de Mouzon J, Erb K, Mocanu E, et al.; European IVF-monitoring Consortium (EIM); European Society of Human Reproduction and Embryology (ESHRE). Assisted reproductive technology in Europe, 2013: results generated from European registers by ESHRE. *Hum Reprod.* 2017;**32**(10):1957–73. doi:10.1093/humrep/dex264.

18. Castilla JA, Hernandez J, Cabello Y, Lafuente A, Pajuelo N, Marqueta J, et al.; Assisted Reproductive Technology Register of the Spanish Fertility Society. Defining poor and optimum performance in an IVF programme. *Hum Reprod.* 2008;**23**(1):85–90. doi:10.1093/humrep/dem361.

19. Wilkinson J, Roberts SA, Vail A. Developments in IVF warrant the adoption of new performance indicators for ART clinics, but do not justify the abandonment of patient-centred measures. *Hum Reprod.* 2017;**32**(6): 1155–9. doi:10.1093/humrep/dex063.

20. van Tilborg TC, Oudshoorn SC, Eijkemans MJC, Mochtar MH, van Golde RJT, Hoek A, et al.; OPTIMIST Study Group. Individualized FSH dosing based on ovarian reserve testing in women starting IVF/ICSI: a multicentre trial and cost-effectiveness analysis. *Hum Reprod.* 2017;**32**(12):2485–95. doi:10.1093/humrep/dex321.

21. van Tilborg TC, Torrance HL, Oudshoorn SC, Eijkemans MJC, Koks CAM, Verhoeve HR, et al.; OPTIMIST Study Group. Individualized versus standard FSH dosing in women starting IVF/ICSI: an RCT. Part 1: The predicted poor responder. *Hum Reprod.* 2017;**32**(12):2496–505. doi:10.1093/humrep/dex318.

22. Oudshoorn SC, van Tilborg TC, Eijkemans MJC, Oosterhuis GJE, Friederich J, van Hooff MHA, et al.; OPTIMIST Study Group. Individualized versus

standard FSH dosing in women starting IVF/ICSI: an RCT. Part 2: The predicted hyper responder. *Hum Reprod.* 2017;**32**(12):2506–14. doi:10.1093/humrep/dex319.

23. Shahangian S, Snyder SR. Laboratory medicine quality indicators: a review of the literature. *Am J Clin Pathol.* 2009;**131**(3):418–31. doi:10.1309/AJCPJF8JI4ZLDQUE.

24. ESHRE Special Interest Group of Embryology and Alpha Scientists in Reproductive Medicine.

The Vienna Consensus: report of an expert meeting on the development of ART laboratory performance indicators. *Reprod Biomed Online.* 2017;**35**(5):494–510. doi:10.1016/j.rbmo.2017.06.015.

25. Levey S, Jennings ER. The use of control charts in the clinical laboratory. *Am J Clin Pathol.* 1950;**20**:1059–66.

26. Westgard JO, Groth T, Aronsson T, Falk H, deVerdler C. Performance characteristics of rules for internal quality control: probabilities for false rejection and error detection. *Clin Chem.* 1981;**27**(3):493–501.

Chapter

9

Monitoring Long-Term Outcomes of ART: Linking ART Surveillance Data with Other Datasets

Barbara Luke, Sheree L. Boulet and Anna-Karina Aaris Henningsen

The findings and conclusions in this report are those of the authors and do not necessarily represent the official position of the Centers for Disease Control and Prevention.

Introduction/Overview

The Importance and Challenge of Evaluating Long-Term Health after ART

Infertility, defined as the inability to conceive within one year of unprotected intercourse, affects an estimated 80 million individuals worldwide, or 10–15% of couples of reproductive age [1, 2, 3, 4, 5]. Assisted reproductive technology (ART), defined as interventions that include the in vitro handling of both human oocytes and sperm or embryos for the purpose of reproduction, includes in vitro fertilization (IVF) and embryo transfer, gamete intrafallopian transfer (GIFT), zygote intra-fallopian transfer (ZIFT), gamete and embryo cryo-preservation, oocyte and embryo donation and gestational carrier cycles [6]. ART does not include intrauterine insemination using sperm from either a woman's partner or a sperm donor. Approximately 12% of couples of reproductive age in the United States (US) have sought medical assistance to achieve conception, and among women 25–44 years of age with current fertility problems, the most commonly used services were medical advice (29%), infertility testing (27%), ovulation drugs (20%), artificial insemination (7.4%), surgery or treatment for blocked tubes (3.2%) and ART (3.1%) [3]. The results of an analysis of women in the Nurses' Health Study who had infertility treatment indicated that 73% of women used ovulation induction with clomiphene as their only form of treatment, 11% had intrauterine insemination and 11% used IVF [7]. Identifying non-IVF fertility treatments is challenging, as there is no US national registry for these therapies. More information on monitoring non-IVF fertility

treatments can be found in Chapter 21, Non-ART Surveillance.

In the US, ART use has risen steadily during the past two decades, primarily because of older age at conception and better insurance coverage [8, 9, 10, 11]. The number of ART cycles performed in the US more than doubled between 2000 and 2015 (from 99,629 to 231,936 cycles per year), with 1.7% of live births the result of ART [12, 13, 14].

Although ART is believed to be safe, our knowledge of the long-term effects of ART on the health of women and children is limited. While rapid technological progress makes it important to continually monitor ART safety for both mothers and infants, studying long-term health outcomes of ART is difficult because both exposure (ART) and some outcomes of interest (e.g. birth defects, cancer and developmental disorders) are rare or distal from exposure. Because national ART registries do not typically collect data beyond delivery, one of the most efficient approaches is to link these registries with other existing specialized health and disease registries [15].

The use of linked health data to study ART outcomes offers numerous advantages over other observational studies, such as large numbers of ART-treated women, detailed treatment data and comprehensive information on validated outcomes [16]. Furthermore, using statewide or national databases provides a comprehensive picture of exposures and outcomes for broad populations where loss to follow-up is likely to be minimal and out-migration is not expected to be greater in any specific group. As such, analyses from linked data registry studies provide an important population-based overview and can help to identify specific areas in need of further clinical research to explore potential mechanisms underlying the reported associations.

Periods of Follow-Up and Health Outcomes of Interest

For the child conceived with ART, the periods of follow-up include fetal period, birth, infancy, childhood, adulthood (potentially including intergenerational reproductive outcomes) and death. For the woman treated with ART, the periods of follow-up include prenatal period, birth, subsequent pregnancies, menopause and death.

The health outcomes of interest may include pregnancy and birth complications, congenital anomalies, growth and development (including psychological) through adulthood, subsequent fertility, risks for cancer, cardiovascular disease, diabetes, metabolic syndrome and developmental origins of health and disease. Information on these health outcomes can be found in specialized registries and databases, such as birth certificates, birth defects registries, cancer registries, hospital discharge data and the US National Death Index.

Selecting the Appropriate Control Group

Choosing an appropriate control or comparison group when studying pregnancy outcomes in women treated for infertility poses a special challenge. The majority of studies compare them to fertile women, but this choice has the limitation that they differ from women treated for infertility by many characteristics, including age, socioeconomic status, education, reproductive history and other underlying or genetic factors. As such, spontaneously conceived births to subfertile women is a more appropriate comparison group than traditionally used non-ART births when studying the effects of ART on maternal and child health. In addition, the use of siblings as the comparison group offers the advantage of eliminating parental characteristics affecting outcomes [17, 18, 19, 20, 21, 22, 23].

Another appropriate control group might consist of women referred for ART but who become pregnant spontaneously while waiting for treatment. However, such a control group of sufficient sample size is difficult to establish.

Linkage Methodologies

In the US, studies of the long-term outcomes of ART involve the challenge of linking databases, in which one database has information on the treatment parameters, and other databases capture the outcomes of interest. Outcomes often include birth factors (collected on the birth certificate), cancer (reported in state or national cancer registries), morbidity (identified using hospital discharge or insurance claims databases) and mortality (reported in the National Death Index, the database of all US deaths). The two primary methods for linking data are deterministic and probabilistic. For deterministic linkages, both datasets contain at least one unique personal identifier (also known as a key) that can be used to match the records. Matches are typically exact or near exact [24, 25]. Probabilistic linkages use multiple identifiers that may not be unique. An algorithm generates a weight for each matching or non-matching value. These weights are then added to calculate a score that reflects the likelihood that the records belong to the same individual. When one unique key is available, deterministic methods are generally preferred; however, when no single identifier can be used, probabilistic methods have been shown to outperform deterministic approaches [24, 25]. The primary linkage variables used in probabilistic linkages of ART data are maternal date of birth, infant date of birth, plurality, maternal social security number (when available), maternal residence zip code and gravidity. Several validation studies of the probabilistic linkage method showed high sensitivity and specificity, and the linkage rates were similar to those obtained from the deterministic linkage methodology [26, 27, 28]. In the Nordic countries, their well-established system of unique personal identification numbers overcomes this issue of linking national and regional databases [29].

Population-Based Linkages in the US

Linkage Studies Using Data from the Centers for Disease Control and Prevention

The Centers for Disease Control and Prevention's (CDC) National ART Surveillance System (NASS) is a web-based reporting system for the federally mandated collection of information on all ART cycles performed in the US. The Fertility Clinic Success Rate and Certification Act (Public Law No. 102–493, 1992) requires that all fertility clinics report cycle-specific data on ART procedures and outcomes to the CDC annually and that the CDC publish clinic-specific success rates. As the intent of the mandate was to provide information on ART success rates for consumers, NASS collects only limited information on treatment and pregnancy outcomes. Data on long-term health outcomes for women undergoing ART and infants conceived using ART are not collected as part of routine surveillance. More information on NASS is available in Chapter 18, ART Surveillance in North America.

Recognizing the importance of having a population-based dataset with information on conception and delivery for ART mother–infant pairs to study ART outcomes, the CDC piloted a project in 2001 linking NASS data with live birth and infant death files from Massachusetts [27]. Approximately 80% of the records were linked using maternal and infant date of birth as primary linking variables, confirming the plausibility of such an approach for population-based research and surveillance of ART-conceived live births. Soon after, the States Monitoring Assisted Reproductive Technology (SMART) Collaborative was established and expanded to include Florida and Michigan [26]. Since its inception, SMART's aim has been to establish, improve and promote state-based surveillance of ART and to monitor and study maternal and infant health outcomes related to ART.

To date, the SMART Collaborative has grown in both size and scope and has resulted in important contributions to the scientific literature. Refinements in the probabilistic linkage methodology and improvements in the quality of birth certificate data led to linkage rates of over 90%, nearly identical to those derived using deterministic methods [26]. Additional health information was added to the linked datasets including birth defects registries and hospital discharge records, and Connecticut joined the SMART Collaborative in 2013. SMART data have been used in studies assessing associations between ART and preterm birth by maternal obesity status [30], accuracy of ART reporting on birth certificates [31], embryo transfer practices and perinatal outcomes for states with and without infertility insurance mandates [32], antenatal hospitalizations among ART-conceived pregnancies [33], ART and birth defects risk [34] and embryo cryopreservation and risk for pre-eclampsia [35].

In the US, vital records are not consistently linked with other datasets at the national level, making it difficult to establish a national cohort of ART-conceived infants and their spontaneously conceived counterparts. While projects such as the SMART Collaborative and the Society for Assisted Reproductive Technology Clinical Outcomes Reporting System (SART CORS) linkages provide valuable information on maternal and child health outcomes of ART, a national dataset inclusive of all US-born infants would provide sufficient sample size to study a host of outcomes, particularly if multiple years of data were included. With this in mind, the CDC is currently working to link NASS data with US period linked birth–infant death files maintained by National Vital Statistics System (NVSS) at the CDC's National Center for Health Statistics. This linkage will facilitate the monitoring of national and state-specific trends in the number of infants conceived with ART for all US states, the potential adverse health risks associated with ART and the impact of ART on adverse maternal and infant outcomes. Additionally, the linkage may be used to validate reporting of ART use on state birth certificates.

Linkage Studies Using Data from the Society for Assisted Reproductive Technology

In 1985, the Society for Assisted Reproductive Technology (SART) was founded to establish standards of treatment and as the basis for a national registry of IVF cycles and outcomes; fewer than 4,000 IVF cycles were reported that year [36]. The first ART success rates report was published by the CDC in collaboration with SART in 1997 [37]. By 2014, SART had 375 member clinics in the US, accounting for 83% of all reporting clinics and 91% of all reported IVF cycles [36]. Currently, data from SART member clinics are collected via the SART CORS and reported to the CDC's NASS [13]. More information on SART CORS is available in Chapter 18, ART Surveillance in North America.

The SART CORS data has two major research advantages over the ART cycles reported to the CDC, which do not include direct patient identifiers. Because the ART cycles in the SART CORS contain protected health information (e.g. woman's first, middle and last names, birth date, social security number, zip code and date of outcome of the cycle), it is possible to use deterministic linkage methods (instead of probabilistic) when matching to other databases (e.g. vital records, cancer registries, birth defects registries, hospital discharge records). In addition, SART CORS data can be used to identify all IVF cycles for a particular woman, which allows researchers to evaluate the cumulative effects of treatment, as well as the effect of prior cycle outcomes on the current cycle outcome [38, 39, 40, 41, 42]. In 2016, the CDC revised its data collection system and is now able to link cycles for individual patients.

SART CORS–PELL Linkage Studies

(Massachusetts Outcomes Study of Assisted Reproductive Technology, MOSART)

The population-based Massachusetts Outcomes Study of Assisted Reproductive Technology (MOSART) links clinical ART data from the SART CORS to Massachusetts vital records and administrative data in the Pregnancy to Early Life Longitudinal (PELL) data system (Fig. 9.1). The project is a collaboration of the Massachusetts Department of Public Health, Boston University School of Public Health and the Centers for Disease Control and Prevention. The core of this data system is the birth and fetal death files that

are linked to the hospital discharge records of mother's delivery and child's birth. In addition, a measure was generated to identify women who did not use IVF for the index birth but had some indication of subfertility. The measure was developed using birth certificate checkbox data on the use of fertility treatments, diagnosis codes for infertility in hospital discharge data and report of prior use of IVF [43].

Two National Institutes of Health (NIH)-funded studies have linked the SART CORS to the Pregnancy to Early Life Longitudinal (PELL) Data System in Massachusetts (*Child Health after Assisted Reproductive Technology: A Population-Based Study*, R01 HD064595, and *Women's Health after Assisted Reproductive Technology: A Population-Based Study*, R01 HD067270, which has been renamed *Subfertility and Assisted Conception Study of Parents and Their Children* in the renewal). These grants resulted in a series of analyses on the effect of infertility diagnoses [44, 45], IVF treatment parameters [22, 46, 47], perinatal outcomes by maternal fertility status [48, 49, 50], severe maternal morbidity and postpartum hospitalization [51, 52, 53] and neonatal and early childhood outcomes [54, 55].

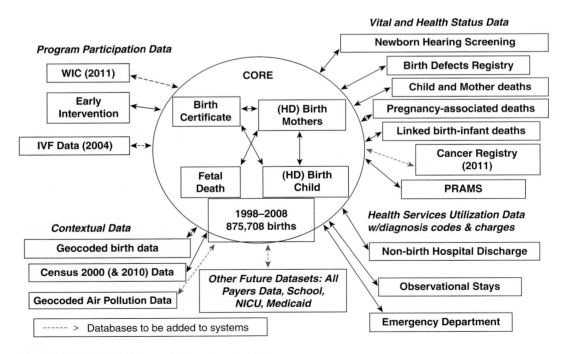

Figure 9.1 The PELL Data System in Massachusetts, USA.

SART CORS–State Vital Records–Cancer Registry Linkage Studies

Three NIH-funded studies have linked the SART CORS to state vital records and cancer registries (R01CA151973 and an administrative supplement, and R01 HD084377). In the grant R01CA151973, *Assisted Reproductive Technology and Risk of Childhood Cancer*, IVF cycles reported to the SART CORS between 2004 and 2012 that resulted in live births in 2004–2013 were linked to the child's birth certificates in 14 states and New York City. All other births of the IVF-treated woman were also identified, as well as a 10:1 sample of non-IVF control children. All three groups of children were linked to their respective state cancer registries and vital records to determine vital status through infancy. The results of this study are currently in press, and include 275,628 IVF children, 42,292 IVF siblings and 2,266,813 control children. As a supplement to this grant (*Assisted Reproductive Technology & Risk of Cancer in Women*), IVF cycles in the SART CORS were linked to the cancer registries in three states (Illinois, Texas and New York), and included 114,601 women (including 1,432 women with cancer prior to IVF and 974 women with cancer after IVF). Three analyses were published from this linkage: cancer prior to IVF [56], the use of embryo banking among women with a cancer diagnosis [57] and cancer after IVF [58].

The most recent study, R01 HD084377, *Assisted Reproductive Technology and Child Health: Risk of Birth Defects, Mortality, and Effect on Grade School Performance*, is continuing to follow IVF children, their siblings and controls born 2004–2013, and adding additional birth cohorts through 2018 in four states (New York, Texas, Massachusetts and North Carolina). This study begins with 106,928 IVF children, 19,490 IVF siblings and 818,474 controls from the prior study on *Assisted Reproductive Technology and Risk of Childhood Cancer*. The purpose of this study is to evaluate the risk of mortality through age 14, birth defects, and grade school performance among children conceived through IVF, their siblings, and non-IVF controls. This study will be based on births from 2004–2018, and will include an estimated 163,000 IVF children, 41,000 IVF siblings and 1,250,000 non-IVF control children.

Future studies will evaluate the health of parents both before and after the IVF-conceived birth, as well as when there was no birth. Additional studies of the growth and development of the IVF-conceived children and their siblings, both before and after birth, are also planned.

Limitations of Population-Based Linkages in the US

Although considerable progress has been made in linking datasets to better study ART outcomes, significant gaps in understanding exist. Notably, nearly all linkages to date rely on vital records data, and therefore exclude women who undergo treatment but do not have a live birth or fetal death. While the current evidence is equivocal, findings from some studies suggest that exposure to fertility medications may increase the risk for certain gynaecological cancers; however, it is unclear to what degree underlying subfertility may contribute to this risk [60, 61, 62]. Even less is known about health risks for oocyte donors, as there is no routine long-term follow-up. This information is important because oocyte donors are otherwise healthy young women who may experience multiple stimulation cycles [63]. While current efforts to link ART surveillance and cancer registry data can shed some light on these questions, other approaches are also needed, such as the addition of questions on past use of fertility medications to cancer surveillance protocols and the development of national egg donor registries.

In addition, while linked data have the potential to provide information on varying periods of follow-up and health outcomes of interest, identifying an appropriate control group continues to be problematic. As adverse outcomes following ART may be attributed in part to the underlying subfertility, accurate identification of subfertile populations is critical [43]. Even when birth data are linked with administrative data, women and couples undergoing other fertility treatments (e.g. using ovulation-inducing medications and/or intrauterine insemination) are still difficult to identify, as these treatments are not reliably reported either in birth certificate data or in administrative claims data [31, 64].

Finally, findings from analyses of linked data are subject to the limitations of observational studies. Observed associations may be explained by selection bias and residual confounding due to missing or poorly measured confounders, and weak associations may reach statistical significance due to large sample size but lack clinical importance. In addition, even among studies with high linkage rates, information on some proportion of the population is missing, and the characteristics of patients whose records cannot be linked may differ from those that are successfully linked. As such, well-designed prospective studies are often needed to confirm associations identified in retrospective studies using linked data.

Future Directions for Population-Based Linkages in the US

In the US, the creation of a comprehensive national database of maternal and child health outcomes for births conceived using ART is challenging because state and local offices are largely responsible for maintaining vital records. The federal government obtains information on vital statistics from the states via cooperative agreements with each individual state [65]. Direct identifiers are not included in these data nor are they routinely collected in national surveillance systems such as NASS; therefore, linkages must be done at the state level using personal identifying information or via probabilistic methods with de-identified data. One way to overcome this issue would be to establish a randomly generated identifier that could be included in state birth certificate data and collected as part of NASS. This variable could then be used to link NASS data with information from the birth certificate, thus eliminating the need for probabilistic methods. Likewise, if this random birth certificate identifier could be collected in other surveillance systems, such as cancer surveillance, integrating health outcome information from a variety of sources would be possible, thereby allowing the assessment of a range of outcomes for ART-conceived births.

Population-Based Linkages in the Nordic Countries

The Nordic countries are world leaders in their foresight of establishing unique personal identification numbers (PINs) to accurately link national databases to track the health of their citizens. The success of these linked national registries was built on several critical factors: free health care, a high degree of public trust in research, core national values of social equality and mutual responsibility and the creation of these unique personal identity numbers [29, 66, 67].

Linkage Studies from Individual Countries: Sweden, Norway, Finland and Denmark

In all of the four Nordic countries, each citizen receives their own unique personal identification number at birth. This personal identification number follows a citizen from cradle to grave and is used in all matters in life such as daycare, school, university, library, health care, dental care, work, income, bank issues and real estate. This means that every time a person is in contact with any kind of health care service, whether it be a general practitioner, outpatient or inpatient health care or any fertility clinic, either public or private, the treatment or service is registered and then subsequently reported to the relevant national health registries.

In all Nordic countries, there has been a long tradition of national health registries with the majority of the large registries having been established in the 1960s and 1970s. Developed in response to the worldwide epidemic of more than 10,000 cases of severe birth defects resulting from the use of thalidomide, the Medical Birth Registry of Norway was established in 1967. The aims of the registry were to conduct surveillance and epidemiological basic research on birth defects and other health problems [66]. In the half century since this population-based registry was established, it has provided data for numerous important studies, including the risk of repeating preterm or low birth weight outcomes [68], risk of recurrence of sudden infant death syndrome [69] and the effect of pre-eclampsia on the subsequent risk of maternal breast cancer [70]. Using similar linked health registries, studies in other Nordic countries examined subsequent maternal cardiovascular disease risk associated with subfertility in Sweden [71] and early or recurrent preterm birth in Denmark [72].

In addition to birth registries, all of the Nordic countries have patient discharge registries, cancer registries, cause of death registries, prescription registries and many others. Furthermore, there are also many national quality registries on factors such as children's diabetes, obstetrical complications and prenatal screening that provide researchers with further data for the investigation of potential consequences of ART. Because reporting to all of these registries is mandatory for all health services and is primarily linked to the financial settlement between the state and the health care system, the reliability of data is high. In countries where all citizens have their own unique personal identification number and where the reporting of all health services, diagnoses and treatment is mandatory, there is good potential for health care research. With the above-described system, a person can be followed throughout life, and data from all of the national health registries can be linked, giving a complete health history for each citizen. The system also allows identification and linkage of children, parents and siblings and allows for intergenerational studies [18, 73, 74]. In the field of ART, therefore, it is possible to identify all women undergoing fertility treatment and then link fertility data to the pregnancy outcome, pregnancy and obstetrical complications and childbirth [75]. Thereafter, the women can be followed through all the other health registries to identify potential side effects of ART. Furthermore, the health of the ART children can be studied thoroughly, not only from neonatal data from the medical birth registry but also through life in regard to both diagnoses and treatment for conditions such as diabetes, congenital malformations, cancer and fertility issues later in life, as well as school performance [76, 77, 78].

In Denmark, Norway and Sweden, detailed information on ART treatment has been collected since the early days of the procedures. In Sweden, the national ART registry was established in 1982, in Denmark this was the case in 1994, and Norway initiated a national ART registry in 1990. Detailed information is gathered on the type of ART treatment, cause of infertility, cycle number and outcome, which facilitates comparison of different types of ART treatments and different types of patients [79, 80]. National studies on ART twins and the risks related to multiple gestations led to a reduction in the rate of twins from 25–30% of children being born after ART being multiples to 5–10%, respectively, between 1995 and 2000 [81, 82]. Still, these large national cohort studies on ART children have been able to show that assisted reproduction is safe for both the women undergoing treatment and their offspring. This has led to both support for and acceptance of ART worldwide.

Consortium Studies Combining Data from Several Countries (CoNARTaS Group)

In 2008, the Committee of Nordic Assisted Reproductive Technology and Safety (CoNARTaS) was established. This is a Nordic collaboration between researchers in Denmark, Finland, Norway and Sweden with the purpose of pooling health data on the ART populations from all four countries. The committee consists of clinicians, epidemiologists, data managers and biostatisticians and has several annual meetings to ensure continuous data collection and initiation of new research projects. The collaboration aims to facilitate investigation of the risk of more rare conditions such as birth defects and cancer and follow-up of the children born after ART through adolescence and adulthood. Furthermore, the Nordic collaboration is intended to surveille new ART methods.

When combining ART data from several countries, it enables the establishment of large ART populations born over several decades [83]. This is unique because it facilitates the investigation of rare outcomes and conditions and allows researchers to follow ART-conceived children over time and thereby analyze potential trends and long-term outcomes in ART [84, 85, 86, 87]. This is crucial to ensure continuous surveillance of both new technology and new clinical protocols that are continuously being implemented in ART [82, 88].

The challenge when pooling data from different countries is first to identify national differences in registration of data and second to identify differences in national health programs, e.g. nationwide prenatal screening programs. These potential technical differences in collection of data can lead to significant differences in prevalence of conditions and complications in both women undergoing ART and children conceived after ART. Still, with the unique personal identification numbers carried by all Nordic citizens, together with all the detailed mandatory health registries, a Nordic collaboration on ART holds new potential and strongly encourages pooling of data from Nordic countries.

Limitation of Population-Based Linkages in Nordic Countries

While the population-based nature of the Nordic registries and their continuous use over decades are major strengths, they have an important limitation: relatively low absolute annual numbers of IVF-conceived births. For example, in 2010 the number of IVF-conceived infants born in Denmark was 3,724; in Finland, 1,873; in Norway, 2,098; and in Sweden, 4,053, for a total of 11,748 infants in these four Nordic countries combined [89]. In contrast, in 2010 there were 61,179 IVF-conceived infants born to women who were US residents, with about half of these infants born in six states: California (7,725), New York (6,304), Texas (4,413), New Jersey (3,856), Illinois (3,714) and Massachusetts (3,404) [90]. As such, multiple years of data may be needed to study emerging treatments or outcomes that are uncommon.

Future Plans or Areas in Need of Further Research

With some of the national Nordic ART registries dating back as far as 1982, it will soon be possible to establish a cohort of men and women, who themselves were conceived after assisted reproduction. This will enable extensive research in many aspects of the potential long-term consequences of ART. It is yet to be investigated whether children conceived after ART have an increased risk of pubertal disorders and whether there are long-term medical consequences of the in vitro technology, such as increased risk of diabetes, cardiovascular diseases or other metabolic diseases. Another interesting question to be answered is whether the population of men and women conceived after ART themselves will have fertility issues and potentially need assisted reproduction.

Conclusions and Recommendations

Although it is now nearly 40 years since the first IVF baby was born, there is a continued need for ongoing surveillance of the ART population for many reasons. First, there are still many as yet unanswered questions on potentially negative, long-term health consequences of these interventions for both parents and children. Second, with the continuous introduction of new treatments and laboratory methods, it is critical to investigate and surveille the safety and efficacy of emerging technologies. Finally, use of ART continues to increase globally with concurrent increases in the number of couples undergoing treatment. Likewise, the number of ART-conceived births is rising and accounting for a growing proportion of the national birth cohort, particularly in countries with high levels of accessibility to ART. Therefore, all countries performing ART may want to consider implementing national ART registries and work to facilitate linkages to population-based health registries, so that potential complications for both women undergoing assisted reproduction and the children conceived after ART can be identified. Because such linkages are possible only when cycle-level data are collected by registries, it is essential that surveillance systems are designed to collect data at the cycle level rather than information reported in aggregate. With continuous surveillance and research in the field of ART, we can effectively monitor the safety and efficacy of ART and use this information to promote the best health outcomes for infertile couples and their offspring.

References

1. Evers JLH. Female subfertility. *Lancet*. 2002;**360**:151–9.

2. Practice Committee of the American Society for Reproductive Medicine. Definitions of infertility and recurrent pregnancy loss: A committee opinion. *Fertil Steril*. 2013;**99**:63. doi:10.1016/j.fertnstert.2012.09.023.

3. Chandra A, Copen CE, Stephen EH. Infertility service use in the United States: data from the National Survey of Family Growth, 1982–2010. *Natl Health Stat Report*. 2014(73):1–21.

4. Mansour R, Ishihara O, Adamson GD, Dyer S, de Mouzon J, Nygren KG, et al. International Committee for Monitoring Assisted Reproductive Technologies world report: assisted reproductive technology 2006. *Hum Reprod*. 2014;**29**:1536–51.

5. Mascarenhas MN, Flaxman SR, Boerma T, Vanderpoel S, Stevens GA. National, regional, and global trends in infertility prevalence since 1990: a systematic analysis of 277 health surveys. *PLoS Med*. 2012;**9**(12):e1001356. Available at: https://doi.org/10.1371/journal.pmed.1001356.

6. Zeger-Hochschild F, Adamson GD, Dyer S, Racowsky C, de Mouzon J, Sokol R, et al. The International Glossary on Infertility and Fertility Care, 2017. *Fertil Steril*. 2017;**108**:393–406.

7. Farland LV, Missmer SA, Rich-Edwards J, Chavarro JE, Barbieri RL, Grodstein F. Use of infertility treatment modalities in a large United States cohort of professional women. *Fertil Steril*. 2014;**101**:1705–10.

8. Mathews TJ, Hamilton BE. *First Births to Older Women Continue to Rise*. NCHS Data Brief No. 152. Hyattsville, MD: National Center for Health Statistics; 2014.

9. Kiatpongsan S, Huckman RS, Hornstein MD. The Great Recession, insurance mandates, and the use of in vitro fertilization services in the United States. *Fertil Steril*. 2015;**103**:448–54.

10. Abramowitz J. Turning back the ticking clock: the effect of increased affordability of assisted reproductive technology on women's marriage timing. *J Popu Econ*. 2014;**27**:603–33.

11. Bitler MP, Schmidt L. Utilization of infertility treatments: the effects of insurance mandates. *Demography*. 2012;**49**:125–49.

12. Wright VC, Schieve LA, Reynolds MA, Jeng G. Assisted reproductive technology surveillance – United States, 2000. *MMWR Surveill Summ.* 2003;**52**(9):1–16.

13. Centers for Disease Control and Prevention, American Society for Reproductive Medicine, and Society for Assisted Reproductive Technology. *2015 Assisted Reproductive Technology National Summary Report.* Atlanta, GA: US Dept of Health and Human Services; 2017.

14. Sunderam S, Kissin DM, Crawford SB, Folger SG, Boulet SL, Warner L, et al. Assisted reproductive technology surveillance – United States, 2015. *MMWR Surveill Summ.* 2018;**67**:1–28.

15. Kissin DM, Jamieson DJ, Barfield WD. Monitoring health outcomes of assisted reproductive technology (Letter to the Editor). *N Engl J Med.* 2014;**371**(1): 91–3.

16. Stern JE, Gopal D, Anderka M, Liberman R, Kotelchuck M, Luke B. Validation of birth outcomes in the SART CORS: population-based analysis from the Massachusetts Outcome Study of Assisted Reproductive Technology (MOSART). *Fertil Steril.* 2016;**106**:717–22.e2.

17. Romundstad LB, Romundstad PR, Sunde A, von Düring V, Skjærven R, Vatten LJ. Increased risk of placenta previa in pregnancies following IVF/ICSI: a comparison of ART and non-ART pregnancies in the same mother. *Hum Reprod.* 2006;**21**:2353–8.

18. Romundstad LB, Romundstad PR, Sunde A, von Düring V, Skjærven R, Gunnell D, Vatten LJ. Effects of technology or maternal factors on perinatal outcome after assisted fertilization: a population-based cohort study. *Lancet.* 2008;**372**:737–43.

19. Shih W, Rushford DD, Bourne H, Garrett C, McBain JC, Healy DL, et al. Factors affecting low birthweight after assisted reproduction technology: difference between transfer of fresh and cryopreserved embryos suggests an adverse effect of oocyte collection. *Hum Reprod.* 2008;**23**:1644–53.

20. Luke B, Brown MB, Spector LG. Perinatal outcomes with and without ART: a population-based study of linked siblings in 12 States. *Fertil Steril.* 2015;**104**:e92.

21. Luke B, Gopal D, Diop H, Stern JE. Perinatal outcomes of singleton siblings: the effects of maternal fertility status and ART treatment. *J Assist Reprod Genet.* 2016;**33**(9):1203–13.

22. Luke B, Brown MB, Wantman E, Stern JE, Toner J, Coddington CC. Increased risk of large-for-gestational age birthweight in singleton siblings conceived with in vitro fertilization in frozen versus fresh cycles. *J Assist Reprod Genet.* 2017;**34**(2):191–200. doi:10.1007/s10815-016-0850-x.

23. Dhalwani, NN, Boulet SL, Kissin DM, Zhang Y, McKane P, Bailey MA, et al. *Fertil Steril.* 2016;**106**: 710–16.

24. Baldwin E, Johnson K, Berthoud H, Dublin S. Linking mothers and infants within electronic health records: a comparison of deterministic and probabilistic algorithms. *Pharmacoepidemiol Drug Saf.* 2015;**24**:45–51.

25. Herman A, McCarthy B, Bakewell J, Ward R, Mueller B, Maconochie N, et al. Data linkage methods used in maternally-linked birth and infant death surveillance data sets from the United States (Georgia, Missouri, Utah and Washington State), Israel, Norway, Scotland and Western Australia. *Paediatr Perinat Epidemiol.* 1997;**11**(Suppl 1):5–22.

26. Mneimneh AS, Boulet SL, Sunderam S, Zhang Y, Jamieson DJ, Crawford S, et al., for the States Monitoring ART (SMART) Collaborative. States Monitoring Assisted Reproductive Technology (SMART) Collaborative: data collection, linkage, dissemination, and use. *J Womens Health.* 2013;**22**:571–7.

27. Sunderam S, Schieve LA, Cohen B, Zhang Z, Jeng G, Reynolds M, et al.; Massachusetts Consortium for Assisted Reproductive Technology Epidemiologic Research. Linking birth and infant death records with assisted reproductive technology data: Massachusetts, 1997–1998. *Matern Child Health J.* 2006;**10**:115–25.

28. Zhang Y, Cohen B, Macaluso M, Zhang Z, Durant T, Nannini A. Probabilistic linkage of assisted reproductive technology information with vital records, Massachusetts 1997–2000. *Matern Child Health J.* 2012;**16**:1703–8.

29. Irgens LM. The Medical Birth Registry of Norway: epidemiological research and surveillance through 30 years. *Acta Obstet Gynecol Scand.* 2000;**79**:435–9.

30. Sauber-Schatz E, Sappenfield W, Grigorescu V, Kulkarni A, Zhang Y, Salihu HM, et al. Assisted reproductive technology, and early preterm birth – Florida, 2004–2006. *Am J Epidemiol.* 2012;**176**:886–96.

31. Cohen B, Bernson D, Sappenfield W, Kirby RS, Kissin D, Zhang Y, et al. Accuracy of assisted reproductive technology information on birth certificates: Florida and Massachusetts, 2004–06. *Paediatr Perina Epidemiol.* 2014;**28**:181–90.

32. Boulet SL, Crawford S, Zhang Y, Sunderam S, Cohen B, Bernson D, et al.; States Monitoring ART Collaborative. Embryo transfer practices and perinatal outcomes by insurance mandate status. *Fertil Steril.* 2015;**104**(2):403–9.

33. Martin AS, Zhang Y, Crawford S, Boulet SL, McKane P, Kissin DM, Jamieson DJ; States Monitoring Assisted Reproductive Technology (SMART) Collaborative. Antenatal hospitalizations among pregnancies

conceived with and without assisted reproductive technology. *Obstet Gynecol.* 2016;**127**(5):941–50.

34. Boulet SL, Kirby RS, Reefhuis J, Zhang Y, Sunderam S, Cohen B, et al. Assisted reproductive technology and birth defects among liveborn infants in Florida, Massachusetts, and Michigan, 2000–2010. *JAMA Pediatr.* 2016;**170**(6):e154934.

35. Sites CK, Wilson D, Barsky M, Bernson D, Bernstein IM, Boulet S, et al. Embryo cryopreservation and preeclampsia risk. *Fertil Steril.* 2017;**108**:784–90.

36. Toner JP, Coddington CC, Doody K, Van Voorhis B, Seifer DB, Ball GD, et al. Society for Assisted Reproductive Technology and assisted reproductive technology in the United States: a 2016 update. *Fertil Steril.* 2016;**106**:541–6.

37. Centers for Disease Control and Prevention, American Society for Reproductive Medicine/Society for Assisted Reproductive Technology, RESOLVE. *1995 Assisted Reproductive Technology Success Rates: National and Summary Fertility Clinic Reports.* Atlanta, GA: US Department of Health and Human Services; 1997.

38. Stern JE, Brown MB, Luke B, Wantman E, Lederman A, Missmer SA, et al. Calculating cumulative live-birth rates from linked cycles of assisted reproductive technology (ART): data from the Massachusetts SART CORS. *Fertil Steril.* 2010;**94**:1334–40.

39. Stern JE, Brown MB, Luke B, Wantman E, Lederman A, Hornstein MD. Cycle 1 as predictor of ART treatment outcome over multiple cycles: analysis of linked cycles from the SART CORS Online Database. *Fertil Steril.* 2011;**95**:600–5.

40. Luke B, Brown MB, Wantman E, Lederman A, Gibbons W, Schattman GL, et al. Cumulative birth rates from linked assisted reproductive technology cycles. *N Engl J Med.* 2012;**366**:2483–91.

41. Luke B, Brown MB, Wantman E, Baker VL, Grow DR, Stern JE. Second try: who returns for additional ART treatment and the effect of a prior ART birth. *Fertil Steril.* 2013;**100**:1580–4.

42. Luke B, Brown MB, Wantman E, Stern JE. Factors associated with monozygosity in assisted reproductive technology (ART) pregnancies and the risk of recurrence using linked cycles. *Fertil Steril.* 2014;**101**:683–9.

43. Declercq ER, Belanoff C, Diop H, Gopal D, Hornstein MD, Kotelchuck M, et al. Identifying women with indicators of subfertility in a statewide population database: operationalizing the missing link in ART research. *Fertil Steril.* 2014;**101**:463–71.

44. Stern JE, Luke B, Tobias M, Gopal D, Hornstein MD, Diop H. Adverse pregnancy and birth outcomes by infertility diagnoses with and without ART treatment. *Fertil Steril.* 2015;**103**:1438–45. PMID:25813277; PMCID:PMC4465778.

45. Luke B, Stern JE, Kotelchuck M, Declercq E, Cohen B, Diop H. Birth outcomes by infertility diagnosis: analyses of the Massachusetts Outcomes Study of Assisted Reproductive Technologies (MOSART). *J Reprod Med.* 2015;**60**:480–90. PMCID:PMC4734384; PMID:26775455.

46. Luke B, Stern JE, Kotelchuck M, Declercq ER, Hornstein MD, Gopal D, et al. Adverse pregnancy outcomes after in vitro fertilization: effect of number of embryos transferred and plurality at conception. *Fertil Steril.* 2015;**104**:79–86. PMID:25956368; PMCID: PMC4489987.

47. Luke B, Stern JE, Kotelchuck M, Declercq E, Anderka M, Diop H. Birth outcomes by infertility treatment: analyses of the Massachusetts Outcomes Study of Assisted Reproductive Technologies (MOSART). *J Reprod Med.* 2016;**61**:114–27. PMID:27172633.

48. Declercq E, Luke B, Belanoff C, Cabral H, Diop H, Gopal D, et al. Perinatal outcomes associated with assisted reproductive technology: the Massachusetts Outcomes Study of Assisted Reproductive Technologies (MOSART). *Fertil Steril.* 2015;**103**: 888–95. PMID:25660721. PMIC:PMC4385441.

49. Luke B, Gopal D, Stern JE, Diop H. Pregnancy, birth, and infant outcomes by maternal fertility status: the Massachusetts Outcomes Study of Assisted Reproductive Technology. *Am J Obstet Gynecol.* 2017;**217**:327.e1–14. doi:10.1016/j.ajog.2017.04.006.

50. Luke B, Gopal D, Stern JE, Diop H. Adverse pregnancy, birth, and infant outcomes in twins: Effects of maternal fertility status and infant gender combination. The Massachusetts Outcomes Study of Assisted Reproductive Technology. *Am J Obstet Gynecol.* 2017;**217**:330.e1–15. doi:10.1016/j.ajog.2017.04.025.

51. Declercq ER, Luke B, Stern JE, Diop H, Gopal D, Cabral H, et al. Maternal postpartum hospitalization following ART births (Research letter). *Epidemiology.* 2015;**26**:e64–5. PMID:26317669.

52. Belanoff C, Declercq ER, Diop H, Gopal D, Kotelchuck M, Luke B, et al. Severe maternal morbidity and the use of assisted reproductive technology. *Obstet Gynecol.* 2016;**127**:527–34. PMID:26855105.

53. Stern JE, Gopal D, Diop H, Missmer S, Coddington C, Luke B. Inpatient hospitalizations in women with and without assisted reproductive technology live birth. *J Assist Reprod Genet.* 2017;**34**(8):1043–9. doi:10.1007/s10815-017-0961-z.

54. Diop H, Gopal D, Cabral H, Belanoff C, Declercq ER, Kotelchuck M, et al. Assisted reproductive technology and early intervention enrollment. *Pediatrics.* 2016;**137** (3):e20152007. PMID:26908668.

55. Liberman R, Getz KD, Luke B, Stern JE, Declercq ER, Chen X, Anderka M. Assisted reproductive technology and birth defects: effects of subfertility and multiple births. *Birth Defects Res.* 2017;**109**(14):1144–53. doi:10.1002/bdr2.1055.

56. Luke B, Brown MB, Missmer SA, Spector LG, Leach RE, Williams M, et al. Assisted reproductive technology use and outcomes among women with a history of cancer. *Hum Reprod.* 2016;**31**(1):183–9. PMCID:PMC4677965.

57. Luke B, Brown MB, Spector LG, Stern JE, Smith YR, Williams M, et al. Embryo banking among women diagnosed with cancer: a population-based study in New York, Texas, and Illinois. *J Assist Reprod Genet.* 2016;**33**(5):667–74. PMID:26843393.

58. Luke B, Brown MB, Spector LG, Missmer SA, Leach RE, Williams M, et al. Cancer in women after assisted reproductive technology. *Fertil Steril.* 2015;**104**:1218–26. PMID:26271227; PMCID: PMC4630138.

60. Skalkidou A, Sergentanis TN, Gialamas SP, Georgakis MK, Psaltopoulou T, Trivella M, et al. Risk of endometrial cancer in women treated with ovary-stimulating drugs for subfertility. *Cochrane Database Syst Rev.* 2017;**2017**:3:CD010931.

61. Kroener L, Dumesic D, Al-Safi Z. Use of fertility medications and cancer risk: a review and update. *Curr Opin Obstet Gynecol.* 2017;**29**(4):195–201.

62. Practice Committee of the American Society for Reproductive Medicine. Fertility drugs and cancer: a guideline. *Fertil Steril.* 2016;**106**(7):1617–26.

63. Schneider J, Lahl J, Kramer W. Long-term breast cancer risk following ovarian stimulation in young egg donors: a call for follow-up, research and informed consent. *Reprod Biomed Online.* 2017;**34**(5):480–5.

64. Luke B, Brown MB, Spector LG. Validation of infertility treatment and assisted reproductive technology use on the birth certificate in eight states. *Am J Obstet Gynecol.* 2016;**215**:126–7.

65. Hetzel AM. History and organization of the vital statistics system. In *U.S. Vital Statistics System: Major Activities and Developments, 1950–95.* Washington, DC: US Department of Health and Human Services, Centers for Disease Control and Prevention, National Center for Health Statistics; 1997. Available at: www.cdc.gov/nchs/data/misc/usvss.pdf.

66. Wilcox AJ. The Medical Birth Registry of Norway – an international perspective. *Norsk Epidemiologi.* 2007;**17**:103–5.

67. Ludvigsson JF, Håberg SE, Knudsen GP, Lafolie P, Zoega H, Sarrkola C, et al. Ethical aspects of registry-based research in the Nordic countries. *Clin Epidemiol.* 2015;**7**:491–508.

68. Bakketeig LS, Hoffman HJ, Harley EE. The tendency to repeat gestational age and birth weight in successive births. *Am J Obstet Gynecol.* 1979;**135**:1086–103.

69. Irgens LM, Skjaerven R, Peterson DR. Prospective assessment of recurrence in sudden infant death syndrome siblings. *J Pediat.* 1984;**104**:349–51.

70. Vatten LJ, Romundstad PR, Trichopoulos D, Skjaerven R. Pre-eclampsia in pregnancy and subsequent risk for breast cancer. *Brit J Cancer.* 2002;**87**:971–3.

71. Parikh NI, Cnattingius S, Mittleman MA, Ludvigsson JF, Ingelsson E. Subfertility and risk of later life maternal cardiovascular disease. *Hum Reprod.* 2012;**27**:568–75.

72. Catov JM, Wu CS, Olsen J, Sutton-Tyrrell K, Li J, Nohr EA. Early or recurrent preterm birth and maternal cardiovascular disease risk. *Ann Epidemiol.* 2010;**20**:604–9.

73. Henningsen AK, Pinborg A, Lidegaard O, Vestergaard C, Forman JL, Andersen AN. Perinatal outcome of singleton siblings born after assisted reproductive technology and spontaneous conception: Danish national sibling-cohort study. *Fertil Steril.* 2011;**95**(3):959–63.

74. Tandberg A, Melve KK, Nordtveit TI, Bjorge T, Skjaerven R. Maternal birth characteristics and perinatal mortality in twin offspring. An intergenerational population-based study in Norway, 1967–2008. *BJOG.* 2011,**118**(6):698–705.

75. Sazonova A, Källen K, Thurin-Kjellberg A, Wennerholm UB, Bergh C. Factors affecting obstetric outcome of singletons born after IVF. *Human Reprod.* 2011;**26**(10):2878–86.

76. Källen B, Finnström O, Nygren KG, Olausson PO. In-vitro fertilization (IVF) in Sweden: infant outcome after different IVF fertilization methods. *Fertil Steril.* 2005;**84**(3):611–17.

77. Kettner O, Matthiesen NB, Ramlau-Hansen CH, Kesmodel US, Bay B, Henriksen TB. Fertility treatment and childhood type 1 diabetes mellitus: a nationwide cohort study of 565,116 live births. *Fertil Steril.* 2016;**106**(7):1751–6.

78. Spangmose AL, Malchau SS, Schmidt L, Vassard D, Rasmussen S, Loft A, et al. Academic performance in adolescents born after ART – a nationwide registry-based cohort study. *Hum Reprod.* 2017;**32**(2):447–56.

79. Malchau SS, Loft A, Henningsen AK, Nyboe Andersen A, Pinborg A. Perinatal outcomes in 6,338 singletons born after intrauterine insemination in Denmark, 2007 to 2012: the influence of ovarian stimulation. *Fertil Steril.* 2014;**102**(4):1110–16.

80. Malchau SS, Henningsen AA, Loft A, Rasmussen S, Forman J, Nyboe Andersen A, Pinborg A.

The long-term prognosis for live-birth in couples initiating fertility treatments. *Hum Reprod.* 2017;32(7): 1439–49.

81. Pinborg A, Loft A, Rasmussen S, Schmidt L, Langhoff-Ross J, Greisen G, Andersen AN. Neonatal outcome in a Danish national cohort of 3438 IVF/ICSI and 10,362 non-IVF/ICSI twins born between 1995 and 2000. *Hum Reprod.* 2004;19(2):435–41.

82. Henningsen AA, Gissler M, Skjaerven R, Bergh C, Tiitinen A, Romundstad LB, et al. Trends in perinatal health after assisted reproduction: a Nordic study from the CoNARTaS group. *Hum Reprod.* 2015 **30**(3):710–16.

83. Henningsen AK, Romundstad LB, Gissler M, Nygren KG, Lidegaard O, Skjaerven R, et al. Infant and maternal health monitoring using a combined Nordic database on ART and safety. *Acta Obstst Gynecol Scand.* 2011 **90**(7):683–91.

84. Hagman A, Loft A, Wennerholm UB, Pinborg A, Bergh C, Aittomäki K, et al. Obstetric and neonatal outcome after oocyte donation in 106 women with Turner syndrome: a Nordic cohort study. *Hum Reprod.* 2013;**28**(6):1598–609.

85. Henningsen AA, Wennerholm UB, Gissler M, Romundstad LB, Nygren KG, Tiitinen A, et al. Risk of stillbirth and infant death after assisted reproductive technology: a Nordic study from the CoNARTaS group. *Hum Reprod.* 2014;**29**(5):1090–6.

86. Sundh KJ, Henningsen AK, Källén K, Bergh C, Romundstad LB, Gissler M, et al. Cancer in children and young adults born after assisted reproductive technology: a Nordic cohort study from the Committee on Nordic ART and Safety (CoNARTaS). *Hum Reprod.* 2014;29(9):2050–7.

87. Opdahl S, Henningsen AA, Tiitinen A, Bergh C, Pinborg A, Romundstad PR, et al. Risk of hypertensive disorders in pregnancies following assisted reproductive technology: a cohort study from the CoNARTaS group. *Hum Reprod.* 2015 **30**(7): 1724–31.

88. Wennerholm UB, Henningsen AK, Romundstad LB, Bergh C, Pinborg A, Skjaerven R, et al. Perinatal outcomes of children born after frozen-thawed embryo transfer: a Nordic cohort study from the CoNARTaS group. *Hum Reprod.* 2013;28(9):2545–53.

89. Dyer S, Chambers GM, de Mouzon J, Nygren KG, Zegers-Hochschild F, Mansour R, et al. International Committee for Monitoring Assisted Reproductive Technologies world report: assisted reproductive technology 2008, 2009 and 2010. *Hum Reprod.* 2016;**31**:1588–609.

90. Sunderam S, Kissin DM, Crawford S, Anderson JE, Folger SG, Jamieson DJ, Barfield WD. Assisted reproductive technology surveillance – United States, 2010. *MMWR Surveill Summ.* 2013;**62**:1–28.

Chapter

10

Use of ART Surveillance by People Experiencing Infertility

Sandra K. Dill, Edgar Mocanu and Petra Thorn

Introduction

Pursuing assisted reproductive technology (ART) is a major life decision. In many countries it is a very costly medical treatment, for which there is limited or no reimbursement through government-provided national health insurance. Therefore, it is vital that individuals and couples considering and undergoing ART make use of comprehensive information regarding treatment options and outcomes. National ART surveillance data are one such option in those countries where these data are publicly available.

Expectations of ART Treatment

The multifaceted ART intervention raises many challenges not only for practitioners but also for patients. Do patients receive sufficient information prior to embarking on treatment, to understand the chances, risks and potential complications of treatment to enable them to make an informed decision to undergo ART? Clinics have a duty to provide comprehensive information about all aspects of treatment, not only orally prior to treatment, but also written, web based or through audiovisual means. A basic understanding of ART should cover what the treatment involves, medications and interventions, under- and over-response to stimulation, adverse reactions to medication used, complications of egg collection, low embryo availability and blastulation rates, low success rates, particularly in women older than 35 years of age, the likelihood and risk of multiple pregnancies and, last but not least, child and pregnancy risks.

More than 25 years' experience from patient support organizations suggests that many patients pursue ART without a full understanding of the risks and potential complications [1]. Therefore, it is imperative that providers ensure adequate patient education to enable them to make an informed decision about undergoing ART. This helps to manage their expectations about commencing and continuing with treatment. However, in addition to the information presented to patients by providers, it is important that publicly available ART surveillance data be available in a format that is unbiased, understandable and meaningful. Most developed countries publish ART registry reports, but the format of these varies considerably and they are usually written for a scientific audience. In the digital age, patients increasingly expect to have access to information on health service outcomes. More research is needed to guide the patient-friendly presentation of ART data collected by national ART registries, including on treatment success rates for different patient groups, risk of complications and different ART treatment modalities.

The chance of an ART cycle being successful varies by prognostic factors including the age of patients, reasons for treatment and, for those who have already commenced treatment, how many failed attempts they have undertaken. These will inform a patient's decision making; however, their final choice will most likely be related to confidence in the treatment and quality of care provided by a particular clinic. They want to know which clinic will give them the best chance of taking home a healthy baby while respecting their particular circumstances and needs. Choosing a clinic based solely on reported success rates either based on ART national registry data or on published clinic data on their websites can create unrealistic expectations about the possibility of having a baby at a particular clinic.

How Can Patients Inform Themselves about National and International Trends in ART Success Rates?

ART statistical data are complex to present and understand even by clinicians and scientists working in the field. A recent review of clinical trials evaluating ART treatment has identified more than 800 reported outcome measures [2]. The reason for the complexity relates to the many numerators and denominators that can be chosen to represent ART success. In addition, ART treatment involves multilevel exposures (e.g. multiple treatments within one woman), multiple stages within an ART cycle (initiated, follicular aspiration, embryo transfer) and multiple end points (implantation, pregnancy, live birth). See more information about variations of ART success rates in Chapter 5, Reporting ART Success Rates. Therefore, where national ART surveillance data are published, it should be in patient-friendly language and include comprehensive information about how to interpret the statistics. In particular, it should be emphasized that the results from national ART registries are population-based averages of all patients who have undergone treatment and may not be applicable to an individual patient's circumstances and chance of success. Such guidance is important because it can help to inform expectations prior to deciding whether to embark on treatment.

Furthermore, available data on which to base a patient's decision to commence or continue with treatment are often lacking and can be biased, as few countries have a compulsory, cycle-by-cycle national reporting system that encompasses all ART therapies performed. Consequently, the burden lies with patients to identify and understand data pertinent to the ART clinic they are considering and any other services or national and international results for comparison purposes.

Using ART Surveillance to Understand Success Rates

How Do ART Surveillance Data Help Patients to Enrich Their Understanding and Ability to Choose?

Standardized data about ART treatment outcomes are difficult for patients to find, despite most developed countries publishing ART registry reports. Due to the competitive nature of these interventions and the continuous enlargement of the 'for profit' ART services globally, there is limited drive for clinics to present uniform, realistic and accurate results of treatments. Having to rely on published clinic-based results, such as those on clinic websites, can be misleading because of the varied way that clinics choose to present their results and the possible omission of some patient groups to artificially improve the published success rates [3].

The only information the vast majority of patients seek is that provided directly by the clinics in their region or country. Information about world regions where surveillance data are available can be found in Section 4 of this book. In order for patients to be aware of national and international registry data that provide overall results in a standardized way, clinics and patient organizations should be encouraged to make this information known, and to encourage ART surveillance reports to be made publicly available with accompanying lay summaries for patients.

At the heart of a patient's question about a clinic's success rates is the need to know whether they can be assured of the best chance of taking home a healthy baby. Some of the more popular means of measuring success rates are live birth rate or positive clinical pregnancy (positive fetal heart showing on ultrasound) per treatment cycles commenced, per egg collection or per embryo transfer. Considerable debate exists on what is the most reliable measure [4, 5]. A discussion on measuring success rates using ART registry data is presented in Chapter 5, Reporting ART Success Rates.

What Counselling Is Available?

Infertility is a major life crisis, and for some the treatment can be somewhat of an emotional roller coaster. Even people who have particularly challenging lives may be surprised by the impact that infertility and its treatment can have on well-being. Under these circumstances, good friends and a supportive family can be important.

Emotional responses to infertility are complex and at times are so strong they can seem overwhelming. Having a professional counsellor available at the clinic can help patients understand that these feelings are normal.

The outcome of ART treatment is not only the possibility of getting pregnant. Emotional support during treatment by an infertility counsellor, friendly opening hours, continuous contact, spontaneous support such as a phone call when the treatment has not worked – all help patients navigate the challenges of ART treatment.

For patients or potential patients reading ART surveillance reports, the stark numbers and percentages presented in multiple tables do not provide any indication of the complex emotions associated with falling on either side of the very binary outcome associated with ART treatment – that is, achieving pregnancy or not.

Measures That Can Be Used to Determine Success Rates

It would be particularly helpful for patients if ART surveillance reports provided more lay vocabulary regarding ART treatment. The following measures explain in patient-friendly language what each of these terms means and give some indication of their respective limitations:

Live birth – this relates to the number of live births per treatment cycle, multiple births being classed as a single live birth. This measure is closest to the intention of the infertile couple; however, collection of data is often slow – at least until all the live births have occurred and been followed up by the clinic and recorded. Live birth figures reflect a number of factors, including the following: age of the female, the number of eggs recovered, fertilization rates, the quality of embryos and embryo transfer technique, not to mention the quality of the laboratory.

Clinical pregnancy – This relates to an ultrasound test, usually at about 7 weeks into the pregnancy when a fetal heart is seen. This is a more rigorous test than that of biochemical pregnancy (the first blood test that shows a positive pregnancy test) and has the advantage that it provides more recent data from the perspective of patients receiving contemporaneous information directly from the clinic rather than from the annual report. However, these data do not show how many of these clinical pregnancies result in a live birth.

Pregnancies/live births per treatment cycles commenced – This relates to the number of pregnancies/live births per cycles where hormonal stimulation of the ovaries has been initiated irrespective of whether any of the cycles were cancelled prior to egg pickup.

Pregnancies/live births per egg collection – This relates to the number of pregnancies/live births per cycles where the woman has proceeded as far as egg collection and would include also all those patients for whom eggs were retrieved but did not result in embryos for transfer.

Pregnancies/live births per embryo transfer – This relates to the number of pregnancies/live births per cycles where the woman has proceeded as far as embryo transfer and would not include those couples for whom the cycle was cancelled, who did not make it to egg pickup, who were overstimulated (ovarian hyperstimulation syndrome (OHSS)) or who did not produce embryos. These data would also include frozen embryo transfers.

Pregnancies/live births per embryo – This refers to the rate of pregnancies/live births per embryo transferred. There is now greater emphasis on transferring a single embryo and reducing the risk of multiple births.

Cumulative pregnancy rates – Some clinics may have data on their cumulative pregnancy rate, which is either pregnancy or live birth per all transfers from one fresh egg collection and includes data from both fresh and frozen cycles.

It is important to realize that as we move down this list, the apparent success rate increases. Armed with this information, it becomes important to ask clinics about the specific per cent figure they are reporting.

An excellent tool in regard to terminology is the International Committee Monitoring Assisted Reproductive Technologies (ICMART) glossary of terms [6]. See Appendix B, International Glossary on Infertility and Fertility Care.

Questions That May Be Useful for Patients to Ask

- *What is the success rate for my particular age group?*
  The age of the woman is a known predictor of the chance of achieving a pregnancy. Patients will find it useful to know what the likely outcome is for their age bracket.
- *What is the success rate for my/our particular case of infertility?*
  Certain etiologies such as endometriosis can reduce the likelihood of pregnancy after ART.
- *What is the risk of a multiple birth?*
  Note: success rates could be higher for clinics that transfer a higher number of embryos, but the multiple pregnancy rate is likely to be higher also. Some clinics may have specific policies on how many embryos should be transferred, so ask them about their policy. In some countries, reimbursement may be linked with the number of embryos transferred, while in other countries, compliance with medical guidelines is required.
  Clinical practice guidelines may restrict the number of embryos transferred to no more than one or two, unless in exceptional circumstances. There is a recommendation in some countries that no more than one embryo be transferred on the

first or second treatment cycle when the egg has been obtained from a woman under 35 [7, 8].

- *How many cycles are conducted per year by the clinic?*

   For smaller clinics, the results can become skewed because of the lack of something called statistical power. This means that their results may look 'good' one year, and then the following year they may look 'bad' but the results cannot be compared. A clinic may have 200 cycles one year and 200 the next; in the first year there were 55 live births and in the second there were 60. The percentages would be 27.5% and 30%, respectively. The percentage difference may look quite marked, but in reality, we are only talking about the difference of 5 live births out of 200. It is important that patients understand such discrepancies.

- *What is the success rate achieved for a so-called gold standard prognosis group?*

   This 'good prognosis' group may be composed of women under 35 years of age who have undergone 3 or fewer cycles. Pregnancy rates vary significantly depending on the type of treatment, the age of the patient and cause of infertility. The success rates achieved by a clinic for the 'good prognosis' group primarily reflect the quality of the clinic rather than the variety of patients.

   A recent advance in the reporting of ART surveillance information is the inclusion of web-based patient prediction calculators, where patients enter individual characteristics about themselves and the treatment they are considering. Two examples are provided by the Society for Assisted Reproductive Technology (SART) based on United States (US) data and using the Human Fertilisation and Embryology Authority (HFEA) data from the United Kingdom (UK) [9, 10, 11, 12]. These prediction tools are based on pooled data from reporting clinics and provide a much more user-friendly way for patients to access information about their chances of ART success, but it is important that these tools be used in conjunction with advice from a patient's clinician.

Opportunities for ART Clinics in Using ART Surveillance Data

Result Presentation

There is an opportunity for clinics and ART registries to drive a new way of reporting their results, one that not only gives live birth rates but also presents the efficient running of the service, protocol personalization, efficiency of stimulation, laboratory quality and utilization of reproductive material, or the ability of the clinic to offer the largest number of good quality embryos from the oocytes and sperm made available to their laboratory.

Presenting results for all patients receiving treatment is informative, particularly at upper age limits, yet the performance of a clinic is best measured by comparing success rates in a standard cohort, for example, 'good prognosis'. Clinics should offer information on their rate of complications during treatment, how efficient they are in creating an embryo from 100 eggs collected, what the likelihood is of a blastocyst forming from 100 fertilized eggs, the percentage of patients who reach an egg collection and an embryo transfer, the percentage of elective single embryo transfers and freeze rates and clinical pregnancy and delivery rates.

One area of interest for patients is represented by the non-in vitro fertilization (IVF) therapies such as ovulation induction with or without intrauterine insemination (IUI), results of which are extremely rarely collected and reported at the national level. In consequence, questions concerning treatment success, treatment safety and cost-effectiveness as well as when one should transit from non-IVF to IVF therapy remain unanswered on large-scale data. From a patient perspective, consideration should be given to collecting such data at national and international levels to aid decision making.

Service Presentation

Reporting of results presents only part of the patient experience during treatment. The idea that patients must pay attention only to the success rates should be challenged. Clinics should describe how they offer a comprehensive treatment to include clinical and laboratory expertise, availability of counselling and out-of-hours contact, friendly hours services and support after the treatment, particularly if it has not worked. Furthermore, clinics have an opportunity to assess the quality of their services through patient satisfaction questionnaires that could be published on an annual basis to reflect the 'non-medical' spectrum of care.

Finally, presenting 'results' creates the opportunity to misinform and mislead vulnerable patients. In contrast, presenting the services provided can help patients to understand how the clinic will support them as they undergo treatment, with realistic expectations about reaching their desired destination. It is important for patients to be confident that the clinic will endeavour to meet their specific needs in a business that offers no guarantees of delivering their dream of a child and in the majority of cases does not.

While correct reporting of results should be a legal obligation for all ART services, correct presentation of services must be a minimal ethical obligation!

Creating Confidence in ART Surveillance Data

When Reporting Success Rates, Should Clinics Be Identified or Anonymous?

An integral function of accrediting bodies and licensing authorities is to collect results for a specific group of patients who have a similar likelihood of having a live birth or pregnancy, in order to compare success rates at different units. Alternatively, or in addition to, results should be risk-adjusted to account for differences in the case-mix of patients attending clinics. The use of these data to measure performance for accreditation purposes is a useful means of identifying ways to improve practice while maintaining confidentiality. A major strength of the data in surveillance reports where clinics are not identified is their anonymity. There is no incentive to manipulate data, so stakeholders can be confident of their reliability [13].

Information that may be provided in national surveillance data identifying clinics can be used to compare the results. But how meaningful is this comparison and do patients truly understand what it represents? It can weaken the quality of the information available for patients because they do not present an accurate picture of an individual's chance of success. This prevents them from making an informed decision about where they choose to undergo treatment.

What is important is not that one clinic's results are better than others, but how their services compare when plotted against all the other clinics in the country. Are the results in the top percentiles or not after risk-adjusting for the prognostics characteristics of patients? When clinics present their results, they should develop a graphical interface that facilitates a transparent and uncomplicated understanding for patients.

National ART surveillance data should be presented in such a way that league tables cannot be created of best- and worst-performing clinics. League tables can be highly misleading. They create incentives for clinics to focus on pregnancy rates at the expense of providing a holistic approach to fertility treatment for patients suffering from infertility. For example, success rates can be optimized by limiting treatment to good prognosis patients and reporting their results while refusing care to harder to treat patients.

Should Clinics Use ART Surveillance to Advertise Their Success Rates?

Advertising on a clinic's website or in other media claiming to have significantly better success rates compared with other clinics or the average of *all* other clinics can be misleading and is arguably deceptive. Unequivocal claims can create unrealistic expectations of live birth rates in vulnerable people needing ART treatment. This may lead them to make financial decisions to choose the clinic that *claims* to give them a better chance of realizing their dream of having a baby. It may also, in some countries, be in breach of the law. However, if patients do not have access to or do not know how to interpret standardized clinic success rates provided by national registries, resorting to website advertisement is the source from which they can make decisions about starting or continuing with treatment.

The Role of Patients' Organizations

The International Alliance of Patients' Organizations (IAPO) has identified key principles of patient-centred health care, including respect for their unique needs, preferences and values, access and support, in addition to choice, empowerment and information [14].

Patients' organizations must be empowered to play meaningful leadership roles in supporting patients to exercise their right to make informed health care choices.

Patient involvement in health policy is supported by the World Health Organization (WHO), which states that patients' organizations should engage in constructive dialogue with health professionals and be represented on appropriate scientific and professional committees. It is the opinion of the authors that ART registries need to involve patients and patients' organizations when making decisions about selecting success rates measures with the hope of providing information that is meaningful to them or use visual presentation of treatment results.

Factual, objective and comprehensive information is essential to enable patients to make informed decisions about health care treatment [15].

International organizations that have recognized and endorsed these principles include the following:

- United Nations Economic and Social Council
- WHO
- International College of Person-Centered Medicine
- World Health Professions Alliance
- International Hospital Federation

These principles, particularly with a focus on information provision, should apply to ART surveillance data, ensuring that the complex ART statistics and success rates are presented in a patient-friendly and meaningful way.

Conclusion

Health services exist because of patients. ART patients are more informed than ever. They read broadly and often challenge practitioners with new data and new therapies, some of which are of value, while others are without any proven benefit. The role of the practitioner and clinics is to assess patients for their suitability for ART, discuss the implications for them and the child to be and ensure that all relevant information has been offered prior to their informed decision to proceed with treatment.

Including a patient representative on licensing bodies in the regulation of ART will ensure transparency and can build public confidence in the accuracy of ART surveillance data. In Australia, this has proved effective and is evidence of the continuing cooperation between all stakeholders: health professionals, government and, most significantly, patients.

Dealing with patients as partners and not passive recipients has been recommended by WHO, which states that there is a need for the profession to have a constructive dialogue with consumer groups in which both sides can listen to each other and talk to each other [16].

In working towards a model that meets the needs of all stakeholders, consumers seek a spirit of cooperation, which will ensure transparency and quality in the delivery of infertility services [17]. This is

appropriate, as it is patients who will live with the consequences of policy and treatment decisions.

References

1. The authors' combined more than 25 years' experience.

2. Wilkinson J, Roberts SA, Showell M, Brison DR. No common denominator: a review of outcome measures in IVF RCTs. *Hum Reprod.* 2016;**31**:2714–22.

3. Hammarberg K, Prentice T, Purcell I, Johnson J. Quality of information about success rates provided on assisted reproductive technology clinic websites in Australia and New Zealand. *Aust N Z J Obstet Gynaecol.* 2018;**58**:330–4.

4. Dickey RP, Sartor BM, Pyrzak R. What is the most relevant standard of success in assisted reproduction?: no single outcome measure is satisfactory when evaluating success in assisted reproduction; both twin births and singleton births should be counted as successes. *Hum Reprod.* 2004;**19**:783–7.

5. Emery M. Which issues concerning multiple pregnancies should be addressed during psychosocial counselling? *Reprod Biomed Online.* 2007; **15**(Suppl 3):18–21.

6. Zegers-Hochschild F, Adamson GD, Dyer S, Racowsky C, de Mouzon J, Sokol R, et al. The International Glossary on Infertility and Fertility Care, 2017. *Hum Reprod.* 2017;**32**(9):1786–801.

7. *Reproductive Technology Accreditation Committee (RTAC) of the Fertility Society of Australia (FSA) Code of Practice.* 2017. Available at: www.fertilitysociety .com/rtac/.

8. Practice Committee of the American Society for Reproductive Medicine. Practice Committee of the Society for Assisted Reproductive Technology. Guidance on the limits to the number of embryos to transfer: a committee opinion. *Fertil Steril.* 2017;**107** (4):901–3.

9. Luke B, Brown MB, Wantman E, Stern JE, Baker VL, Gibbons W, et al. A prediction model for live birth after assisted reproductive technology. *Fertil Steril.* 2014;**102**:744–52.

10. Society for Assisted Reproductive Technology. What are my chances with ART? Society for Assisted Reproductive Technology. Available at: www .sartcorsonline.com/predictor/patient, accessed April 2018.

11. McLernon DJ, Steyerberg EW, Te Velde ER, Lee AJ, Bhattacharya S. Predicting the chances of live birth after one or more complete cycles of in vitro fertilization: population based study of linked cycle data from 113,873 women. *BMJ.* 2016;**355**:i5735.51.

12. University of Aberdeen. Outcome prediction in subfertility. Available at: https://w3.abdn.ac.uk/clsm/opis, accessed April 2018.

13. Fitzgerald O, Harris K, Paul RC, Chambers GM. *Assisted Reproductive Technology in Australia and New Zealand 2015*. Sydney: National Perinatal Epidemiology and Statistics Unit, the University of New South Wales Sydney; 2017.

14. International Alliance of Patients' Organizations home page. Available at: www.iapo.org.uk.

15. Vayena E, Rowe PJ, Griffin PD (eds.). *Current Practices and Controversies in Assisted Reproduction: Report of a Meeting on 'Medical, Ethical and Social Aspects of Assisted Reproduction'*. Geneva: WHO; 2001.

16. Fathalla MF. Current challenges in assisted reproduction. In E Vayena, PJ Rowe, PD Griffin (eds.), *Current Practices and Controversies in Assisted Reproduction: Report of a Meeting on 'Medical, Ethical and Social Aspects of Assisted Reproduction'*. Geneva: WHO; 2001.

17. Dill S. Consumer perspectives. In E Vayena, PJ Rowe, PD Griffin (eds.), *Current Practices and Controversies in Assisted Reproduction: Report of a Meeting on 'Medical, Ethical and Social Aspects of Assisted Reproduction'*. Geneva: WHO; 2001.

Chapter

11

Global ART Surveillance: The International Committee Monitoring Assisted Reproductive Technologies (ICMART)

G. David Adamson

History of ICMART's Global Art Surveillance

The Early Years[*]

The first meeting of professionals responsible for existing or planned national registries was arranged by Paul Lancaster (Australia) and Jacques de Mouzon (France) in Oxford in 1990, resulting in the creation of the International Working Group for Registers on Assisted Reproduction (IWGROAR). The first real world report was given by Paul Lancaster at the 7th World Congress on In Vitro Fertilization and Assisted Procreations in Paris in June 1991 concerning procedures performed in 1989. The scientific committee for the 1993 Eighth World Congress asked Jean Cohen from France to prepare a world report for procedures for 1991.

In order to make the report as complete as possible, it was decided there would be a collaboration between Dr Cohen and representatives of IWGROAR, namely, Drs Lancaster, de Mouzon and Fernando Zegers-Hochschild from Chile. For the 1991 data, a questionnaire was established from the one that had already been used by IWGROAR for 1989 data. This questionnaire was distributed to the responsible individuals of existing national or supranational registries, 31 countries reporting to 18 registries. In countries in which such registries did not exist, contacts were made with different known doctors asking them to provide a list of units doing ART procedures in their countries, resulting in completed questionnaires from 61 units in 15 countries [1].

The IWGROAR continued to collect international data and obtained an agreement with Dr Cohen, then President of the International Federation of Fertility Societies (IFFS), to publish a report on procedures performed in 1993 during the IFFS World Congress on ART in Montpellier in 1995 [2].

The 1995 data were then presented at the World Congresses on ART in Vancouver in 1997 and for the first time in a report published in a journal [3]. In 1997, Dr Karl Nygren from Sweden joined IWGROAR. The 1996 data were presented at the 16th World Congress on Fertility and Sterility, a combined American Society for Reproductive Medicine (ASRM)/IFFS meeting in San Francisco in 1998 [4].

Dr Karl Nygren was elected Chair of IWGROAR in 1997. In 1999, Dr David Adamson, a reproductive endocrinologist from the United States (US), joined IWGROAR. All the individuals joining IWGROAR had extensive experience with registries in their own country/region: Dr Lancaster with the Australia/New Zealand registry, Drs Nygren and de Mouzon with Europe, Dr Fernando Zegers-Hochschild with Latin America and Dr Adamson with the US.

Data for the 1998 world report were collected by two different mechanisms: directly from regional reports already existing in Australia/New Zealand, Latin America, the US and Europe, and indirectly from those countries not covered by regional reports. Lists of countries were kept by Jacques de Mouzon and also by Bernard Hedon from IFFS. Data collection forms were created by IWGROAR based on those used by the European Society of Human Reproduction and Embryology (ESHRE) and the other registries; ESHRE forms were particularly helpful because more than 50% of cycles were reported on their forms. A letter explaining why this world effort to collect data was being done and how the forms should be filled in was written by Karl Nygren. Special emphasis was placed on the necessity for precise definitions. At the IFFS meeting in Melbourne in 2001, IWGROAR presented the 1998 data [5].

---

[*] The early history of international registries is provided in more detail in Chapter 2.

By 2001, IWGROAR had also developed standardized international definitions to be presented at the World Health Organization (WHO) in September 2001. It also had developed guidelines for countries that wished to establish and/or improve their own ART registries. The adopted strategy was that in vitro fertilization (IVF) centres should report data only once and that the international reports should be compiled from national or regional reports.

In 2001, IWGROAR requested funding from IFFS, and also from the Bertarelli Foundation, for its work. Consideration was also given to requesting funds from other professional organizations such as ASRM, the Society for Assisted Reproductive Technology (SART) and ESHRE. However, as an informal group, no funding was received. IWGROAR continued its work on a completely voluntary basis, with the IWGROAR members responsible for all the costs associated with their work.

Formation and Organization of ICMART

In 2001, IWGROAR simplified its name somewhat to IWGRAR. Since there had been no funding from other organizations, IWGRAR also decided to begin the process to become an independent non-profit organization. The new organization was named the International Committee Monitoring Assisted Reproductive Technologies (ICMART). ICMART was incorporated in California on 29 January 2003 by Dr David Adamson and was organized as a 501(c)(3) non-profit organization. This incorporation was ratified at the first Board meeting of ICMART in Cairo, Egypt, on 8 October 2003. Dr Karl Nygren was elected Chairman of the Board and Chief Executive Officer, and Dr David Adamson became Chief Financial Officer and Secretary. Board members elected were Drs Jacques de Mouzon, Paul Lancaster, Fernando Zegers-Hochschild and Professor Elizabeth Sullivan (Australia). ICMART engaged an accounting firm and a legal firm to provide necessary advice and guidance in these activities.

Dr Ragaa Mansour (Egypt) became a board member in 2004. Subsequently, Osamu Ishihara joined as a Regional Representative in 2005 and became a board member in 2015. Manish Banker (India) became a Regional Representative in 2012. Elizabeth Sullivan retired from the board in 2015 and Georgina Chambers became the Regional Representative for Australia/New Zealand. Paul Lancaster retired from the board in 2009 and was recognized as Honorary Past Chair.

In 2011, Dr Nygren became Past Chair, Dr Adamson became Chair and Professor Elizabeth Sullivan became Secretary Treasurer. In 2015, Dr Karl Nygen retired from the Board as Honorary Past Chair. In 2015, Dr Jacques de Mouzon became Secretary Treasurer. In 2017, the position was divided, with Dr de Mouzon remaining Secretary and Professor Osamu Ishihara becoming Treasurer.

In its incorporation, ICMART defined its mission to collect, analyze and publish data from ART registries globally on utilization, effectiveness and safety; help standardize the practice of ART through standardized definitions; increase the number and quality of registries globally; and increase global awareness and acceptance of ART.

Over the ensuing years, ICMART pursued its mission with the unrestricted financial assistance of the following professional organizations: ASRM, SART, ESHRE, Red Latinoamericana de Reproducción Asistida (REDLARA), Fertility Society of Australia (FSA), Japan Society for Reproductive Medicine (JSRM), Japan Society of Fertilization and Implantation (JSFI), Asia Pacific Initiative Reproduction and Embryology (ASPIRE) and Middle East Fertility Society (MEFS). In addition, ICMART received restricted funds from the Bertarelli Foundation, the government of Canada for projects, the World Health Organization for expenses in WHO projects and, more recently, ongoing unrestricted financial support from Ferring. It would have been impossible for ICMART to enjoy the success it has had without the generous support of these organizations, for which it is profoundly grateful.

ICMART Activities

In 2004, ICMART collaborated with the Bertarelli Foundation and received financial support to biennially produce and disseminate a world report using an international register monitoring the procedures and outcomes of ART using standardized forms. Two years later, ICMART had accomplished these goals. It had published its IVF world report in *Fertility and Sterility*; re-published its glossary, previously published with WHO, in both *Human Reproduction* and *Fertility and Sterility*; presented preliminary world data for 2002 at ESHRE and ASRM annual meetings; held 'Contributors' Meetings' at these two meetings; started data collection for the next world report; prepared a symposium, in cooperation with WHO, for the 2007 IFFS meeting in Durban; and started contacts for possible data collection in Japan, Vietnam, India and China.

ICMART continued its focus on activities of data collection, both the actual collection as well as improvement in participating registries and initiation of registries in countries that did not yet have them. An important aspect of this was development of the ICMART Toolbox, an online website tool that provided step-by-step details for collecting and submitting national and regional registry data to ICMART. In addition, starting in 2010 ICMART began annual presentations of preliminary results at ESHRE. It also began publishing its annual report alternately in *Human Reproduction* and *Fertility and Sterility* [6, 7, 8, 9, 10, 11, 12, 13, 14]. Reports and other information about ICMART were placed on its website (www.icmartivf.org).

In 2009, ICMART was invited to participate in the First International Forum on Cross-Border Reproductive Care: Quality and Safety, sponsored by Assisted Human Reproduction Canada, in Ottawa, Canada. ICMART was commissioned to provide data on this topic and received a Government of Canada grant to do so. Karl Nygren presented the paper 'Fertility Patients' Experiences of Cross-Border Reproductive Health Care' [15]. This work with the government of Canada was followed by another research grant: 'Cross-Border Reproductive Care in North America: A Pilot Study Testing a Prospective Data Collection Program for IVF Clinics in Canada and the United States'. This research project was carried out with a second Government of Canada grant and the results of the research presented to the government and published [16].

Additionally, ICMART increased its collaboration with national and regional registries, helping to improve and expand registries within countries and regions, as well as internationally. The focus was and is on developing countries and regions. ICMART activities included publishing articles and book chapters, presenting abstracts at various congresses, and organizing major symposia and workshops including in Cairo, Tokyo, Thessaloniki (in cooperation with ESHRE) and Durban.

These activities were quite successful, resulting in the organization or further development of national and regional registries. These and subsequent activities have been led by Fernando Zegers in Latin America (REDLARA), Karl Nygren with the

European IVF Monitoring Consortium (EIM), Jacques de Mouzon with EIM and Groupe Interafricain d'Etude, de Recherche et d'Application sur la Fertilité (GIERAF), Silke Dyer with the South African Register of Assisted Reproductive Techniques (SARA) and the African Network and Registry for ART (ANARA), Ragaa Mansour with the MEFS, Manish Banker with the National ART Registry of India (NARI), Osamu Ishihara in Japan with JSRM and JSFI, and Elizabeth Sullivan and Georgina Chambers with the Australia/New Zealand Registry. In particular, REDLARA and Fernando Zegers gave exceptional assistance and support to the development of ANARA. David Adamson helped direct the activities globally.

Meetings of the many contributors who manage the national and regional registries were begun at ESHRE and ASRM annual meetings in 2005. These have been very successful in bringing the interested and working parties together. Sharing of information has led to much faster progress and the building of professional relationships. Additionally, these meetings have encouraged many of the contributors to continue and expand their efforts in their own countries.

Finally, ICMART Board members and Regional Representatives have given many presentations globally over the past 29 years to increase understanding of ART on a global basis.

ICMART has maintained a constructive and collaborative relationship with the IFFS, with Dr Adamson serving on the Board of IFFS as the ASRM representative from 2007 to 2014 and ex officio executive committee member since 2014. ICMART has also participated with the IFFS, ASRM, ESHRE and FIGO in meetings to promote collaboration and integration of global initiatives in women's reproductive health.

On an organizational basis, ICMART partnered with the Uppsala Clinical Research Center (UCR) at the University of Uppsala in Uppsala, Sweden, in 2007. They have a large, internationally recognized epidemiological and research centre with a great deal of experience in registries. After ICMART collects the international data annually, UCR formats and checks the arithmetic of the data so that errors can be identified and fixed. UCR creates a final corrected dataset that is reviewed by all ICMART members and then closed. ICMART members prepare the manuscript for publication with a rotating authorship, alternating publication between *Fertility and Sterility* and *Human Reproduction*.

As ICMART's activities have expanded, it has become necessary to increase logistical support. Historically, all aspects of organization support were provided by the Board members and their staff in their institutions. However, in 2015 an organization support company was engaged to provide additional support for ICMART. Eventually, the intention is for International Convention Services (ICS) to provide all the logistical support needed by ICMART.

ICMART Relationship with the World Health Organization (WHO)

By 2001, IWGROAR had also developed standardized international definitions. Due largely to Dr Zegers' relationships at the WHO with Drs Paul van Look, Paddy Rowe and Ian Cooke, a consultant to the WHO from the United Kingdom (UK), it was arranged to present these definitions at a WHO meeting in Geneva, Switzerland, 17–21 September 2001. This meeting on medical, ethical and social aspects of assisted reproduction involved the Department of Reproductive Health and Research (RHR) including UNDP/UNFPA/ UNICEF/WHO/World Bank Special Programme of Research, Development and Research Training in Human Reproduction (HRP). This meeting and subsequent discussions resulted in collaboration between RHR and IWGRAR to develop guidelines for national registries; these were implemented in subsequent world reports. At the 12th World Congress on IVF and Molecular Reproduction, another meeting elaborated details of the collaboration and work plan. Studies on increased malformation rates of ART babies underlined the critical role of ART data collection in determining both the efficacy and safety of ART, and its potential to become a public health problem [17]. However, it was noted that not all countries where ART was practised had established a reporting system.

IWGRAR had already established techniques for data collection, published five world reports on the outcomes of ART and identified globally important regions to expand its network. IWGRAR produced a template for a registry based on its existing data collection forms, which were then tailored to the needs of individual countries and used for the development of a national registry.

RHR's role was seen in the review of the template and its dissemination in the countries which needed it. RHR was not involved with the actual data collection or with the development of a worldwide database. It was felt RHR's extensive network of collaborative centres, regional institutions and professionals would enable it to play a crucial educational role in the dissemination of a validated mechanism for the collection of data.

It was decided that resources would be best used if a workshop were held in one of the regions that was interested in establishing registries. The workshop would help with the assessment of local needs and support the implementation of the registry. Such activity could be organized in collaboration with the local professional society/ministry.

A work plan was established in which IWGRAR prepared the template, which included an introduction stressing the importance of establishing a national registry and an actual format for data collection and included the ART definitions modified after the September 2002 meeting at ESHRE in Vienna. Outside reviewers were included in collaboration with RHR. The final document was produced by IWGRAR by the end of August 2002. The workshop venue was chosen to be the Middle East Fertility Society in Cairo in October 2003. Generous sponsors of the meeting were Ferring, along with the sponsors of ICMART – ASRM, ESHRE, SART and REDLARA.

The meeting, organized under the leadership of Dr Ragaa Mansour, was a major success. Titled 'Strategies for National Registers to Monitor the Efficacy and Safety of ART', several hundred clinical and laboratory representatives from almost all countries in the Middle East attended, as well as the Egyptian Minister of Health, the President of the Egyptian Medical Syndicate, Effy Vayena from WHO and other important representatives such as Mohamed Aboulghar and Gamal Serour.

During the early 2000s, WHO, specifically Effy Vayena and Paddy Rowe, participated in a number of international symposia and workshops with ICMART, described as a 'technical cooperation'. These opportunities were used to describe the WHO position on infertility care worldwide and to promote the importance of infertility as a global health problem [18]. This WHO participation and collaboration was very helpful in promoting improvement and expansion of registries.

ICMART worked with WHO to publish a glossary simultaneously in *Human Reproduction* and *Fertility and Sterility* in 2006 [19, 20]. Further collaboration resulted in a revised 2009 glossary [21, 22]. Of particular note in the 2009 glossary was the new definition of 'infertility', in which it is defined as a disease for the first time.

In 2009, ICMART had continued its many relationships with WHO and decided to apply for non-governmental organization (NGO) status. In this regard, it was directed and helped by Dr Sheryl van der Poel, who had become ICMART's contact person at WHO. In its application it was stated, "The specific purpose of this corporation is to research and collect data, prepare reports and analyze information regarding Assisted Reproductive Technologies and to function as a technical advisor to other organizations, such as the World Health Organization, in connection with Assisted Reproductive Technologies." At the 126th session in January 2010, the WHO Executive Board admitted ICMART into official relations with the WHO. ICMART's relationship as an NGO, later changed to non-state actor (NSA), has continued since that time. In the intervening years, ICMART has participated as Co-chair of the Rapid Assessment Task Force with Ian Cooke, as well as on the Infertility Guidelines project and the ICD-11 project (the International Classification of Diseases, 11th edition). The glossary was then revised again, with much assistance but without the formal endorsement or inclusion of WHO as an author, in 2017 [23, 24]. In all of these activities, ICMART received very significant support and direction from Dr Sheryl van der Poel at WHO, and also assistance from Dr Marlene Temmerman, Dr Igor Toskin and Dr Stephen Nurse-Findlay. More recently, ICMART has had the opportunity to work with Dr Ian Askew, Dr James Kiarie and Dr Thabo Matsaseng, who are giving strong support to new initiatives on infertility guidelines and access to infertility care.

The Global Art Glossary

Glossaries are important because terms, especially if not carefully constructed, can have different meanings in different settings and with different people. For example, non-biological terms such as 'conception' can have many arguable connotations and ramifications, inaccurate terms such as 'spontaneous' can imply non-realistic events (e.g. 'spontaneous' pregnancy requires an act of coitus) or words can be potentially pejorative if they make a desirable opposite, for example 'natural' versus

'unnatural'. The terminology we use defines how we think about all aspects of our professional work, including clinical, scientific, ethical, legal, sociological and psychological issues. Important characteristics of a glossary are that it is empirically and scientifically based, created through general consensus, unambiguous and comprehensive for all cases. A glossary determines the breadth of our field of interest and standardizes and harmonizes the terms. This benefits clinicians, laboratory scientists, researchers, professionals, policy makers, other stakeholders and the public. Such harmonization is essential for accurate and effective communication, writing, research, policy and advocacy. It is essential to our assessment of diagnosis, treatment interventions, utilization, effectiveness and safety of infertility and fertility care and ART.

Furthermore, the way terms are defined can sometimes affect their psychological impact and social acceptance, and this can affect how reproductive medicine is practised in a region or country. For example, the difference between a zygote and an embryo can be significant, as can the term 'spontaneous abortion' versus 'miscarriage'. The gestational age at which a miscarriage/abortion becomes a stillbirth affects individual case documentation and subsequent calculations of miscarriage and perinatal mortality rates. Similarly, by defining infertility as a disease of the reproductive system that can lead to disability, equity of access to fertility treatments has been facilitated during debate and decision making at regional and national levels.

ICMART's activities in glossary development have been led by Dr Fernando Zegers-Hochschild since 2000. The first international standardized definitions for reporting ART procedures were published by the International Committee Monitoring Assisted Reproductive Technologies (ICMART) in 2006 as the 'ICMART Glossary on ART Terminology' [19, 20]. This document resulted from an ICMART initiative, presented and documented within the meeting report 'Medical, Ethical and Social Aspects of Assisted Reproduction' and published by WHO, in 2002. In 2008, WHO, together with ICMART, the Low-Cost IVF Foundation and the International Federation of Fertility Societies (IFFS), organized an international consensus consultation on 'Assisted Reproductive Technologies: Common Terminology and Management in Low-Resource Settings', again held at WHO in Geneva, Switzerland. WHO was responsible for steering and management of the consensus consultation, with expert technical lead provided from ICMART, which resulted in the first revision of the glossary [21, 22].

The 2017 glossary revision was led by Dr Fernando Zegers-Hochschild and ICMART, with participation of WHO and the support and collaboration of 108 international experts, including clinicians, basic scientists, epidemiologists and social scientists, along with national and regional representatives of infertile persons. Collectively, these individuals represented almost all major reproductive medicine organizations in the world [23, 24]. They collaborated in a consensus process to develop the evidence-based, revised and greatly expanded glossary. Thus, the reproductive medicine community now has a comprehensive, expert, consensus-based, standardized and harmonized set of definitions by which all global stakeholders can communicate. Importantly, this glossary is now being translated into multiple languages, including Spanish, Portuguese, Russian and others.

The ICMART World Reports

The Value of Global Data Collection

Individual ART centres collect data to monitor their own procedures, improve their results, perform research, inform their patients and provide data for publications. International research programs are generally multicentre epidemiological studies rather than a multinational registry program and primarily serve to identify rare but important events. Global data collection such as that done by ICMART has the goal of describing the worldwide use of ART, identifying access, effectiveness and safety, and identifying similarities, differences and trends. ICMART is the only global ART registry, and so has many unique characteristics, attributes and challenges.

Data collection, analysis and reporting of global ART activity are important for multiple reasons. For providers, the data provide an external quality control to compare themselves with others in the same region, enable the region to compare itself with others in the world and enable monitoring to improve quality. For patients, the data give information about reasonable expectations, enhance treatment decision making and inform about services possibly not available in the local jurisdiction. For policy makers, the data inform about utilization and access, provide information on which to base

health care policy and enhance the ability to provide appropriate regulatory oversight. For society, the data educate about the capabilities of fertility treatments, reduce ignorance and fear of ART and increase public support for infertility care.

ICMART has standardized data collection forms that are now in an electronic online portal. The following data are collected: type of registry, number and size of clinics and proportion reporting; type (fresh, frozen, donor, preimplantation genetic testing (PGT)) and number of ART procedures by cycle start and aspiration for IVF and intracytoplasmic sperm injection (ICSI); pregnancy outcomes by clinical pregnancy, miscarriages, premature delivery, live births, stillbirths and perinatal mortality; number of embryos transferred and pregnancy rates, delivery rates, twins and triplets by number of embryos transferred; pregnancy rates and delivery rates by IVF, ICSI, frozen embryo transfer (FET) and donor egg; number of babies reported and estimated; distribution of female age; pregnancy outcomes by women's age; bleeding and ovarian hyperstimulation syndrome (OHSS) complications; availability of in vitro maturation (IVM), fetal reduction and gestational carrier; oocyte donation results; preimplantation genetic testing results; results by age of intrauterine insemination with husband/partner sperm; results by age of intrauterine insemination with donor sperm; cross-border reproductive care.

Types of Registries

Different regions of the world have different types of registries. Some are voluntary and some mandatory or obligatory, either by government regulation (with potential societal legal sanctions) or by professional requirements (with potential professional sanctions). Mandatory registries almost always have complete or almost complete data, while voluntary registries often do not. Mandatory registries generally make more data public than do voluntary registries, including clinic-specific and identifiable outcomes. This has led in some environments to competition among clinics and clinical and reporting activities that enhance published results [25].

ICMART collects data generally from large multinational registries such as EIM (Europe), REDLARA (Latin America), FSA (Australia/New Zealand) and now ANARA (Africa). However, it also collects data from national registries such as SART and NASS (US), JSRM (Japan), ISAR (India) and many others.

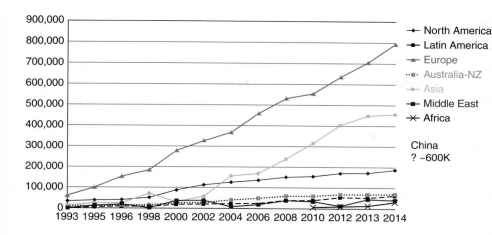

Figure 11.1 Growth of ART cycles by region. A colour version of the figure is provided in the plate section.

In a few cases in which countries don't have national or regional registries, ICMART collects data from individual clinics.

There are at least two methodologies to collect data. Data can involve national/regional collection and analysis of clinic result summaries: each clinic gives an annual summary report of all their cycles; these data from reporting clinics are then aggregated to a national report. The advantage of this method is that it is relatively simple and inexpensive, but the major disadvantage is that it is less informative. The second method involves centralized individual-based data collection (cycle-based or case-by-case). These individualized data from the clinics constitute the national/regional registry data. In the second method, the entire cycle can be followed, and the treatment interventions can be connected to the outcomes, so research can be done on multiple factors influencing selected outcomes of interest. This is not possible with summary/aggregated datasets, so the data in them are less useful. However, such registries are more difficult to maintain, are more expensive and require a uniform data collection system.

Of note, most cycle-based registries still cannot link all the cycles to a single patient's treatment over time and so cumulative pregnancy rates from multiple cycles, fresh and/or frozen, can only be estimated for the population. The optimal registry that collects individual cycle data that can also be linked to each patient throughout all of their treatment, and even treatment for subsequent pregnancy attempts, is exceptionally difficult to create and manage because of privacy rules, changes in treatment location, changes in names, incomplete patient history, cross-border care, lack of

electronic records and other problems. Such a registry is currently only a future goal in almost all countries.

Utilization of ART

In 1991, there were 25 countries that reported 140,000 ART cycles. By 2014, there were 77 countries and 2,734 clinics reporting 1,648,000 cycles [26] (Fig. 11.1). The 10 largest contributors, in order, were Japan, US, Spain, Russia, France, Germany, Italy, Australia, UK and Israel. Europe contributed 47% of the cycles, Asia 30%, North America 12%, Latin America 5%, Middle East 3%, Australia 3% and Africa 1%. Europe has been the largest contributor of cycles, but Asia is increasing quickly, and does not include China, which does not currently report and is thought to perform over 500,000 cycles of ART per year. It is estimated that, excluding China, approximately 2.3 to 2.6 million cycles were performed in 2014 and, including China, approximately 3 million.

The percentage of the population with access to ART varies greatly globally. For example, Denmark has approximately 6% of the population born from ART, Australia/New Zealand about 4%, Japan about 3%, UK and France about 2%, US about 1.5%, and most countries well under 1%. The factors affecting access to ART are complex. They involve affordability, availability and acceptability [27, 28]. Affordability varies greatly among countries [29]. ICMART data provide availability information through documenting the number of clinics. The geographic distribution within a country is also important. Acceptability is a bilateral relationship; the patient must be acceptable to the service (ART), and in turn the service must be acceptable to the patient. For example, ART is more acceptable to some people than others, and certain types of ART services are not acceptable to providers and/or patients in some countries and/or cultures [30]. When infertile people cannot obtain care in their own country because of regulatory limitations, cultural boundaries, affordability, quality of care or other reasons, they often pursue cross-border reproductive care [31]. These factors all affect national and regional utilization rates of ART.

Profile of Procedures and Patients

The types of ART procedures performed have changed over time. For example, gamete intrafallopian transfer (GIFT) represented 4.6% of cycles in 1995 but only 0.3% in 2002. ICSI, however, increased from 0% in 1990 to 52.0% in 2000, 60% in 2004 and 66.6% in 2007, from which time it has been fairly constant, at 70.6% in 2014. These data show that clinicians have been quick to adopt effective new technologies and also are prepared to abandon those that aren't useful. Similarly, FET has also increased significantly from 8.8% of fresh and frozen cycles in 1991 to 32.0% in 2014. Oocyte donation cycles increased from 2.0% of cycles in 1991 to 7.1% of cycles in 2014.

However, these trends are not evenly distributed globally. ICSI is performed in almost all cases in the Middle East, 90.5% in Africa, 85.5% in Latin America and over 75.8% in North America, 71.5% in Europe, 66.0% in Australia/New Zealand and 63.6% in Japan. The reasons for these differences are not well defined, but are likely related to sociocultural aspects, economics of health care and other unknown factors.

In addition to changes in types of ART procedures over time, the characteristics of patients have changed. One of the most significant is age of patients. In 1991, only 9.1% of women undergoing ART were 40 years of age or older; in 2014, 27.1% of women were. This is likely due to a combination of improved technology and success rates, increasing affordability through insurance/government coverage in more affluent countries, societal trends accepting older motherhood and perhaps other reasons.

Effectiveness of ART

Infertility is now defined as "a disease characterized by the failure to establish a clinical pregnancy after 12 months of regular unprotected sexual intercourse or due to an impairment of a person's capacity to reproduce either as an individual or with his/her partner. Fertility interventions may be initiated in less than 1 year based on medical, sexual and reproductive history, age, physical findings and diagnostic testing. Infertility is a disease, which generates disability as an impairment of function" [23, 24]. As a result, different outcomes need to be measured following fertility interventions depending on the intention/desire of the patient(s) or other stakeholder(s): these include desired end results such as live birth of a singleton, live birth of twins (often a patient desire), number of eggs/embryos frozen, cumulative live birth rate, healthy babies, absence of complications, long-term health of children and cost. Society has an interest in cost-effectiveness, value of babies to society and adherence to social norms. Therefore, it is difficult to define ART 'success' in simple terms. Furthermore, intermediate outcomes can be important, because they provide helpful information to inform patients and providers regarding clinical care and further treatment interventions. They also enable some comparisons and standardization of embryology, technology and pregnancy metrics: these include number of eggs retrieved, number of embryos transferred or cryopreserved, number of apparently 'normal' embryos, biochemical pregnancy, clinical pregnancy, ongoing pregnancy, and so forth. Hence, when defining 'effectiveness', let alone the commonly used but very non-specific term 'success', it is necessary to state which metric measures the desired outcome of the intervention being performed and state both numerator, denominator and any other qualifying factors. The most desirable outcome measure is cumulative singleton live births per initiated cycle. Total singleton live birth rate per initiated cycle takes into account not only first but also subsequent pregnancies; but data on this metric are rarely available. The most commonly available and used metric is clinical pregnancy per egg retrieval or per frozen-thawed transfer. Cumulative and total rates add less absolute and relative value with increasing age.

Globally, pregnancy rates with ART have increased from deliveries per egg retrieval cycle of 13.9% in 1991 to 18.9% in 2014. While the cumulative live birth rate is not known for 1991, it is clear from the increase in percentage of embryo freezing cycles and improved cryopreservation technology that it has increased, and in 2014 it was 28.6%.

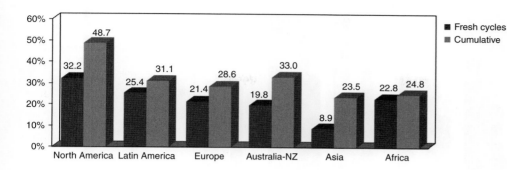

Figure 11.2 Fresh and cumulative delivery rate per aspiration for IVF/ICSI by region 2014. A colour version of the figure is provided in the plate section.

Pregnancy rates vary widely globally. There are many reasons for this in addition to quality of laboratory and clinical care. Patient populations can be very different; this is affected by demographics, sociological drivers of parenthood and health care, economics of the country, affordability of health care, insurance coverage, country perceptions of benefit (pregnancy) versus risk (complications, including multiple pregnancies), treatment protocols such as number of embryos transferred, embryo stage at transfer, use of preimplantation genetic testing (PGT), regulatory and legal environment, training and experience of personnel, quality of facilities and others. While it can be very instructive to compare countries to identify similarities and differences to be emulated or avoided, it is not easy to identify 'better' or 'worse' countries. North America has the highest live birth rate per cycle start at 32.2% and Asia the lowest at 8.9% (Fig. 11.2). North America has the highest cumulative live birth rate per cycle start at 48.7% and Asia the lowest at 23.5%. The low Asia rates are due to the large number of cycles from Japan and their extensive use of single embryo transfer, including in older patients.

Safety of ART

The first two decades of ART were largely focused on increasing the effectiveness of ART. As this occurred, it became apparent that an increased emphasis was needed on safety of ART. The major safety issues that are controlled by IVF clinics are multiple birth and ovarian hyperstimulation syndrome (OHSS); the latter is severe in less than 1% of patients and can be managed by patient selection and clinical protocols. Surgical haemorrhage, infection and anaesthesia complications are less controllable and rare, but any of these complications can result in significant morbidity or even mortality. Lack of standardized definitions and reporting mechanisms has limited the

collection of good data on ART complications. It is hoped the glossary and continued emphasis will improve these data.

Questions have also arisen regarding the safety of ICSI and abnormalities in ART babies [32, 33, 34, 35]. Outcomes may potentially be affected by epigenetics, cryopreservation, ovarian stimulation, culture time and other factors that might affect embryos, endometrium and other aspects of implantation and pregnancy. While the population of women and men undergoing ART likely represents the most significant factor in the increase in adverse outcomes, impact of ART technology intervention almost certainly has some deleterious effects, although the absolute impact is likely low.

Of note, the most important controllable factor, by far, that affects safety is the number of embryos transferred. With the rare exception of identical twinning, the number of embryos transferred determines the multiple pregnancy rate [36]. The past two decades have seen an increasing emphasis on reducing the number of embryos transferred, preferably to single embryo transfer in the great majority of cases. The percentage of cycles with two or fewer embryos transferred has increased significantly in all regions of the world since 1998 (Fig. 11.3). The average number of embryos transferred in 2014 was 1.73. At the same time, the delivery rate has increased, and the twin rate has decreased in most regions (Fig. 11.4). The triplet rate has decreased to 1% or substantially less in all regions of the world except for Latin America. Single embryo transfer is increasingly being performed, constituting 31.4% of all fresh transfers and 51.6% of all frozen transfers in 2011. More recent national and regional data confirm the trend to single embryo transfer (SET) is continuing. Japan, Australia/New Zealand and the Nordic countries have led the way in single embryo transfer.

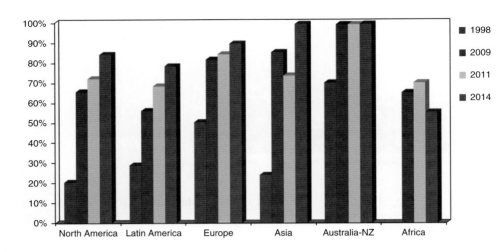

Figure 11.3 Transfers of ≤2 embryos by region, 1998 to 2014. A colour version of the figure is provided in the plate section.

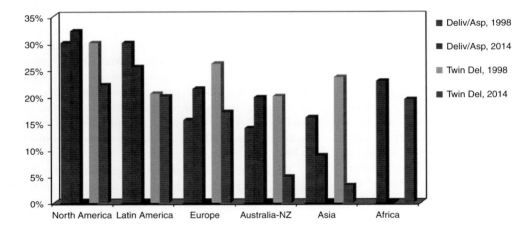

Figure 11.4 Delivery and twin delivery rate (fresh transfer/aspiration) by region, 1998 compared with 2014. A colour version of the figure is provided in the plate section.

Global practice differences are influenced by the perspective of most patients and many clinicians who believe that twin live birth is a better outcome than no live birth, and that not all singletons are healthy while approximately 90% of twins are healthy. Each child brings a cost to be created, with or without medical intervention, and to be delivered and cared for, over the short and long term. This cost must be balanced against the monetary and social value that is determined by cultural, economic and other characteristics of society. These complex factors will almost certainly continue to drive national and regional differences, but good embryo transfer policies need to be developed taking these factors into consideration and then applying good clinical judgement and informed patient consent.

Current Data Collection Challenges

ICMART and its predecessors have been collecting, analyzing, reporting and publishing global ART utilization, effectiveness and safety data since 1989. Original data collection was very rudimentary, using the collection of written reports and hand calculators. The ICMART world reports have become much more inclusive, comprehensive, accurate, sophisticated, used and useful through the application of standardized definitions, formats and computers. Nevertheless, reporting global ART is a challenging undertaking and limitations remain a reality.

The first issue is that it is not possible at this time to collect data on all ART cycles performed in the world, simply because some clinics and countries do not document all the cycles performed. Some

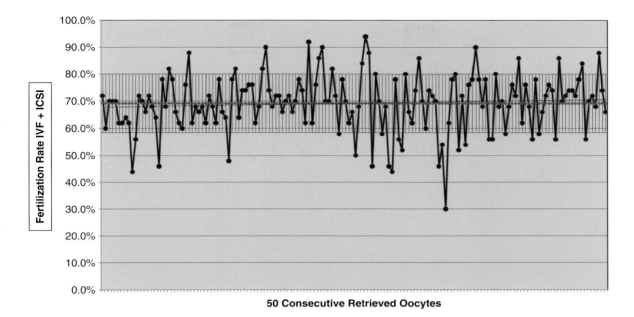

Figure 8.4 Fertilization control chart: each dot represents 50 consecutive retrieved oocytes exposed to sperm by either conventional insemination or ICSI. (Doody KJ, unpublished data)

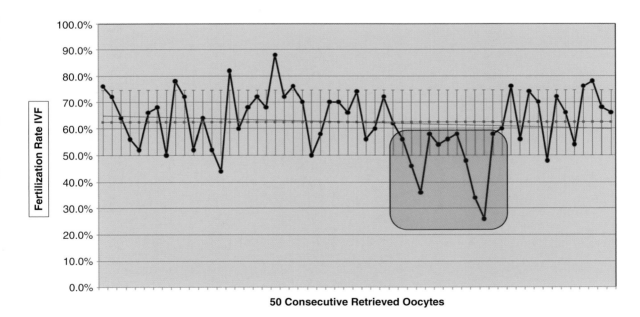

Figure 8.5 Fertilization control chart: each dot represents 50 consecutive retrieved oocytes exposed to sperm by conventional insemination with identified performance issue. (Doody KJ, unpublished data)

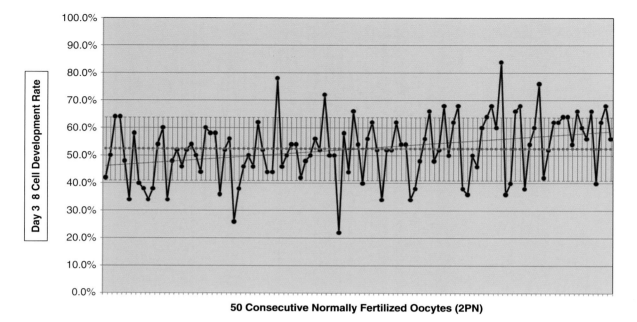

Figure 8.6 Early embryo development control chart: number of 8 cell embryos per 50 consecutive normally fertilized eggs (two-pronuclear (2PN) zygotes). (Doody KJ, unpublished data)

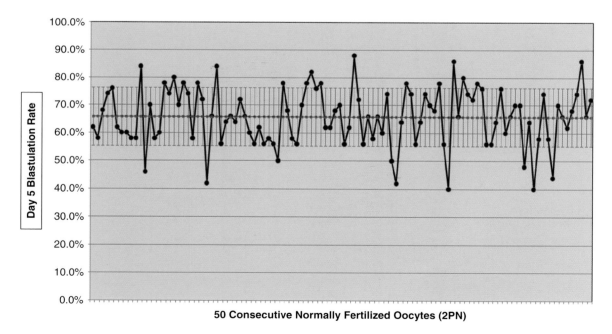

Figure 8.7 Performance graph demonstrating performance with early and late embryo culture: blastulation rate per 50 consecutive fertilized oocytes. (Doody KJ, unpublished data)

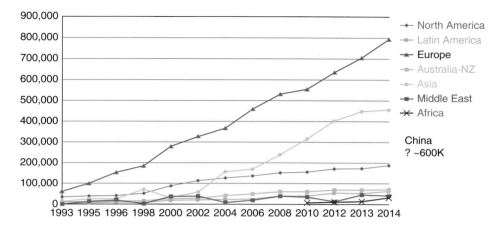

Figure 11.1 Growth of ART cycles by region.

- North America
- Latin America
- Europe
- Australia-NZ
- Asia
- Middle East
- Africa

China
? ~600K

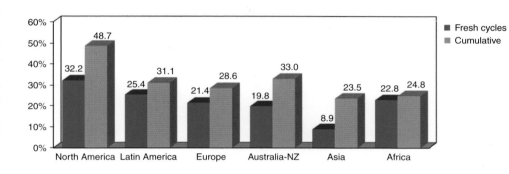

Figure 11.2 Fresh and cumulative delivery rate per aspiration for IVF/ICSI by region 2014.

- Fresh cycles
- Cumulative

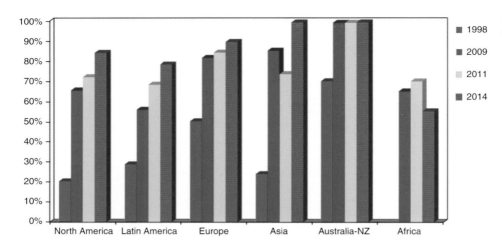

Figure 11.3 Transfers of ≤2 embryos by region, 1998 to 2014.

Legend: 1998, 2009, 2011, 2014

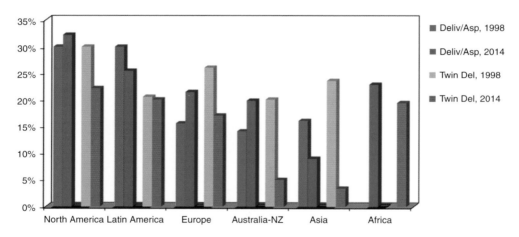

Legend: Deliv/Asp, 1998; Deliv/Asp, 2014; Twin Del, 1998; Twin Del, 2014

Figure 11.4 Delivery and twin delivery rate (fresh transfer/aspiration) by region, 1998 compared with 2014.

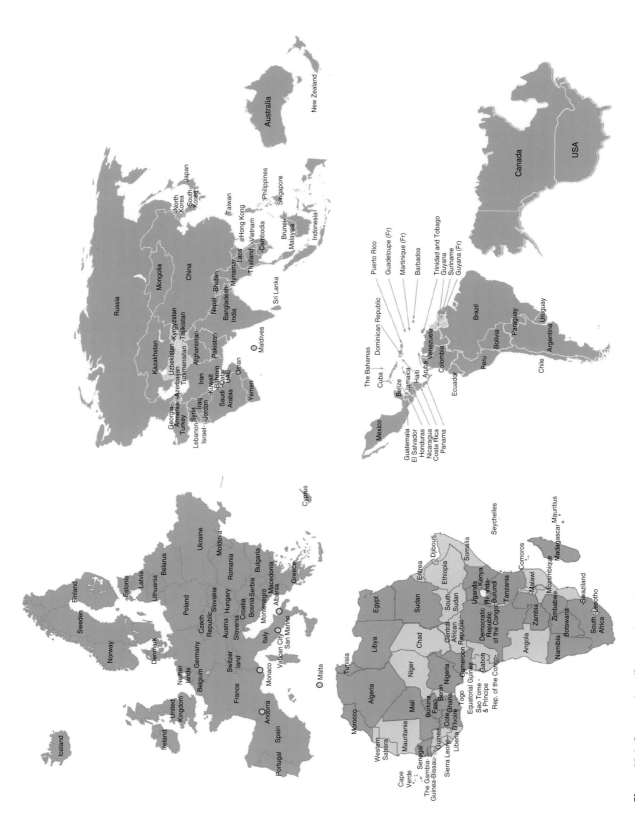

Figure 12.1 Countries that offer assisted reproductive tehnology (green).

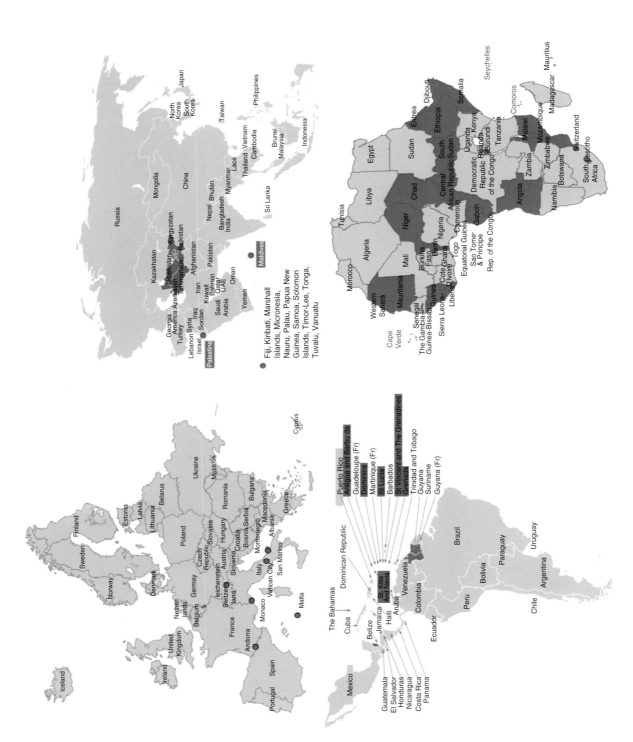

Figure 12.2 Countries that provide no assisted reproductive technology services (red).

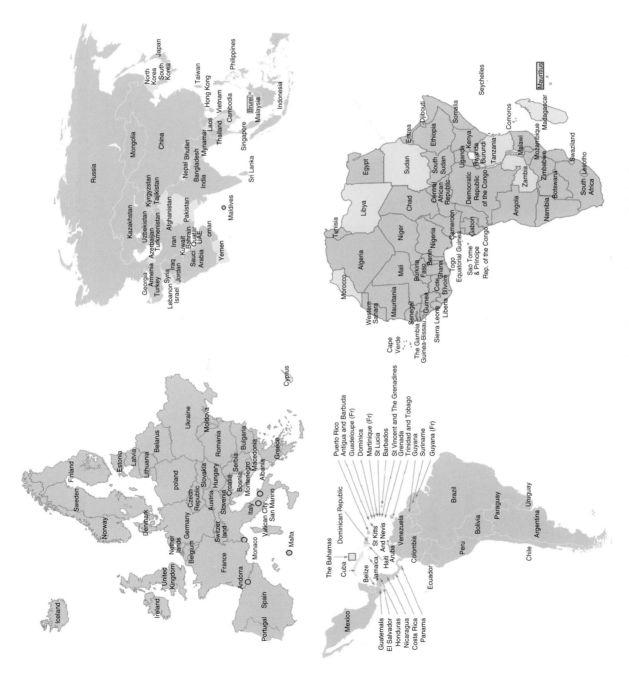

Figure 12.3 Countries with unknown status about provision of assisted reproductive technology services (light blue).

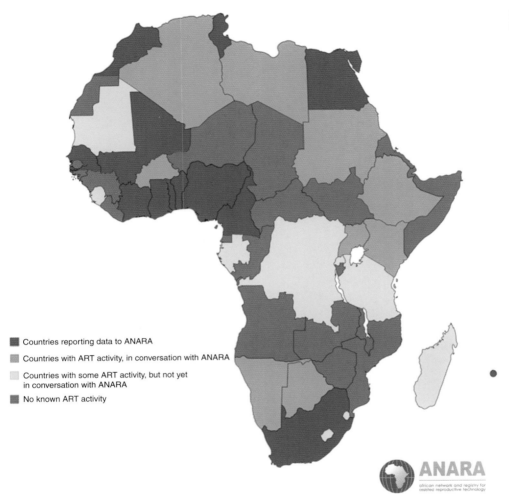

Figure 13.2 ANARA activity in Africa.

Countries reporting data to ANARA

Countries with ART activity, in conversation with ANARA

Countries with some ART activity, but not yet in conversation with ANARA

No known ART activity

ANARA
african network and registry for assisted reproductive technology

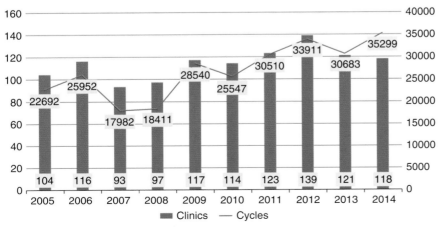

Figure 14.3 Numbers of registered clinics and cycles of ART in India.

■ Clinics ── Cycles

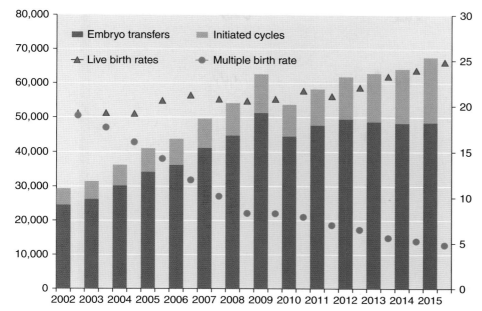

Figure 15.2 Trends in autologous ART treatment, Australia, 2002–2015.

Source: Australian and New Zealand Assisted Reproduction Database (ANZARD)

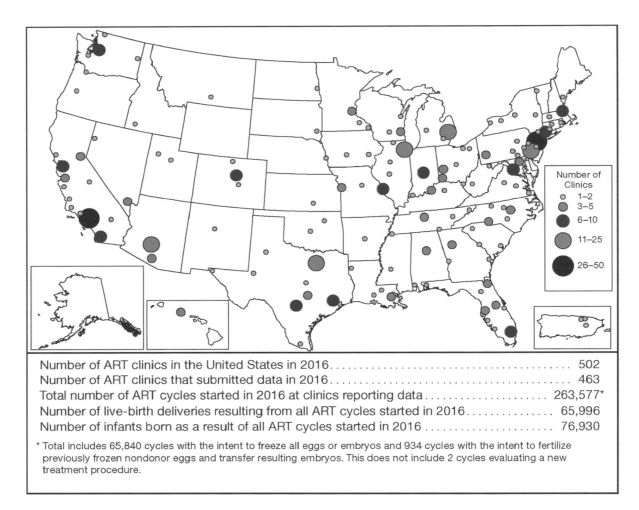

Number of ART clinics in the United States in 2016. 502
Number of ART clinics that submitted data in 2016. 463
Total number of ART cycles started in 2016 at clinics reporting data. 263,577*
Number of live-birth deliveries resulting from all ART cycles started in 2016. 65,996
Number of infants born as a result of all ART cycles started in 2016 76,930

* Total includes 65,840 cycles with the intent to freeze all eggs or embryos and 934 cycles with the intent to fertilize
  previously frozen nondonor eggs and transfer resulting embryos. This does not include 2 cycles evaluating a new
  treatment procedure.

Figure 18.1 Locations of ART Clinics in the US and Puerto Rico, 2016.

Source: Centers for Disease Control and Prevention, American Society for Reproductive Medicine, Society for Assisted Reproductive
Technology. *2016 Assisted Reproductive Technology National Summary Report.* Atlanta, GA: US Department of Health and Human Services; 2018.

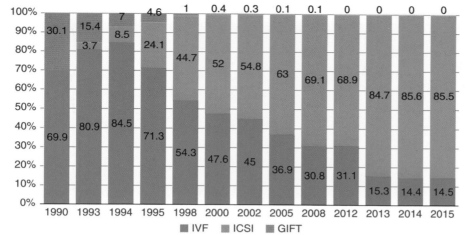

Figure 19.3 Trends in type of fertilization: retrievals.

RLA 1990–2015.

IVF, in vitro fertilization; ICSI, intracytoplasmic sperm injection; GIFT, gamete intrafallopian transfer

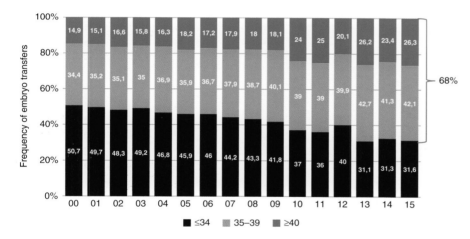

Figure 19.4 Frequency of embryo transfers in IVF/ICSI according to a woman's age.

RLA 2000–2015.

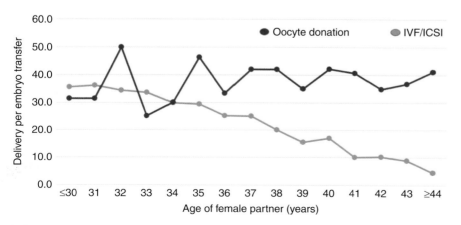

Figure 19.5 Delivery rate per embryo transfer in IVF/ICSI and OD cycles.

RLA 2015.

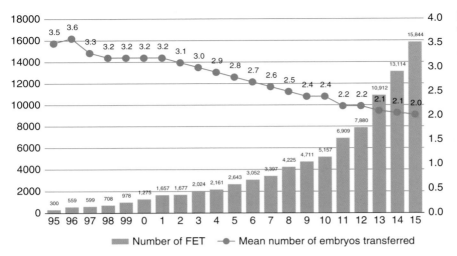

Figure 19.6 Mean number of embryos transferred and number of FET cycles.
RLA 1995–2015.

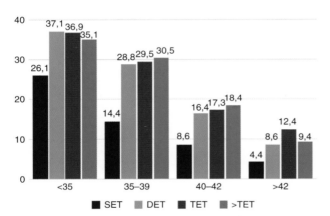

Figure 19.7 Delivery rate according to the number of embryos transferred by age of women in IVF/ICSI.
RLA 2015.
DET, double embryo transfer; SET, single embryo transfer; TET, triple embryo transfer

countries do have registries but do not report their data to ICMART, for example, Singapore. Some countries are developing registries but are not yet prepared to report to ICMART, for example, China. ICMART has limited participation from the Middle East. While it has historically been difficult to collect data in Africa, ANARA, with the strong support of REDLARA and ICMART, is making good progress promoting and developing African registries.

Many countries do not have mandatory reporting systems, so often less than 100% of the clinics report in those countries. In those countries, ICMART estimates the number of clinics reporting and the number of cycles not reported. This is done through consultation with same-country registry experts, publications and other sources of information [10].

The ICMART world reports are compiled and analyzed from regional, national and, in a few cases, individual clinic reports. Data validity is checked by ICMART with respect to arithmetic calculations and personal inquiries of the country, but ICMART has no capability to check further. Some countries and regions, such as the US, UK, Australia/New Zealand, Belgium, France, Switzerland and Latin America, have robust validation systems, but other countries do not. Until they do, which will take years in some cases, ICMART necessarily must rely on the data submitted. However, continuing improvement in overall data validity is expected, especially because ICMART's new electronic data portal, released in 2018, has enhanced data validation, which will continue to be improved in the future.

Some important variables are not collected by all countries, including intention to treat (cycle starts), use of ICSI versus IVF, day of transfer of embryos and complete data on pregnancy outcomes. While the detailed data requested by ICMART are identical for all countries, it is not possible for ICMART to report data that are not collected by countries. Intention-to-treat data are often not collected and outcomes after the first trimester are difficult because these data often must be collected by professionals who are not part of the ART clinic. However, ICMART will continue to include these important variables while recognizing the difficulties many registries face providing them.

Global ART datasets are large but also heterogeneous. Some variables are complicated to track because of treatment options and other variabilities. These include egg freezing cycles both during infertility treatment concurrently and for fertility preservation and use in later years. Embryos from a single retrieval might be used fresh and then frozen. 'Freeze-all' embryo cycles can be particularly problematic because multiple embryo transfers may subsequently occur and not even in the same reporting year, and with or without PGT. Furthermore, the best embryo(s) will generally be transferred first.

Preimplantation genetic testing (PGT) complicates the reporting of outcomes. When it is done for specific diseases (PGT-M), a statistical percentage will not be used (although those embryos diagnosed to have just carrier status might be) and so the number of embryos that can be used is likely reduced significantly. When PGT is performed for aneuploidy (PGT-A) and/or structural rearrangements (PGT-SR), some embryos will be diagnosed as abnormal/mosaic and this will reduce the number available for transfer, even though some tested abnormal/mosaic might actually be normal. Embryos tested normal, however, have higher implantation rates. Therefore, reporting PGT cycles can be complex because different outcomes and pregnancy rates are to be expected. Different PGT platforms can give different results, different practices use different protocols regarding interpretation of results (e.g. mosaic embryos), and so pregnancy rates would understandably vary. While PGT appears to help increase the selection of an embryo with a higher chance of implantation, overall the reproductive potential of the cycle is reduced because of damage during biopsy, platform testing errors, mosaicism and mis-categorization of embryos.

Complex and standardized rules for linking retrievals with transfers need to be developed and then followed by all registries to increase interpretability of reported results. On a global basis, these difficult issues are just beginning to be addressed. Safety variables such as ovarian hyperstimulation syndrome and maternal and neonatal outcomes have been variably reported in the past, although the revised glossary has attempted to standardize these. Further, until individual longitudinal, patient-identifiable and cycle-based data are collected universally, it will not be possible to calculate individual patient cumulative outcomes. New methods of doing so are being created by different national and regional registries. Currently, ICMART approximates these outcomes with estimates and algorithms [10].

Another issue is that many countries still collect only aggregate, not individual, patient-level cycle data. This limits the ability to conduct more detailed analyses. However, even countries that do collect and report individual data to their national registries are generally prevented by both jurisdictional and sometimes commercial law from sharing individual patient data outside of their country.

ICMART continuously assesses the best way to collect data given new technologies and new clinical practices in ART. Changes made in some of the more advanced national registries help inform ICMART as it continues to modify its registry to optimize global ART data collection.

ICMART has as a major goal the reporting of global data within four years of the ART procedures. This four-year delay is necessary to allow a year each for clinics to collect and report live birth outcomes; national registries to analyze and report their own data; regional registries to report; and, finally, ICMART to collect, validate, analyze, write and publish its report. Generally, country and regional registries want to report their own data before ICMART does. The timeliness of this process will be enhanced with the new electronic data portal.

Additional Value Created by the ICMART Global ART Registry and National and Regional Registries

In addition to the value brought to stakeholders through the information derived from the global registry, participation in the global registry brings multiple additional 'softer', but no less important, benefits. Individual providers, professional societies, health departments and the health care system are enabled to develop capabilities they did not previously have. New relationships are formed through cooperation and collaboration, bringing innovation, capacity building and synergistic progress.

The ICMART registry has provided useful data to explore other aspects of infertility treatment, such as affordability, number of babies born and gender inequality. It has also stimulated research on birth outcomes through linkage of national ART registries with other medical registries.

The pillars of freedom to access health care are affordability, availability and acceptability [27]. ICMART data provide availability of information through documenting the number of clinics. As more professionals and stakeholders use registries to make ART more visible, understandable, accountable and

transparent to policy makers and society, there is increasing trust, which leads to acceptability and support for access to ART as a reproductive right.

While access to care is multidimensional and not directly measurable, ICMART provides the only global proxy marker to estimate access to infertility care, namely, ART utilization. ICMART also disaggregates this proxy marker by country and region. Our data thus highlight some global inequalities in access to infertility care. We have also recently explored other associations with ART utilization and, using ICMART data in conjunction with WHO, the World Bank and other data showed that low rates of ART utilization correlated with greater gender inequality [26]. ICMART agrees with the concept that data are essential to make the invisible visible.

Finally, we believe that global ART data collection strongly influences ART practice in a country and region. This has been seen, for example, in Latin America (REDLARA) and Africa (ANARA). In both situations, the development of ART registries has brought clinicians, laboratories and other professionals together, increased cooperation among clinics and countries, increased standardization and improved quality of care through measurement, management and the development of new quality improvement systems. Cooperation, advice and support from ICMART and REDLARA through assisting ANARA with annual publications have not only increased awareness of the value of the data but also identified areas needing improvement. Such collaboration has also increased the visibility of clinics and countries performing ART, which in turn has increased the number of clinics reporting within countries and the number of countries reporting. All these consequences of data collection bring better quality of care, greater societal acceptance and increased access.

The Future of Global Art Reports

ICMART believes the future of clinic, national, regional and global ART reporting is bright. We expect the trend of more clinics and countries reporting will continue until it is almost universal, although this will take time. ICMART is continuously working towards more timely and comprehensive reports. This will require more sophisticated electronic data collection systems and robust data entry portal.

We will also continue to develop the global ART registry and assist in the development of national and regional registries so that we can increase both access to and quality of ART procedures for all those who can benefit.

ICMART will continue to address the challenges noted above. These include better understanding and adherence to standardized data collection and more harmonization of all the data in the registries. They also include more granular data from real time electronic medical records, including data that enable linkage of individual eggs/embryos/cycles/intended parents/gamete sources/gestational carriers to treatment outcomes over time and in different locations, including cross-border care.

To achieve these goals, ICMART will need to build capacity through increased infrastructure and enhanced organizational capabilities. This will be made possible through bringing value to other stakeholders. This will also include more developed relationships with professional, WHO, industry and other stakeholders to bring synergy to our common goals.

Information on cost and cost-effectiveness, impact of funding on access to treatment, costs and societal value of ART treatment and babies needs to be collected through linkage of ICMART data with other datasets. Linkage with other health care registries will increase capacity to understand fertility and infertility in the context of overall life health, and its relationship to genetics, the microbiome, the environment and other psychosocial factors.

Large, comprehensive, harmonized registries will facilitate development of improved algorithms to identify useful but 'hidden' information in the registries. Artificial intelligence will almost certainly be useful for aggregating national and regional ART datasets.

The future should include more research from ICMART global ART data, more publications and presentations, not just in the infertility sector but also in reproductive medicine and general medicine. More use of ICMART world reports and other scientific work products by stakeholders should help increase recognition that infertility treatment involves reproductive rights that are human rights. This will, it is hoped, result in increased access to quality health care globally.

Acknowledgements

I would like to acknowledge especially the contributors, ICMART Board members, the WHO, the professional organizations and industry who have supported ICMART in its mission over the past 29 years.

References

1. IWGROAR, prepared by Cohen J, de Mouzon J, Lancaster P. World collaborative report on in vitro fertilization, 1991. *VIIIth Congress on In Vitro and Alternate Assisted Reproduction, Congress Booklet, Kyoto, 12–15 September 1993.*

2. IWGROAR, prepared by de Mouzon J, Lancaster P. World collaborative report on in vitro fertilization, 1993. *Congress Booklet, Montpellier, 17–22 September 1995.*

3. IWGROAR, prepared by de Mouzon J, Lancaster P. World collaborative report on in vitro fertilization. Preliminary data for 1995. *J Assist Reprod Gen.* 1997;**14**:251s–65s.

4. IWGROAR, presented by de Mouzon J, Lancaster P, Nygren K-G, Zegers-Hochschild F. World report: preliminary data for 1996. *16th World Congress on Fertility and Sterility, IFFS San Francisco USA, 4–9 October 1998.*

5. IWGROAR, prepared by Adamson D, Lancaster P, de Mouzon J (co-coordinator), Nygren K-G (chairman), Zegers-Hochschild F. World collaborative report on assisted reproductive technology, 1998. IFFS, Melbourne, November 25–9, 2001. In DL Healy, GP Kovacs, E McLachlan, O Rodriguez-Armas (eds.), *Reproductive Medicine in the 21st century.* London: Parthenon Publishing Group; 2001. pp.209–19.

6. International Committee Monitoring Assisted Reproductive Technology, Adamson GD, de Mouzon J, Lancaster P, Nygren K-G, Sullivan E, Zegers-Hochschild F. World collaborative report on in vitro fertilization, 2000. *Fertil Steril.* 2006;**85**(6):1586–622.

7. de Mouzon J, Lancaster P, Nygren K-G, Sullivan E, Zegers-Hochschild F, Mansour R, et al. World collaborative report on assisted reproductive technology, 2002. *Hum Reprod.* 2009;**24**(9):2310–20. doi:10.1093/humrep/dep098.

8. Nygren K-G, Sullivan E, Zegers-Hochschild F, Mansour R, Ishihara O, Adamson GD, et al. International Committee for Monitoring Assisted Reproductive Technology (ICMART) world report: assisted reproductive technology 2003. *Fertil Steril.* 2011;**95**(7):2209–22, 2222.e1–17. Epub 2011 May 4.

9. Sullivan E, Zegers-Hochschild F, Mansour R, Ishihara O, de Mouzon J, Nygren K-G, Adamson GD. International Committee for Monitoring Assisted Reproductive Technology world report: assisted reproductive technology 2004. *Hum Reprod.* 2013;**28**(5):1375–90.

10. Zegers-Hochschild F, Mansour R, Ishihara O, Adamson GD, de Mouzon J, Nygren K-G, et al. International Committee for Monitoring Assisted Reproductive Technology: world report on assisted

reproductive technology, 2005. *Fertil Steril.* 2014;**101**: 366–78.

11. Mansour R, Ishihara O, Adamson GD, de Mouzon J, Nygren K-G, Sullivan E, et al. International Committee for Monitoring Assisted Reproductive Technologies world report: assisted reproductive technology 2006. *Hum Reprod.* 2014;**29**(7):1536–51. doi:10.1093/humrep/deu084.gd. Epub 2014 May 2.

12. Ishihara O, Adamson GD, de Mouzon J, Sullivan E, Zegers-Hochschild R, Mansour R. International Committee for Monitoring Assisted Reproductive Technologies: world report on assisted reproductive technologies, 2007. *Fertil Steril.* 2015;**103**(2): 402–13.e11. doi:10.1016/j.fertnstert.2014.11.004. Epub 2014 Dec 13.

13. Dyer S, Chambers GM, de Mouzon J, Nygren K-G, Zegers-Hochschild F, Mansour R, et al. International Committee for Monitoring Assisted Reproductive Technologies world report: assisted reproductive technology 2008, 2009 and 2010. *Hum Reprod.* 2016;**31**(7):1588–609. doi:10.1093/humrep/dew082. Epub 2016 May 20.

14. Adamson GD, de Mouzon J, Chambers GM, Zegers-Hochschild F, Mansour R, Ishihara O, et al. International Committee for Monitoring Assisted Reproductive Technologies: world report on assisted reproductive technology 2011. *Fertil Steril.* 2018;**110**(6):1067–80. doi:10.1016/j.fertnstert.2018.06.039.

15. Nygren K, Adamson D, Zegers-Hochschild F, de Mouzon J, on behalf of the International Committee Monitoring Assisted Reproductive Technologies. Cross-border fertility—International Committee Monitoring Assisted Reproductive Technologies global survey: 2006 data and estimates. *Fertil Steril.* 2010;**94**(1):e4–e8. doi:10.1016/j.fertnstert.209.12.049.

16. Hughes E, Adamson GD. Cross-border reproductive care in North America: a pilot study testing a prospective data collection program for IVF clinics in Canada and the United States. *Fertil Steril.* 2016;**105**(3):786–90. doi:10.1016/j.fertnstert.2015.11.048. Epub 2015 Dec 13.

17. Hansen M, Kurinczuk JJ, Bower C, Webb S. The risk of major birth defects after intracytoplasmic sperm injection and in vitro fertilization. *N Engl J Med.* 2002;**346**:725–30. doi:10.1056/NEJMoa010035.

18. Vayena E, Peterson H, Nygren K-G, Adamson GD. Assisted reproductive technologies in developing countries; are we caring yet? *Fertil Steril.* 2009;**92**(2):413–16. Epub 2009 Mar 25.

19. Zegers-Hochschild F, Nygren K-G, Adamson GD, de Mouzon J, Mansour R, Lancaster P, et al. The ICMART Glossary on ART Terminology. *Fertil Steril.* 2006;**86**(1):16–19 (Simultaneous publication with *Human Reproduction*).

20. Zegers-Hochschild F, Nygren K-G, Adamson GD, de Mouzon J, Mansour R, Lancaster P, Sullivan E. The ICMART Glossary on ART Terminology. *Hum Reprod.* 2006;**21**:1968–70 (Simultaneous publication with *Fertility and Sterility*).

21. Zegers-Hochschild F, Adamson GD, de Mouzon J, Ishihara O, Mansour R, Nygren K-G, et al. International Committee for Monitoring Assisted Reproductive Technology (ICMART) and the World Health Organization (WHO) Revised Glossary of ART Terminology, 2009. *Fertil Steril.* 2009;**92**(5):1520–4 (Simultaneous publication with *Human Reproduction*).

22. Zegers-Hochschild F, Adamson GD, de Mouzon J, Ishihara O, Mansour R, Nygren K-G, et al.; International Committee for Monitoring Assisted Reproductive Technology; World Health Organization. The International Committee for Monitoring Assisted Reproductive Technology (ICMART) and the World Health Organization (WHO) Revised Glossary on ART Terminology, 2009. *Hum Reprod.* 2009;**24**(11):2683–7. doi:10.1093/humrep/dep343 (*Human Reproduction* advance access originally published online on 4 October 2009; simultaneous publication with *Fertility and Sterility*).

23. Zegers-Hochschild F, Adamson GD, Dyer S, Racowsky C, de Mouzon J, Sokol R, et al. The International Glossary on Infertility and Fertility Care, 2017. *Fertil Steril.* 2017;**108**(3):393–406. doi:10.1016/j.fertnstert.2017.06.005. Epub 2017 Jul 29.

24. Zegers-Hochschild F, Adamson GD, Dyer S, Racowsky C, de Mouzon J, Sokol R, et al. The International Glossary on Infertility and Fertility Care, 2017. *Hum Reprod.* 2017;**32**(9):1786–801. https://doi.org/10.1093/humrep/dex234.

25. Abusief ME, Hornstein MD, Jain T. Assessment of United States fertility clinic websites according to the American Society for Reproductive Medicine (ASRM)/Society for Assisted Reproductive Technology (SART) guidelines. *Fertil Steril.* 2007;**87**(1):88–92.

26. Adamson GD, Zegers-Hochschild F, Dyer S, Chambers G, Ishihara O, Mansour R, et al., for the International Committee for Monitoring Assisted Reproductive Technologies. *International Committee for Monitoring Assisted Reproductive Technologies (ICMART) World Report on ART, 2014. Session 38: European and Global ART Monitoring Session.* ESHRE Annual Meeting. Barcelona, Spain, 3 July 2018.

27. Thiede M, McIntyre D. Information, communication and equitable access to health care: a conceptual note. *Cad Saude Publica.* 2008;**24**(5):1168–73.

28. Adamson GD. Global cultural and socioeconomic factors that influence access to ART. *Women's Health (Lond).* 2009;**5**(4):351–8.

29. Chambers G, Phuong Hoang V, Sullivan E, Chapman M, Ishihara O, Zegers-Hochschild F, et al. The impact of consumer affordability on access to assisted reproductive technologies and embryo transfer practices: An international analysis. *Fertil Steril.* 2014;**101**(1):191–8.

30. Präg P, Mills MC. Cultural determinants influence assisted reproduction usage in Europe more than economic and demographic factors. *Hum Reprod.* 2017;**32**(11):2305–14.

31. Hudson N, Culley L, Blyth E, Norton W, Rapport F, Pacey A. Cross-border reproductive care: a review of the literature. *Reprod Biomed Online.* 2011;**22**(7):673–85. doi:10.1016/j.rbmo.2011.03.010. Epub 2011 Mar 13.

32. Pandey S, Shetty A, Hamilton M, Bhattacharya S, Maheshwari A. Obstetric and perinatal outcomes in singleton pregnancies resulting from IVF/ICSI: a systematic review and meta-analysis. *Hum Reprod Update.* 2012;**18**(5):485–503. https://doi.org/10.1093/humupd/dms018.

33. Woo I, Hindoyan R, Landay M, Ho J, Ingles SA, McGinnis LK, et al. Perinatal outcomes after natural conception versus in vitro fertilization (IVF) in gestational surrogates: a model to evaluate IVF treatment versus maternal effects. *Fertil Steril.* 2017;**108**(6):993–8. doi:10.1016/j.fertnstert.2017.09.014.

34. Pinborg A, Wennerholm UB, Romundstad LB, Loft A, Aittomaki K, Söderström-Anttila V, et al. Why do singletons conceived after assisted reproduction technology have adverse perinatal outcome? Systematic review and meta-analysis. *Hum Reprod Update.* 2013;**19**(2):87–104. doi:10.1093/humupd/dms044. Epub 2012 Nov 14.

35. Davies MJ, Moore, VM, Willson KJ, Van Essen P, Priest K, Scott H, et al. Reproductive technologies and the risk of birth defects. *N Engl J Med.* 2012;**366**:1803–13. doi:10.1056/NEJMoa1008095.

36. Gerris J, de Sutter P, Racowsky C, Adamson GD (eds.). *Elective Single Embryo Transfer.* Cambridge: Cambridge University Press; 2009.

Chapter

12

Global Variations in ART Policy: Data from the International Federation of Fertility Societies (IFFS)

Steven J. Ory and Kathleen Miller

History of the International Federation of Fertility Societies (IFFS)

The first attempt to undertake a compilation of international assisted reproductive technology (ART) practices was initiated in 1997 by Drs Howard Jones and Jean Cohen with a written questionnaire of more than 200 questions as a project of the International Federation of Fertility Societies (IFFS), originally established in 1951 as the International Fertility Association (Association Internationale de Fertilité). The IFFS is a union of more than 65 independent fertility societies representing individual countries, which have served as the initial and ongoing sponsor of the survey. The IFFS is a non-state actor (NSA) that promotes and develops educational initiatives in the field of reproductive health in support of World Health Organization (WHO) aims and objectives in response to WHO's renewed focus and prioritization of infertility as a disease [1]. The IFFS meets in a different host city every 3 years and the results of the questionnaire are presented in the course of the scientific meeting. The findings of the initial survey were presented in San Francisco in 1998 and subsequently published as *IFFS Surveillance 01* with the expressed purpose "to document the current status of the various issues in the hope that it is a further step along the road to a scientifically based consensus" [2]. They noted, "The development of [in vitro fertilization] IVF and its subsequent variations and extensions, all now included under the umbrella of assisted reproductive technology (ART), seems to have generated more interest and concern among religious leaders, bioethicists, and the general public than any other medical procedure. This widespread interest and concern attracted the attention of, or was called to the attention of, the political process, not only by ethicists and moral theologians but by consumer groups, some members of which expressed dissatisfaction with one or another aspect of their treatment or lack of access thereto. As a result of these events, many committees and commissions, some governmental, some not, have examined the ethical, legal, religious, medical, and public policy aspects of ART, resulting in the establishments of guidelines and/or government regulations in many sovereign states practicing ART." The original publication described the practices of 39 countries as they pertained to the adoption of guidelines and regulations and methods of surveillance of a number of ART practices such as micromanipulation, number of embryos transferred and preimplantation genetic testing (PGT). Related issues including accessibility, donation, welfare of the child, embryo reduction, surrogacy and cloning were also addressed. *Surveillance* does not collect or report clinical outcome data such as that collected by ICMART (see Chapter 11, Global ART Surveillance: The International Committee Monitoring Assisted Reproductive Technologies (ICMART)).

IFFS Surveillance has subsequently become a triennial survey and the most recent publication, *IFFS Surveillance 2016*, was released in September 2016 [3]. Preparation of the eighth iteration, *Surveillance 2019: Global Trends in Reproductive Policy and Practice*, 8th edition, is now under way. The reports were previously published in *Fertility and Sterility* and *Human Reproduction* but are now published solely in the official IFFS electronic journal, *Global Reproductive Health*. Although most of the original topics and format have been retained, it has been reorganized and several new sections have been added to reflect newer ART practices, and some topics, such as gamete intrafallopian transfer (GIFT), have been deleted. The questionnaire itself is now completed online and consists of 97 questions organized to facilitate completion by an international group of collaborators. The questionnaire can be accessed in several languages. It has been extensively modified over the past 20 years to promote clarity, eliminate redundancy and facilitate accurate, efficient completion. An online survey consultant has been engaged for product development.

Methodology of *IFFS Surveillance*

Compiling a detailed analysis of international ART practices is a formidable challenge. Respondents for *Surveillance* are all unpaid volunteers and the project has a modest budget appropriated only for information technology (IT) support and design in addition to implementation and conducting of the online questionnaire. Funding has been provided through the IFFS operating budget and, occasionally, from unrestricted educational grants provided by industry. The biggest challenge for *IFFS Surveillance* has been in engaging knowledgeable, committed respondents in each country to complete the approximately one-hour task. Accuracy has been addressed by enlisting multiple participants for countries, when feasible, and comparing their answers and checking results with other related publications reviewed by the Editorial Board, when practical. However, there are no comprehensive resources available for validation of the data submitted and lack of validation remains an inherent weakness. As *IFFS Surveillance* has reached a broader audience and has assumed greater importance for health ministries, policy planners and other stakeholders, it has received greater scrutiny and the readership has been relied upon to report new developments and errors. Recording ART policies and practices is a dynamic, ongoing endeavour and another inherent weakness is that the publication may not reflect changes occurring after completion of the survey.

Respondents have usually been officers, leaders or designees in their respective country's fertility societies and they have relied on a variety of resources to complete their reports. In countries with several jurisdictions (states and provinces), multiple respondents or multiple sources for a single respondent have been employed. In smaller countries and with less developed ART resources, completion is usually much quicker and simpler. Respondents are not given explicit instructions for the completion of the survey and may rely on a variety of resources and methods for completion.

Development of *Surveillance* is an ongoing project. The Editorial Board monitors relevant scientific and legislative literature continuously to identify relevant trends and developments in the field of ART. Compilation of the potential respondent list is a continuous process and is constantly modified as new candidates are identified and individuals no longer able to participate are deleted. The Editorial Board meets twice yearly at international meetings to review relevant topics and develop the next questionnaire. Development of the new questionnaire is completed approximately 18 months prior to publication, and the survey is launched online about a year prior to publication. It is accessible online for two months. The data are made available to the members of the Editorial Board within a month of completion and assigned to the various authors for chapter development. The editorial process is completed two to three months prior to the triennial IFFS World Congress meeting and the findings are presented at a plenary session at the congress. The publication is simultaneously released online and in print after oral presentation. The Editorial Board meets at the World Congress and then begins the process anew.

ART Reporting Mechanisms

Reporting mechanisms have evolved considerably over the past 20 years and vary widely among countries in terms of focus, scope, resources and mechanisms for collection and validation. As noted in *Surveillance*, they record performance and trends over time and changes in practice. The ongoing assessment of outcome may be utilized to assess the effect on overall safety and relevant epidemiological evidence may become part of the analysis [4]. Monitoring mechanisms have also been utilized for legislating, licensing and credentialing ART centres and individual practitioners. They have been used as an integral part of quality control and quality assurance programs and are essential for long-term follow-up of patients undergoing ART and children conceived with various ART techniques [5]. Responding countries have employed diverse means for collecting and reporting their data, including obligatory, legally sanctioned requirements and voluntary reporting to non-governmental organizations and professional organizations. Several countries have no regulatory requirements.

The 2016 publication noted that the majority of countries surveyed (49/70, 70%) required some form of reporting [3]. This was especially true in Europe, Australia, Canada, Israel, South Africa and some Middle East and Asian countries, where the practice of ART is legislated. In 10 countries (Australia, Austria, Bulgaria, Canada, Germany, Indonesia, Italy, Russian Federation, Sweden, Switzerland), legislative oversight is provided by multiple jurisdictions including national, provincial and/or municipal entities. The United States (US) has multiple statutes (e.g. national, state and municipal) addressing ART, and oversight varies widely among the states. Twenty countries have no regulations regarding reporting mechanisms, including some in Latin America (Chile, Colombia, Ecuador, El Salvador,

Honduras, Mexico, Paraguay, Venezuela), the Caribbean (Barbados, Trinidad and Tobago), Africa (Cameroon, Nigeria, Kenya, Senegal), India, and Asia (Myanmar, Philippines, Sri Lanka, Japan). In Europe, Ireland alone lacks a reporting mechanism. Argentina enacted an expanded, more detailed ART bill which included provisions for reporting mechanisms after an insurance coverage law was passed in 2013. In 16 countries (Australia, Brazil, Bulgaria, China, Denmark, Estonia, Finland, France, Germany, Greece, Guatemala, Indonesia, Iran, Portugal, Romania, the US), reporting is made directly to a governmental agency. In 31 countries, reports are submitted to a discrete licensing organization, and some countries have overlapping reporting requirements. The most prevalent reporting mechanism, utilized by 46 countries out of the 70 surveyed (65.7%), involves submitting a report to a professional organization or scientific society. The majority of countries surveyed (64.2%) have monitoring mechanisms in place for governance or credentialing of ART centres, and 26 countries (37.1%) have monitoring mechanisms applied for individual professionals. This requirement included three countries that do not monitor ART centres (Canada, Mali, the Netherlands). Separate monitoring of ART laboratory facilities is undertaken by 36 countries, including 35 of the 45 countries reporting as having ART centre monitoring. The Netherlands, which does not monitor ART centres per se, does monitor laboratory facilities and some personnel.

Adherence to monitoring mechanisms by ART centres is usually achieved by government officials or a combination of officials and agencies (54.2%). In 9 countries (Austria, France, Greece, Iraq, Ireland, Myanmar, Portugal, South Africa, the United Kingdom (UK)), control was delegated to independent agencies (12.8%), and in Denmark and Japan, by medical officials. Eleven countries (15.7%) have no mechanisms in place for monitoring compliance (Bangladesh, Barbados, Cameroon, El Salvador, Guatemala, Malaysia, Nigeria, Senegal, Sri Lanka, Trinidad and Tobago, Venezuela). Adherence in the ART Lab was similarly distributed, with 41.4% relying on agents or a combination of government officials and agencies, 10% independent agencies and 18.6% reported no mechanisms for ensuring adherence. A similar trend was noted in the monitoring of adherence control of clinicians with 27.1% using governmental officials, independent agencies or a combination to monitor adherence to regulation, 8% through independent agencies,

8% with medical officials, and 22.8% lacking any mechanism for monitoring adherence. Regarding the monitoring of adherence of lab personnel, 24.3% regulate via governmental officials, independent agencies or a combination, 8% use independent agencies, 5.7% rely on medical officials, and 22.8% have no regulations.

ART outcome monitoring was also queried. The most commonly employed method (40%) relied on the use of governmental officials and independent agencies for outcome assessments. Four countries utilize medical officials for monitoring outcomes, and 20% reported having no requirement for follow-up. In many countries, outcomes were also monitored by professional organizations or scientific societies (including most Latin American countries which report to REDLARA; see Chapter 19, ART Surveillance in Latin America) and specially created licensing and/or regulatory agencies (UK and Australia). Monitoring of ART centres was carried out with a variety of mechanisms. Five countries (7.1%) report to an international registry (Colombia, Estonia, Guatemala, Ireland, Venezuela), and 18 countries (25.7%) send results to national registries. Six countries utilize periodic reporting and on-site inspection only (Australia, Bulgaria, Kazakhstan, Singapore, Slovak Republic, South Korea), and two countries (Philippines, Senegal) use only periodic reporting. Bangladesh, Belarus, Ecuador, India, Iran, the Netherlands and the Russian Federation, have only on-site inspection. Canada has voluntary reporting to a national database. Monitoring of reproductive endocrinologists and other physicians practising ART was performed through national registries in 11 cases (15.7%), in 17.1% thorough on-site inspection or periodic reporting is performed (in some cases jointly with an accreditation process), and in 10% through a recertification process. Monitoring of the ART laboratories followed the same overall trend as ART centres, with 18.6% reporting to a national registry and undergoing on-site inspections and periodic reporting; 7.1% report to international registries, and 31.4% have only on-site inspections, periodic reporting or both. Sixteen countries (22.8%) reported that violations of national policies pertaining to the practice of ART had occurred (Australia, Belgium, Brazil, Canada, China, Czech Republic, Germany, Greece, Iran, Israel, Japan, Kazakhstan, Panama, Romania, Russian Federation, the US). Forty countries (57.1%) noted that no violations had occurred. Forty countries (57.1%) noted that specific penalties exist for violations, and these potential sanctions include financial penalties, loss of accreditation or licence to practise, closure of the centre and criminal charges including fines and imprisonment.

In essence, monitoring and reporting mechanisms are in place in most of Europe, Australia, the US, South East Asia and Latin America. Countries have implemented a diverse array of mechanisms to accomplish monitoring and ensure enforcement. They include reliance on government officials and establishment of or delegation to independent agencies. The most commonly employed practice involves the use of professional organizations and scientific societies. These groups also play a prominent role in auditing clinical and laboratory outcomes, as well as licensing and certifying ART procedures. Publication of the eighth edition of *Surveillance* is under way and its anticipated release date is April 2019.

The content of *Surveillance 2019: Global Trends in Reproductive Policy and Practice,* 8th edition, will include the following:

1. Number of centers
2. Legislation, policy, guidelines/reporting mechanisms
3. Insurance coverage
4. Marital status/same sex/single parenting policy
5. Number of embryos for transfer in ART
6. Fertility cryopreservation
7. Posthumous insemination
8. Donation and anonymity of donors
9. Micromanipulation/oocyte maturation
10. Welfare of the child and identity rights
11. Fetal reduction and sex selection
12. Preimplantation genetic testing
13. IVF surrogacy
14. Cross-border reproductive care
15. Research and experimentation on the embryo/cloning
16. Status of the embryo

Overview of Global ART Policy

The online questionnaire, the data source for *Surveillance 2019,* ended in April 2018. *Surveillance 2016* produced more data from a larger proportion of countries actively providing ART services than did previous surveys, and preliminary results from the 2018 project suggest an even greater participation rate with more than 90 countries responding. It is estimated that about 130 countries offer ART (Fig. 12.1). For the first time, in 2018, an attempt was made to identify and note the countries that provide no ART services, and it

was estimated that there are more than 60 of these countries (Fig. 12.2). The ART status of a much smaller remainder of countries is unknown (Fig. 12.3). Analysis of the 2018 data in anticipation of the publication of *Surveillance 2019* is now under way. It is expected that the 2019 publication will reveal a continuation of trends noted in 2016.

Although *Surveillance 2016* documented a trend of continued congruence of attitudes and approaches, significant disparities exist among countries offering ART around the world [3]. Respondents from most countries reported a modest growth in the number of ART centres, suggesting further acceptance and maturation of ART as a clinical service. In 2016, it was estimated that there were approximately 5,300 ART centres in the 74 countries responding.

At that time, more than 80% of countries relied on legislation, guidelines or a combination to ensure safety, efficacy, standardization and access to ART. Monitoring and reporting mechanisms existed in most of Europe, Australia, the US, South East Asia and Latin America. Over a third of respondents noted the enactment of new legislation after 2012, which was generally perceived as salutary. A majority of countries had implemented legislation or guidelines restricting the number of embryos permissible for embryo transfer.

Preimplantation genetic testing (PGT), primarily for aneuploidy (PGT-A), was noted to constitute an increasing proportion of IVF cycles. A variety of ART techniques was available in most countries for fertility preservation, including gamete and embryo cryopreservation, and they are widely performed. Practices such as cryopreservation, posthumous reproduction and gamete donation received greater attention from participants and were more commonly done. However, significant regional differences in practice, access, and frequency of application exist. Intracytoplasmic sperm injection (ICSI) was reported to be almost universally available and performed. Access to and utilization of donor gametes and embryos and gestational carriers increased but was restricted in many countries by legal, ethical and religious constraints. Significant differences in available options and restrictions were reported to exist even among countries in proximity to each other. This latter phenomenon contributed to a greater demand for cross-border reproductive services, raising new ethical concerns [6].

Additional trends noted in 2016 included increased attention to social aspects of ART such as the pretreatment assessment for the potential welfare

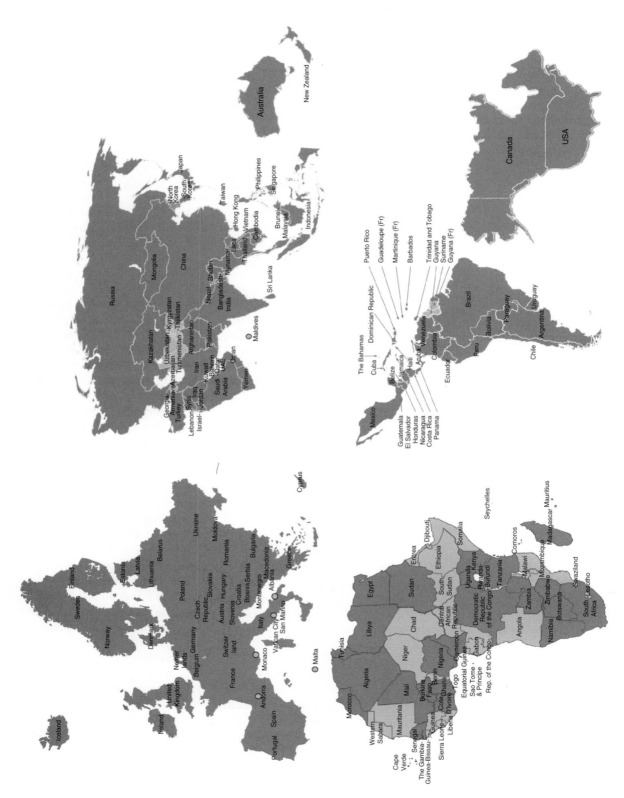

Figure 12.1 Countries that offer assisted reproductive technology (darker colour). A colour version of the figure is provided in the plate section.

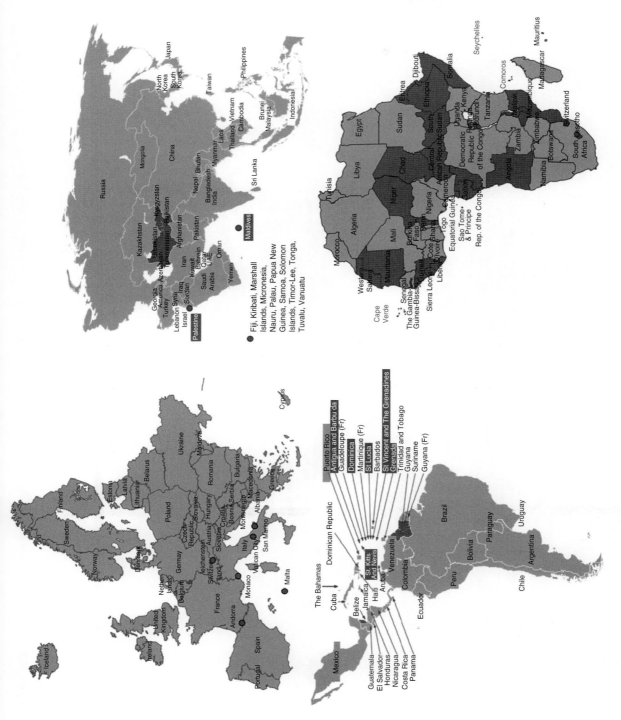

Figure 12.2 Countries that provide no assisted reproductive technology services (darker colour). A colour version of the figure is provided in the plate section.

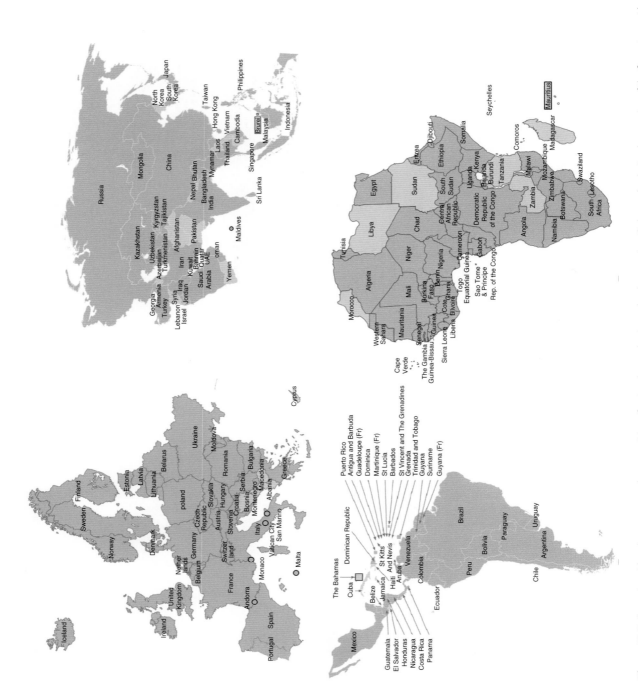

Figure 12.3 Countries with unknown status about provision of assisted reproductive technology services (lighter colour). A colour version of the figure is provided in the plate section.

of the child, concerns regarding issues of anonymity and disclosure for families utilizing donor gametes, and the status accorded the embryo. A wide variety of new measures had been suggested and undertaken to address these issues, but these subjects were regarded as highly contentious and no universal recommendations had been endorsed. There were incremental increases in utilization of some ART applications such as oocyte maturation and assisted hatching, but no new significant trends were identified.

Experimentation on embryonic cells was allowed to a very limited extent. Stem cell research on embryonic cells was permitted in fewer than half of countries but with rigid guidelines in place. The amount of research performed had apparently increased. Therapeutic cloning research was being performed in very few countries.

Conclusions

Surveillance was established by the IFFS in 1998 as an effort to chronicle the progress and trends pertaining to ART internationally with the objective of engaging as many of the countries offering ART services as possible. The seven editions of *Surveillance* have noted consistent growth of ART reflected in the number of countries actively participating in ART services, number of centres and number of treatment cycles performed. Overall, *IFFS Surveillance 2016* depicted greater accessibility of worldwide ART services to a larger number of individuals. Barriers to ART services based on location, marital status and gender still existed. There were also reports of ongoing efforts to curtail the practice of ART in some locations. However, the expanding application of ART services and greater involvement of a host of interested parties seemed to affirm ART's great clinical value. Much of the legislation and other initiatives recently undertaken have promoted safety, efficacy and availability. Each issue of *IFFS Surveillance* has attested to an expanding scope of ART practices, policies and activities among nations around the world but highlighted significant and important differences.

References

1. Zegers-Hochschild F, Adamson GD, Dyer S, Racowsky C, de Mouson J, Sokol R, et al. The International Glossary on Infertility and Fertility Care, 2017. *Fertil Steril*. 2017;**108**(3):393–406.

2. Jones H, Cohen J. IFFS Surveillance 01. *Fertil Steril*. 2001;**76**(5):5–36.

3. IFFS Surveillance 2016. *Glob Reprod Health*. 2016; e1:1–143.

4. EIM; ESHRE; Kupka MA, D'Hoogh T, Ferraretti AP, de Mouson J, et al. Assisted reproductive technology in Europe, 2011: results generated from European registers by ESHRE. *Hum Reprod*. 2016:**31**(2):233–48.

5. Belva F, Roelants M, Painter R, Bonduelle M, Devroey P, De Schepper J. Pubertal development in ICSI children. *Hum Reprod*. 2012;**27**(4):1156–61.

6. Ethics Committee of American Society for Reproductive Medicine. Cross-border reproductive care: a committee opinion. *Fertil Steril*. 2013;**100**(3):645–50. doi:10.1016/j.fertnstert.2013.02.051.

Chapter 13

ART Surveillance in Africa

Silke Dyer, Paversan Archary and G. David Adamson

History of ART in Africa

Assisted reproductive technology (ART) was initiated in Africa within several years of its introduction into clinical practice. The first ART baby in Africa was born in 1984 in South Africa (Kruger, personal communication). This success is attributable to Thinus Kruger, working at Tygerberg Hospital, University of Stellenbosch. Kruger also pioneered the strict criteria for sperm morphology in collaboration with the Jones Institute, Norfolk, Virginia, USA, which were later adopted by the World Health Organization (WHO) [1, 2]. Twelve years later, the first intracytoplasmic sperm injection (ICSI) baby in South Africa was born following treatment at the same institution (Kruger, personal communication).

In North Africa, in vitro fertilization (IVF) technology was brought to Egypt from the Ohio State University, Columbus, Ohio, by Ragaa Mansour, who returned from the United States (US) in 1986. She collaborated with Gamal Serour and Mohamed Aboulghar to establish the first IVF centre in Egypt (Egyptian IVF Centre). The centre recorded its first baby born in 1987 [3]. A few years later, other ART centres were established in neighbouring countries in Libya, Sudan, Tunisia, Algeria and Morocco.

In Central Africa, ART was pioneered at Lagos University Teaching Hospital, Nigeria, by Oladapo Ashiru, who started research on laboratory animals in 1981 [4]. Subsequent work on human gametes and embryos resulted in the first live birth following IVF in 1989 [5]. Oladapo Ashiru subsequently also pursued clinical and academic practice in the US before returning to Nigeria in 2004.

In several other African countries, ART only started taking root at the end of the twentieth and beginning of the twenty-first centuries. The technology was introduced either by African specialists who brought back the necessary experience, primarily from Europe but also India and the US, or by immigrating non-Africans.

In Ghana, the first IVF baby was born in 1995 following the establishment of an ART centre by Dr Joe Mainoo, who brought back skills and technology after training in Germany [6]. In Cameroon, ART began in 1997 with two centres in Douala, the economic capital of the country. In Togo, the first IVF baby was born in 1997 following the establishment of ART by Dr Moïse Fiadjoe. Rajat Goswamy, originally from India but with clinical and research experience gained in the United Kingdom (UK), set up the first comprehensive ART centre in Mauritius in 2002. Previously, limited services were provided via an ART laboratory on Reunion Island, and most couples could access ART only through cross-border care. In Uganda, IVF was introduced in 2004. Pioneers included local specialist Edward Tamali Sali, who acquired training in the UK and the Middle East, together with support from visiting or temporarily resident international clinical and laboratory experts [7]. The first live birth was reported in 2005. In Mali, the first ART births were documented in 2010 [8].

Then and now, the vast majority of ART centres were established and operate in the private health sector. Reasons for this relate predominantly to a lack of funding and prioritization by governments, as infertility has traditionally not been considered a health priority or even a disease. Until recently, there has been a similar lack of prioritization by WHO, transnational health non-governmental organizations (NGOs) and similar health initiatives. Additional and compounding reasons include the overall high burden of disease in Africa and the frequent lack of human resources and health infrastructure to deliver more advanced clinical and technological services in the public health sector. As a result, to date only a handful of ART centres, located in South Africa, Egypt and Nigeria, have existed in the public sector. Fortunately, there are encouraging signs that the situation may have begun to change. In Cameroon, a public centre opened in 2016, and similar activity is under way in Benin, Congo and Uganda.

As ART began to establish itself, fertility societies gradually emerged. At the regional level, this was led by the founding of the Groupe Interafricain d'Etude, de Recherche et d'Application sur la Fertilité (GIERAF) in 2009 in Lomé, Togo, with Moïse Fiadjoe as the founding president. The objectives of GIERAF are to promote the "reduction of preventable causes of infertility; encourage training and interaction with international organizations; promote research into infertility in Africa; and to act with medical and political authorities for the preservation of fertility in Africa".

A fertility society for Africa was launched in 2015 at the European Society of Human Reproduction and Embryology (ESHRE) conference in Lisbon, although plans were begun some five years earlier. Interim leadership of the African Fertility Society (AFS) was provided by Oladapo Ashiru (Nigeria, President) and James Olobo-Lalobo (Uganda, Vice President), which was subsequently ratified through elections and an inaugural meeting at the Association for Fertility and Reproductive Health (AFRH) conference in Nigeria later in 2015. AFS has stated that its mission is "to promote safe and quality reproductive health care in Africa; to promote the acquisition of knowledge, training and research in support of fertility care provision; and to minimize and eliminate the stigma and psychosocial consequences of infertility". AFS is still developing some of its organizational structures, which include the need to clarify whether it will evolve as a federation of fertility societies like the International Federation of Fertility Societies (IFFS) or a society based on individual membership similar to ESHRE or the American Society for Reproductive Medicine (ASRM). Delegates from both AFS and GIERAF participated in generating the International Glossary on Infertility and Fertility Care [9], under the leadership of the International Committee Monitoring Assisted Reproductive Technologies (ICMART), and in the development of WHO Infertility Guidelines.

At the national level, several fertility organizations and societies currently exist: the Southern African Society of Reproductive Medicine and Gynaecological Endoscopy (SASREG), established in 1988 as the South African Society of Reproductive Medicine; the Egyptian Fertility and Sterility Society, formed in 1994; the Sudan Human Reproduction and Embryology Society, founded in 2008; the Association for Fertility and Reproductive Health (AFRH), established in 1992 as the Nigerian Fertility Society, then incorporated as AFRH in 2010; the Uganda Fertility Society, established

2014; and the Fertility Society of Ghana (FERSOG), established in 2016. Similar societies exist in Morocco, Tunisia and Algeria.

Concurrently, some patient advocacy organizations have emerged to provide support to couples with reproductive health issues through education, counselling, advocacy and awareness programs. The Joyce Fertility Support Centre, established in 1998 in Uganda by Rita Sembuya following a personal struggle with infertility, has been active at the community level and has also engaged with national and international organizations to further infertility awareness and treatment in Africa. Similarly, the Infertility Awareness Association of South Africa (IFAASA), established in 2013, promotes infertility awareness while lobbying for medical insurance coverage of fertility treatment in South Africa.

This overview of the history of ART in Africa is fragmented and incomplete. It is largely based on personal communications (see acknowledgements) and supplemented by what published data there are. The latter emphasize the diverse pathways through which ART established itself in Africa and the equal diversity of countries in which skills and knowledge were exported, spanning, among others, to the north of Africa, the UK, Germany, Belgium, France and Sweden; to the east, the former USSR (today Ukraine) and India; and to the west, the US and Cuba [7, 8]. In addition, the many challenges related to the import of equipment, lack of continuity of medical supply chains, unstable supply of electricity and early community antagonism have been documented [7]. While the latter narrative applies to the origins of ART in Uganda, one might hypothesize that it is applicable to many other countries. Finally, the very scant or absent ART activity in several of Africa's 55 countries must be acknowledged (Fig. 13.1). No formal or comprehensive evaluation of countries with and without ART in Africa exists, but to the authors' knowledge there is some ART activity in Botswana, Democratic Republic of the Congo, Gabon, Libya, Madagascar and Mauritania; but none in Angola, Burundi, Central African Republic, Chad, Congo, Equatorial Guinea, Eritrea, Gambia, Guinea, Guinea-Bissau, Liberia, Malawi, Mozambique, Niger, Somalia, South Sudan and Zambia.

The Beginning of ART Surveillance in Africa

ART surveillance in Africa was initiated through three different avenues that continued independent of each

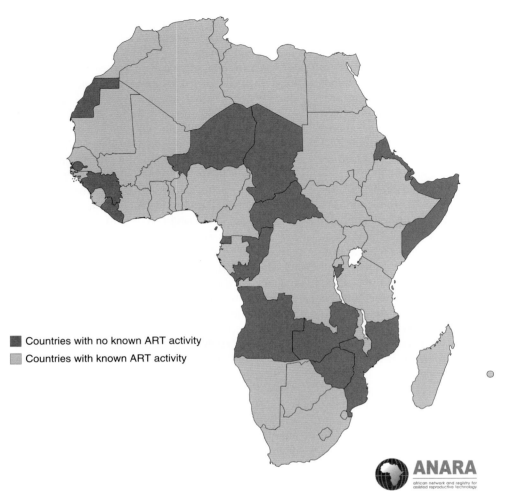

Figure 13.1
Distribution of ART services in Africa. (Figure created with mapchart.net ©)

■ Countries with no known ART activity
■ Countries with known ART activity

other for several years. All avenues were, however, initiated together with ICMART.

Starting in 1989 in Egypt, ART data were sent annually from the founding centre (Egyptian IVF Centre) to ICMART, which was then called the International Working Group on Assisted Reproduction (IWGOAR). The first IVF registry in Egypt was started by Ragaa Mansour in 2001, collecting data from cycles done in 1999 [10]. The Egyptian IVF Registry data were sent annually to ICMART. In October 2003, a workshop was held in Cairo, organized by ICMART in collaboration with WHO and facilitated by Ragaa Mansour, to establish the first Middle East IVF Registry. This workshop was under

the auspices of the Egyptian Ministry of Health and the Egyptian Medical Syndicate. It was attended by 139 infertility specialists from 97 ART centres in 14 countries [11]. The workshop was very successful, and 98% of the participants agreed to start the Middle East IVF Registry under the direction of Ragaa Mansour. This regional registry collected data starting with cycles done in 2000 in which 31 centres participated from 8 countries reporting on 16,523 cycles [11]. The registry continued to report data to ICMART annually until 2011, when reporting started to become irregular and sporadic due to political instability in the region [12, 13, 14]. Egypt, however, maintained annual data collection and reporting to ICMART [14, 15]. In 2017, Egyptian centres decided to report as part of Africa rather than the Middle East, and joined ANARA, the African Network and Registry for ART that had since emerged. First data, pertaining to cycles performed in 2013, were sent to ANARA at the end of 2017 and will be part of ANARA's inaugural publication.

In the francophone countries of West Africa, ICMART, represented especially by Jacques de Mouzon from France, liaised with individual ART centres as well as with representatives of GIERAF. As a result, Cameroon and Togo sent first data to the ICMART world report in 2009, joined by Mali and then Benin and Ivory Coast in 2010 and 2011, respectively. Only single ART centres exist in most of these countries, reflecting the relatively sparse availability of ART.

In anglophone sub-Saharan Africa, ART monitoring was initiated in South Africa at the 19th World Congress of IFFS held in Durban, South Africa, in 2007. As part of this meeting, ICMART scheduled an ART data symposium to invite feedback from African delegates regarding national and regional ART data collection [16]. In the absence of any such data collection, the feedback provided was embarrassingly meagre. The symposium, however, prompted the Southern African Society of Reproductive Medicine and Gynaecological Endoscopy (SASREG) to form a task group, under the leadership of Silke Dyer, to initiate national, voluntary and anonymous data collection and monitoring. It took two years of preparatory work to motivate ART centres to participate in the South African Registry for ART (SARA) and to reach a first consensus as to what data variables to collect and how. In 2010, SARA made a first call for data using a basic Microsoft Excel* spreadsheet to collect rudimentary data. Centres sent de-identified retrospective summary data to the SASREG secretariat, who pooled the data, maintaining strict anonymity of all centre-specific data; the pooled data were then made available to the SARA chair for analysis and reporting. *Ab initio*, SARA received major developmental assistance and support from the Latin American Register of Assisted Reproduction (RLA), represented by its founder and director, Fernando Zegers-Hochschild, as well as ongoing guidance from ICMART. In parallel to the first data collection, RLA adapted its own data software to South African needs and made this available to South African ART centres free of charge via its own online data

submission platform. This electronic interface was then used to collect annual data for 2011 to 2014.

Establishing the African Network and Registry for ART

Following the successful establishment of a national ART registry in South Africa, ICMART encouraged thinking towards a regional registry in sub-Saharan Africa. The thinking was driven not only by the overwhelming absence of ART data from sub-Saharan Africa but also by the understanding that African countries had to come together in order to put Africa on the map of global ART and infertility-related reproductive health; and that data would be needed to create visibility and engagement. In December 2014, at a WHO-ICMART Infertility Guidelines and ART Glossary meeting in Geneva, David Adamson (Chair of ICMART), Fernando Zegers-Hochschild (Vice Chair of ICMART and Director of RLA), and Silke Dyer (board member of ICMART and SARA Chair), further conceptualized the idea and named it ANARA (African Network and Registry for ART). Silke Dyer wrote a project proposal modelling ANARA on the Latin American Network and Register of Assisted Reproduction (REDLARA). Approval for both the project and registry was obtained from the Ethics Committee of the Faculty of Health Sciences, University of Cape Town, and has since been maintained. First emails were sent in 2015, initially inviting ART leaders from anglophone sub-Saharan African countries to a conversation on ART data collection, and first positive replies were received. Regional and international meetings provided opportunities for face-to-face meetings, strengthening both relationships and the conversation. The fact that ART monitoring in Africa was far outside mainstream thinking was exemplified at the regional meeting of the International Federation of Gynecology and Obstetrics (FIGO) Africa in Addis Ababa in October 2015. On request, the conference organizers had announced a lunchtime meeting to discuss data collection on ART in sub-Saharan Africa. Approximately 25 delegates arrived. All but one left when realizing that the meeting was not about HIV and antiretroviral therapy. The one remaining, Rudolph Kantum Adageba, however, became an advocate for data collection in Ghana and helped to form the Fertility Society of Ghana in 2016.

By 2016, ANARA had a logo and a website (www .anara-africa.com). More important, ANARA also had its own software. The Latin American Register had converted from retrospective summary data to the collection of cycle-by-cycle data and had built a user-friendly, state-of-the art program (see Chapter 19, ART Surveillance in Latin America). This was duplicated and given to ANARA as a gift. ANARA reached an agreement with the software developer to continue maintaining both registries, which thus are closely related yet function separately from each other. Moreover, RLA and ANARA agreed to remain in close communication and to make any beneficial changes in the one registry data program available to each other.

The growing conversation around infertility, ART and data collection gave clarity to ANARA's vision and mission. The vision was developed "to reduce the high burden of infertility in sub-Saharan Africa through ART that is available, effective and safe". This vision clearly required data on availability, effectiveness and safety of ART as the cornerstone of all development strategies, and the collaboration between ART centres within and across countries. The unification of both people and data thus became ANARA's mission.

These developments were paralleled by creating a hub and infrastructure to support the registry and network within the Clinical Research Centre (CRC) of the Faculty of Health Sciences at the University of Cape Town. ANARA is constituted as a research network and registry, and relevant terms of reference as well as standard operating procedures were developed. The CRC continues to provide assistance in project management and administration and all financial transactions are handled by the research finance section of the faculty.

In November 2015, the first ANARA workshop was held in Pretoria, South Africa. With the help of two industry grants, a selected group of ART centre directors plus embryologists from other African countries was sponsored to attend, resulting in participation from Botswana, Cameroon, Ghana, Kenya, Nigeria, Mauritius, Uganda and Togo. The meeting was vibrant, successful and indicative of what was to follow. To date, workshops have been held at Ivory Coast (at the bi-annual meeting of GIERAF), in Nigeria (at the annual Association for Fertility and Reproductive Health conference), Ghana (at the launch of the Fertility Society of Ghana), Togo (again in conjunction with GIERAF), Uganda (at the AFS/IFFS meeting in 2018) and Cairo (in conjunction with the Egyptian IVF Registry) – and more will follow.

The objective of these workshops is to build capacity in data collection including hands-on training in the use of ANARA's software. It is equally about meeting people, building and strengthening relationships and understanding the diverse and collective context in which infertility care is rendered with its many opportunities and challenges – both being plentiful in Africa.

By the end of 2017, Egypt had joined ANARA. A few months later, the president of GIERAF, Mohamed Latoundji, and the Director of ANARA, Silke Dyer, signed a Memorandum of Understanding, reflecting a spirit of collaboration. This growing acceptance of and belonging to ANARA implied that the initial focus on anglophone countries in sub-Saharan Africa had shifted to encompass North and francophone African countries, thus making ANARA a truly African registry and network.

First Regional Data and Methodology of Data Collection

In 2017, ANARA responded to ICMART's call for the 2013 world data and, in conjunction with ICMART, collected data from 40 centres in 13 countries. As the data preceded the launch of ANARA and its data software, data were collected by means of the ICMART data spreadsheets, capturing retrospective summary data pertaining to ART utilization, effectiveness and safety. In addition, several centres submitted centre-specific data formats. Data quality was diverse, but most centres and countries were not able to provide all information requested by ICMART. Missing data related not only to techniques that were not available or utilized, such as preimplantation genetic testing, but more often to lack of data per se, particularly pertaining to deliveries and births. Pooled data were analyzed after data errors were resolved through queries with ART centres and, where this was not possible, by eliminating errors through triangulation or dismissing a subset of data that were not plausible.

These first data were presented at the 2017 AFRH conference in Nigeria. Ibrahim Wada, Deputy President of AFRH, presented the first data for Nigeria; Moïse Fiadjoe, Founding President of GIERAF, presented the first data for francophone African countries; and Silke Dyer, Director of ANARA, presented the first data for Africa. The data are currently being written up for publication and, once released, will be the final sign of the successful establishment of ANARA. In acknowledgement, all participating centres received certificates of participation from both ICMART and ANARA.

Going forward, the ANARA software will enable a better process for collecting information as well as better data. Participating centres are given free access to the registry software. Upon registration with ANARA, centres receive login credentials with which to access their own, centre-specific and confidential home page within the registry. Data are captured cycle by cycle pertaining to six ART techniques and procedures: fresh IVF/ICSI, frozen embryo transfers, frozen-thawed oocyte transfers, oocyte donation, fertility preservation and intrauterine insemination. Collected data can be viewed through interactive reports and graphs that, for example, show pregnancy and delivery rates by age or number of embryos transferred. Centres have access to three levels of information: their own centre's data; their own country's data; and the regional African data. Both patient confidentiality and centre confidentiality are strictly maintained: all patient data are de-identified, and no centre can see the data of another centre. In addition, no country can see the data from another country, although all countries can see the data for Africa. ANARA also protects data ownership: centres continue to own their own data, countries own their national data and ANARA owns the regional data. Terms and conditions of data submission are captured in a Memorandum of Understanding that is signed by ANARA and each participating centre. See Figure 13.2 for ANARA's activity in Africa.

Data Scope and Validity

The scope of data is of critical importance. Each data point must be pertinent. Too many data points make the system laborious and time-consuming without adding relevant benefit to stakeholders, thus risking non-compliance in a setting where data collection is still being established and voluntary. There is an international expert debate on the width and depth of registry data, informed by the large registries such as ICMART, EIM, REDLARA and SART, which is beyond the scope of this chapter. Suffice to say that ANARA's data software, being identical to REDLARA's, benefits enormously from REDLARA's years of experience on what data to collect and how. Moreover, Africa as a region is often compared with Latin America and shares a more similar context of data collection than with, for example, Europe or the

US. ANARA's software offers a robust yet elegant, cycle-by-cycle-based method of data collection that is comprehensive without being time-consuming, and it is easy to use. Homogeneity of how and what data are collected across an entire region strengthens the process of data collection as well as the resultant data – and further fosters a collective spirit within the network. That said, ANARA's mission does not lie in the promotion or implementation of a particular software but in the bringing together of people and of data. It is open to interact with and receive data from other software programs, whether these are used by individual ART centres or an entire country. In the case of the latter, the process of data collection, anonymity, data protection and feedback at the level of individual centres and a country does not rest with ANARA, but ANARA will receive such data for integration into the regional African data and will provide anonymity, data protection and feedback at the regional level.

Data validity is as important as the scope of data collected. For now, ANARA has, however, prioritized the building of trust and relationships over the investigation of data validity. Currently, all data that are mathematically correct are accepted at face value. Because data are pooled and no data from individual centres are ever disclosed, there is, in principle, no reason for or benefit in the submission of biased data. It will be for the network part of ANARA, meaning its people, to decide if and when data submitted to the Registry will be validated and if so, how. When this point is reached, REDLARA again provides an attractive model. Briefly, ART centres are accredited in three stages (temporary, partial and full accreditation) and part of this process involves checking the quality and validity of data submitted. REDLARA has an accreditation committee and members who are trained and qualified to undertake accreditation visits. Inspections are performed by persons from another country to provide an additional layer of confidentiality and hence acceptability for the centre undergoing accreditation [17].

Success, Challenges and Future Plans

Success

ANARA has enjoyed considerable success in a relatively short time. This success has several roots. The many benefits of national, regional and global ART registries were already established and

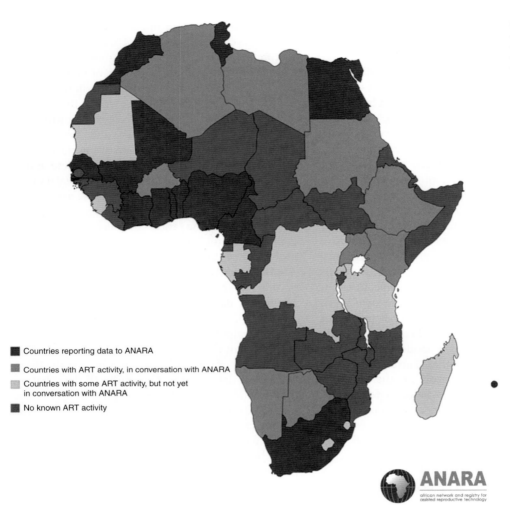

Figure 13.2 ANARA activity in Africa. A colour version of the figure is provided in the plate section. (Figure created with mapchart.net ©)

Countries reporting data to ANARA

Countries with ART activity, in conversation with ANARA

Countries with some ART activity, but not yet in conversation with ANARA

No known ART activity

ANARA
african network and registry for
assisted reproductive technology

recognized, providing the foundation for ANARA. ANARA's vision and mission were equally important, as they linked the need for a registry with the goal of creating togetherness and building an African stewardship with and around data, aimed ultimately at reducing the burden of infertility on the continent. The vision and mission were most readily received by centres and fertility organizations, resulting in a new spirit of collaboration. Such collaboration had been previously lacking, as ART centres were historically more likely to develop partnerships with centres in Europe and North America than within or between countries in Africa [5, 8].

From the beginning, ANARA focused on building relationships with individual centres, which are ANARA's primary stakeholders, as well as with the regional and national fertility organizations.

The latter required an understanding and acceptance of the differences between a fertility organization and a registry. Briefly, the former is characterized by elected and changing office bearers, membership structures and mandates relating to the interests of its members and, beyond this, to developing or informing policies, regulations and overall capacity building for ART service delivery. ANARA, in contrast, is a research network aimed at collecting data and maintaining data integrity. This aim is best served by the consistency provided by a small operational core group that is not involved with the politics of fertility organizations and its changing office bearers. Both sides stand to benefit from the relationship and from mutual assistance in achieving set goals. Specifically, ANARA benefits if fertility societies encourage their members to participate in data collection, while ANARA makes the data freely available to the fertility organizations to help them achieve their respective mandates.

ANARA's successful establishment would not have been possible without the enormous developmental assistance provided by the Latin American Register. This assistance included not only the initial sharing and subsequent donation of software, but also the equal sharing of invaluable experience concerning how to build a regional registry and network. In addition, ANARA received ever-present guidance from ICMART that provided a global perspective and insight relating to data registries. ICMART has a strong reputation in Africa; the ability to contribute data to ICMART for the annual ART world report, and in turn receive recognition from ICMART, continues to be a motivating force. Equally important was the collaborative spirit in which individual ART centres as well as national and regional fertility societies in Africa were willing to engage. Receipt of some funding from the South African National Research Foundation provided financial support as well as recognition of the importance of ANARA's research. Industry stakeholders also contributed to ANARA's success through their supportive attitude, spreading of the word and providing financial assistance for workshops and some of ANARA's infrastructure.

Challenges

Challenges remain. Barriers to the sharing of data are not unique to Africa. They include reluctance of centres to share data, often driven by a fear of disclosure of their own individual data; undue competitiveness between centres; as well as lack of a process or infrastructure for data collection and relative inexperience with the collection of scientific data. These barriers were similarly encountered in the early years of the Latin American Register but successfully overcome [17]. Some of these barriers are driven by the lack of resource allocation to infertility in general and ART specifically by governments and medical aid schemes. Overcoming these barriers requires the building of trust and relationships and recognition that collectively and with sound data more can be achieved to promote availability and utilization of safe and effective ART with multiple resultant benefits. To date, the majority of countries providing ART in Africa have joined ANARA, but the majority of centres have yet to do so. According to the curve of adoption of new technology, ANARA is, however, past the tipping

point. Briefly, according to this theory, the majority of potential users (68%) will not accept innovation or new technology until the innovators (2.5%) and the early adopters (13.5%) have done so – at which point the system tips in favour of the new technology [18]. In 2017, in those countries that participated, 19.1% of centres that were reported to exist shared their data. This percentage lies beyond the tipping point of 16%.

Another challenge will be maintaining financial stability and sustainability. To date, ANARA has provided its software and processes of data collection and reporting for free to participating centres and intends to continue doing so in the future. Its own operational requirements, aimed at creating maximal effectiveness with minimal means, have been supported by two modest industry grants as well as a national research foundation grant.

Future Plans

ANARA's five-year goal is to continue growing the network and invite participation in the Registry. This goal will be pursued through the avenues of active engagement with all stakeholders, participation in scientific meetings on the continent and further afield, facilitation of data workshops, expanding e-Learning material and the annual publication of regional data. ANARA will seek to develop its software for data collection, keeping it abreast of new developments in ART and capable of capturing these. While not without challenges – as many registries are currently exploring, for example, how to capture ART outcomes by woman rather than by cycle – the close relationship with REDLARA will allow for mutual exchange of new registry developments in the developing Global South. Moreover, both registries and networks have similar goals, such as the reduction of multiple pregnancies and improving access to care. Although access to care is in itself not a measurable entity, ART utilization is one of very few proxy indicators for access to infertility care that exist [19, 20]. Latin America and Africa have by far the lowest rate of ART utilization globally (150 and 84 cycles/million population/annum [21]), with the estimated global need for ART being 1,500 cycles/million population [22]. Thus, reporting of this indicator year after year is arguably the only monitor of inequalities and inequities in access to infertility care in these regions.

In order to make impact, ANARA will make its data widely available and will seek to work with fertility organizations and other stakeholders in Africa to optimize ART accessibility, effectiveness and safety. Last but not least, ANARA will seek to further build on the existing relationships with global fertility organizations such as ICMART, IFFS and FIGO, and with other regional registries, with the aim of strengthening Africa's contribution in global monitoring of ART as well as progress towards universal access to infertility care, which underpins the human right to establish a family.

Acknowledgements

The authors wish to gratefully acknowledge Professor Oladapo Ashiru (Nigeria), Ms Afua Dadzie (Ghana), Dr Moïse Fiadjoe (Togo), Dr Rajat Goswamy (Mauritius), Dr Bell Bea Gwet (Cameroon), Dr Ernestine Gwet Bell (Cameroon), Professor Thinus Kruger (South Africa), Dr Ragaa Mansour (Egypt) and Dr James Olobo-Lalobo (Uganda) for providing information pertaining to the history of ART in Africa.

References

1. Kruger TF, Menkveld R, Stander FS, Lombard CJ, Van der Merwe JP, Van Zyl JA, et al. Sperm morphologic features as a prognostic factor in in-vitro fertilization. *Fertil Steril.* 1986;**46**(6):1118–23.

2. Kruger TF, Acosta AA, Simmons KF, Swanson RJ, Matta JF, Oehninger S. Predictive value of abnormal sperm morphology in in-vitro fertilization. *Fertil Steril.* 1988;**49**(1):112–17.

3. Mansour RT. The establishment of the first IVF registry in Egypt. *Middle East Fertil Soc J.* 2003;**8**(2):97–102.

4. Ashiru OA, Akinola LA. Emerging roles of anatomists: development of assisted reproductive technology in West Africa. *Anatomy J Africa.* 2013;**2**(1):84–96.

5. Giwa-Osagie OF. ART in developing countries with particular reference to sub-Saharan Africa. In E Vayena, PJ Rowe, D Griffin (eds.), *Current Practices and Controversies in Assisted Reproduction: Report of a Meeting on 'Medical, Ethical and Social Aspects of Assisted Reproduction' Held at WHO Headquarters in Geneva, Switzerland, 17–21 September 2001.* Geneva: WHO; 2002. pp.22–7.

6. Gerrits T. Assisted reproductive technologies in Ghana: transnational undertakings, local practices and 'more affordable' IVF. *Reprod Biomed Soc Online.* 2016(2): 32–8.

7. Platteau P, Desmet B, Odoma G, Albano C, Devroey P, Tamale Sali E. Four years of IVF/ICSI experience in Kampala (Uganda). *ESHRE Monographs.* 2008(1):90–2.

8. Hörbst V. 'You cannot do IVF in Africa as in Europe': the making of IVF in Mali and Uganda. *Reprod Biomed Soc Online.* 2016(2):108–15.

9. Zegers-Hochschild F, Adamson D, Dyer S, Racowsky C, de Mouzon J, Sokol R, et al. The International Glossary on Infertility and Fertility Care, 2017. *Hum Reprod.* 2017(32):1786–801.

10. Mansour RT, Abou-Setta AM. Assisted reproductive technology in Egypt, 2001: results generated from the Egyptian IVF Registry. *Middle East Fertil Soc J.* 2005;**10** (2):87–93.

11. Mansour R. The Middle East IVF Registry for the year 2000. *Middle East Fertil Soc J.* 2004;**9**(3):181–6.

12. International Committee for Monitoring Assisted Reproductive Technology (ICMART), Adamson GD, de Mouzon J, Lancaster P, Nygren KG, Sullivan E, Zegers-Hochschild F. World collaborative report on in-vitro fertilisation, 2000. *Fertil Steril.* 2006;**85**(6): 1586–622.

13. Mansour RT, Abou-Setta AM. Results of assisted reproductive technology in 2001 generated from the Middle East IVF Registry. *Middle East Fertil Soc J.* 2006;**11**(3):145–51.

14. Mansour RT, Abou-Setta AM, Kamal O. Assisted reproductive technology in Egypt, 2003–2004: results generated from the Egyptian IVF Registry. *Middle East Fertil Soc J.* 2011(16):1–6.

15. Mansour RT, El-Faissal Y, Kamal O. The Egyptian IVF Registry report: assisted reproductive technology in Egypt 2005. *Middle East Fertil Soc J.* 2014 (19):16–21.

16. Dalmeyer P. Reproductive medicine in South Africa and IFFS 2007 – Durban. *S Afr J Obstet Gynaecol.* 2007;**13**(2):34–5.

17. Zegers-Hochschild F, Schwarze JE, Galdames V. Assisted reproductive technologies in Latin America: an example of regional co-operation and development. *ESHRE Monographs.* 2008(1):42–7.

18. Berwick DM. Disseminating innovations in health care. *JAMA.* 2003;**289**(15):1969–75.

19. McIntyre D, Thiede M, Birch S. Access as a policy-relevant concept in low and middle income countries. *Health Econ Policy Law.* 2009(4):79–193.

20. Botha B, Shamley D, Dyer S. Availability, effectiveness and safety of ART in sub-Saharan Africa: a systematic review. *Hum Reprod Open.* 2018(2):hoy003.

21. Dyer S, Chambers GM, de Mouzon J, Nygren KG, Zegers-Hochschild F, Mansour R, et al. International Committee for Monitoring Assisted Reproductive Technologies world report: assisted reproductive technology 2008, 2009 and 2010. *Hum Reprod.* 2016;**31** (7):1588–609.

22. ESHRE Capri Workshop Group. Social determinants of human reproduction. *Hum Reprod.* 2001;**16**(7): 1518–26.

ART Surveillance in Asia

Osamu Ishihara, Manish Banker and Bai Fu

Introduction

Asia is composed of more than 40 countries, containing about 60% of the global population. Because Asia is the largest continent, geographically variable and culturally and socially diverse, it is almost impossible to describe the whole area in one chapter. Rapid decline of birth rates in multiple countries, particularly in eastern Asia, drew wide public attention and promoted the treatment of and care for infertile couples. In particular, assisted reproductive technology (ART) has spread significantly in many Asian countries and its growth is still ongoing. Although ART registries were established in several Asian countries many years ago, there is no Asian regional registry because the area is so diverse. In this chapter, therefore, we will describe ART surveillance in China, India and Japan.

Art Surveillance in China

Introduction

In China, ART refers to all medical treatments or procedures that include the in vitro handling of human oocytes or sperm, zygotes and embryos for the purpose of establishing a pregnancy. This includes artificial insemination (AI) and in vitro fertilization and embryo transfer (IVF-ET) and the various derived technologies.

The first IVF-ET baby in China was born at Peking University Third Hospital in March 1988 [1]. The first intracytoplasmic sperm injection (ICSI) baby was born in April 1996 at the First Affiliated Hospital of Sun Yatsen University (Zhongshan Hospital), Guangdong province, which was also the birthplace of the first preimplantation genetic diagnosis (PGD) baby in 2000 [2].

Infertility is defined as the failure to achieve a clinical pregnancy after 12 months or more of regular unprotected sexual intercourse. The prevalence of infertility in China is about 7–10% [3]. Since 1988, China has made great progress in reproductive medicine. Core assisted reproductive technologies have been practised comprehensively in China. The number of accredited ART centres has increased rapidly, especially in the past decade, from 37 in 2004 to 451 in 2016. The number of IVF/ICSI cycles is now more than 200,000 each year, and the clinical pregnancy rate is about 40% [4].

Registry of ART Service Providers in China

A registry of ART service providers began in the mid-1990s. In 1994, the State Council of the People's Republic of China promulgated the Regulations on Administration of Medical Institutions (RAMI), which were formally implemented on 1 September 1994. Medical institutions must be registered and obtain a practice licence for a medical institution, as clearly specified in RAMI. The main registered items include the following: name of the registered medical institutions, address, and principal person in charge, forms of ownership, health care subjects, number of beds and the registered capital. Medical institutions that provide ART services were registered as 'Reproductive health and infertility treatment subject' under the obstetrics and gynaecology health care subject registry. ART registry was combined with medical institution registry during that period.

Centre-Based ART Surveillance and Registry

In 2001, the Ministry of Health (now the National Health Commission, NHC) promulgated the Regulations for Management of Human Assisted Reproductive Technology and Regulations for Management of Human Sperm Bank. These two policies marked a significant milestone in assisted

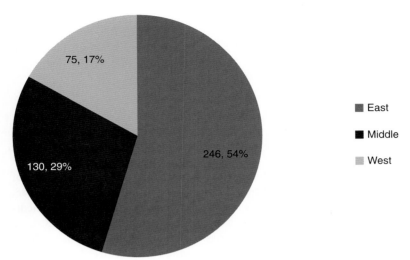

Figure 14.1 Regional distribution of ART clinics in China.

- East
- Middle
- West

reproductive technology management. As clearly stipulated in the regulations for ART application, medical institutions should be preapproved by the health administrative department of the people's governments of provinces, autonomous regions and municipalities directly under the central government. The preliminary provincial opinion is essential for the final approval of the Ministry of Health [5].

The approved institutions providing ART services should conform to the provisions concerning the technical personnel, site condition, equipment and facilities, medical ethics committee and other technical specifications and basic standards. In 2007, the administrative approval of ART was adjusted by the State Council to the provincial health administrative department. The NHC is responsible for the dynamic supervision of ART services approval and implementation nationwide and for the registration of approved ART centres. The purpose of registration is to provide guidance for infertility health care seekers by regularly providing the list of ART centres to the public. The variables are as follows: name of ART centre, address, ART services provided (artificial insemination homologous (AIH), artificial insemination by donor (AID), IVF/ICSI-ET, PGD, sperm bank), practice state (trial or formal) and approval date.

In 2004, there were a total of 37 ART centres in China; in 2007 and 2012, there were 102 and 358 ART centres, respectively. By the end of 2016, the total

number of ART centres increased significantly to 451. ART centre distributions and ART services being provided in eastern, central and western regions are shown in Figures 14.1 and 14.2.

Cycle-Based ART Surveillance System in China

Since 1988, ART has gradually become an important medical measure for infertile couples, bringing hope to tens of thousands of families grappling with infertility. ART, however, involves many medical, social, ethical and legal issues, and therefore belongs to a special section of medical technology that should be practised under scientific data-supported supervision and evaluation [6].

A collection form has been used for reporting yearly statistical data of the cycles completed in ART centres. In 2012, the total number of initiated cycles was 507,190 (including 103,730 artificial insemination cycles), with 162,585 clinical pregnancies and 158,287 live births. The clinical pregnancy rate per 100 initiated cycles was 32%.

NHC sponsored a public welfare scientific research program, 'Establishment of Quality Control System of Assisted Reproductive Technology', in 2014. The National Center for Women and Children's Health (NCWCH) was responsible for one of the tasks – 'Research and Development of the Cycle-Based China ART Surveillance System (CASS) Platform'. CASS was designed as a quality

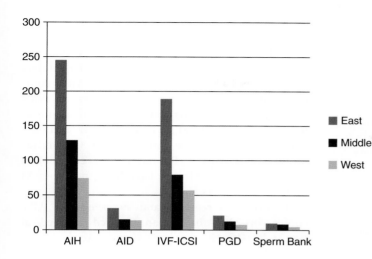

Figure 14.2 Services provided at ART clinics in China.

surveillance, data collecting platform that covers all ART categories (AIH/AID/IVF/ICSI/frozen embryo transfer (FET)/PGD) and all cycles initiated. Key variables collected are listed as follows: cycle ID number, age, cause of infertility, ART category, oocyte source, ovulation induction regimens, sperm source, sperm retrieval, number of oocytes retrieved, number of fertilized oocytes, number of embryos transferred, pregnancy outcome (clinical pregnancy/abortion/ectopic pregnancy), delivery outcome (live birth/single-infant birth/multiple-infant birth/birth defect), mild and severe ovarian hyperstimulation syndrome (OHSS). By July 2017, CASS had been successfully developed.

Successes and Challenges

As one of the world's most populous nations, China has made great strides in health improvement and health service provision. The past three decades have also witnessed the amazing advances in ART. China is making efforts to standardize ART monitoring and evaluation. The successful development of CASS is one milestone along the way.

The Network Security Law of the People's Republic of China has officially been implemented since 1 June 2017. The ART database should completely comply with the requirements of the Network Security Law of the People's Republic of China and the Measures for the Management of Information Security Protection. The ART data should be transmitted and stored in a secure limited-access, digital certificate authentication and password-protected environment with the purpose of information security protection.

Art Surveillance in India

Introduction

Infertility causes intense mental agony and trauma to the couple. Although there are no detailed figures of the extent of infertility prevalence in India, a multinational study carried out by the World Health Organization (WHO) [7], which included India, places the incidence of infertility between 10 and 15%. By extrapolating the WHO estimate, approximately 13–19 million couples are likely to be infertile in the country at any given time.

The world's first IVF baby, Louise Brown, was born 25 July 1978 in the United Kingdom (UK) through the efforts of Dr Robert G. Edwards and Dr Patrick Steptoe. Sixty-seven days later, the world's second and India's first IVF baby, Kanupriya, alias Durga, was born 3 October 1978, in Kolkata, through the efforts of Dr Subhas Mukherjee. Unfortunately, the state authorities prevented him from presenting his work at scientific conferences, although he had published a brief report on the work done in the *Indian Journal of Cryogenics* [8]. Therefore, it was much later that India had the first scientifically documented IVF baby, Harsha, who was born in Mumbai on 6 August 1986, through the collaborative efforts of the Indian Council of Medical Research (ICMR) Institute for Research in Reproduction and King Edward's Memorial Hospital.

ART Registry in India

World data on the availability, effectiveness and safety of ART have been published beginning in 1989 [9]. The first initiative to establish an Indian ART registry was taken by the Indian Society for Assisted Reproduction (ISAR) in 2000. It involved voluntary contributions by ART clinics, wherein forms were sent to all ISAR members and ART clinics. The first edition of the National ART Registry of India (NARI 2000) had 43 clinics submitting their data. Information was collected under 6 categories: fresh ovarian stimulations and embryo transfer, thawed embryo transfers, egg donation cycles, egg sharing, embryo donation and surrogacy. Annual summary data collection included information about total number of cycles, indications for ART, type of stimulation protocols, drugs used (urinary or recombinant), number of eggs collected, number of embryos transferred, pregnancy rate and pregnancy outcome (singleton/multiple gestation, abortions, ectopic pregnancy). Data were scrutinized for obvious discrepancies and omissions and the respective clinics were asked to correct for them if there were any. Because ISAR does not have any statutory powers, it could neither verify the authenticity of the data nor force all clinics to participate. It was difficult to convince clinics to send their data. However, the number of clinics increased gradually to 116 in 2006. Total stimulations increased from 7,273 in 2001 to 21,408 in 2006. The major drawback was that there was no control to check authenticity of data, poor documentation by many centres and lack of information on complications, delivery outcomes and neonatal outcomes.

Web-Based Registry

In order to increase participation and make ART registry more robust, NARI was converted to an online web-based registry in April 2010. The software was licensed from the Society for Assisted Reproductive Technology (SART). Each clinic was given its own ID and password to enter the data. The registry maintained confidentiality, as only the clinic was able to access its own data. Yearly national summaries were published. It gave clinics the advantage of analyzing their own data and comparing them with the national averages. However, the online web-based system of collecting data did not succeed and ISAR had to revert to manual data collection two years later. Every year, NARI's compiled data are mailed to all contributors, all ISAR members and presidents and secretaries of all obstetric and gynaecological societies of India. Data are also submitted to the International Committee Monitoring Assisted Reproductive Technologies (ICMART) every year and have been incorporated in its world reports.

In order to regulate and supervise the ART clinics, in 2005 the Indian Council of Medical Research (ICMR) and National Academy of Medical Sciences (NAMS) formulated guidelines for accreditation, supervision and regulation of ART clinics [10]. The drafting committee was composed of 19 members from government nominees, ART specialists, lawyers and non-governmental organizations (NGOs). The guidelines defined categories of infertility care units, indications, minimum requirements of ART clinics, complications of ART and code of practice, ethical considerations and legal issues.

ART Bill in India

Based on these guidelines, the Indian Council of Medical Research and the Ministry of Health and Family Welfare developed a draft, the Assisted Reproductive Technology (Regulation) Bill, in 2008. This draft was subjected to extensive debate and, based on the comments and recommendations of the drafting committee, the draft Assisted Reproductive Technology (Regulation) Rules were revised and finalized. The finalized version of the draft Assisted Reproductive Technology (Regulation) Bill-2010 was sent to the Ministry of Health and Family Welfare and has now been placed on the government's website as the Assisted Reproductive Technology (Regulation) Bill-2017 for final comments from all stakeholders [11]. The Regulation Bill also proposed the formation of the National Registry of Assisted Reproductive Technology Clinics and Banks in India (NRACBI), which would act as the central database for all the assisted reproductive technology clinics and banks in India and would help the state boards and the national board in accreditation, supervision and regulation of ART clinics and banks and also would contribute in policy making.

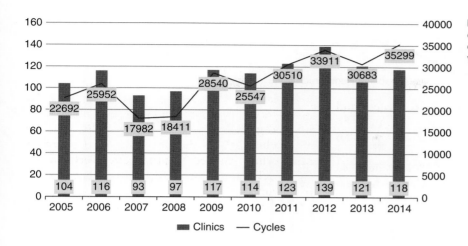

Figure 14.3 Numbers of registered clinics and cycles of ART in India. A colour version of this figure is provided in the plate section.

Current reporting of NARI takes into account the type of the cycle. In a fresh cycle, indication of ART, methods of stimulation protocol, number of eggs retrieved, number of embryos transferred, outcome of pregnancy and multiple pregnancies are noted. In frozen-thawed cycles, type of protocol, number of embryos transferred, outcome in terms of pregnancy and multiple gestation are noted. In egg donation cycles, the age of recipients, indications, number of eggs used for sharing, number of embryos transferred and the outcome are noted. In embryo donation cycles, number of embryos and outcome are noted. In surrogacy, indications, number of embryos transferred and pregnancy outcome are noted. To date, no data collection has been reported for intrauterine insemination.

Future Perspective

The most recent data published in 2015 included the reports from 2013 and 2014. Fresh embryo transfers rose from 15,508 in 2013 to 16,856 in 2014, with pregnancies from 5,900 to 6,905, respectively. Frozen-thawed embryo transfers increased from 6,179 in 2013 to 7,046 in 2014 (Fig. 14.3).

The major problem today is the absence of legislation, making the contribution voluntary. There is also a lack of awareness of NARI among the general public. This can be overcome by linking to as many websites as possible as well as releasing information to media that would subsequently put pressure on ART clinics. Financial issues need to be addressed, which can be overcome by collecting token fees from participating clinics as well as asking for help from industry.

Art Surveillance in Japan

Introduction of Registry

In response to the birth of the first IVF baby in 1983 at Tohoku University, the Japan Society of Obstetrics and Gynecology (JSOG) introduced a guideline of IVF-ET in October 1983 [12]. This guideline was composed of the indications, the requirements for couples and participating doctors and the minimal requirements concerning ethical and legal perspectives for practising IVF-ET. Subsequently, the first Japanese registry for ART (IVF and GIFT) was established by JSOG in March 1986. This mandatory registry was operated by the ART registry committee of JSOG according to the separate JSOG guideline asking for registration by every ART clinic [13].

This first registry required registered clinics to report yearly their annual numbers of patients, laparoscopic egg collections, collected eggs, frozen eggs and embryos, transferred cycles and transferred embryos; 24 clinics were included in the first annual registry report [14]. Treatment outcomes including pregnancy, miscarriage and delivery were also requested from each clinic.

In 1989, the registry introduced a more detailed, cycle-based questionnaire consisting of 39 items including information about patients and infants. However, the response rate dropped to approximately 70% of the 125 registered clinics, partly owing to the cumbersome paperwork. Therefore, the registry started to organize two separate systems simultaneously beginning in 1990, i.e. a compulsory clinic-based annual data collection previously used and

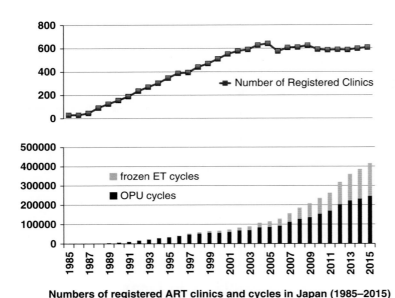

Figure 14.4 Numbers of registered clinics and cycles of ART in Japan.

Numbers of registered ART clinics and cycles in Japan (1985–2015)

a voluntary cycle-based data collection that started in 1989. In 1990, 142 out of 156 registered clinics (91%) responded, reporting 7,405 cycles resulting in 1,178 pregnancies, 771 live births and 1,031 babies [15]. From 1992, the JSOG Ethics Committee became responsible for the compulsory clinic-based data collection and began collecting ICSI data as well. Because of JSOG's reorganization, its Registry and Investigation Committee became responsible for the registry beginning in 1999. It started to collect the data of donor insemination cycles practised at 19 clinics, although there has been no data collection for intrauterine insemination to date. Meanwhile, more detailed information was collected by the voluntary group, as mentioned above; however, the response rate was far from satisfactory.

Advances and Drawbacks of ART

The number of ART clinics and cycles continued to increase during the 1990s in Japan, just as in other countries (Fig. 14.4). The upper limit of transferred embryos was set at 3 according to a 1996 JSOG guideline, which was fairly advanced at the time. However, the high multiple pregnancy rate (MPR) after ART, approximately 20%, resulted in large numbers of pre-term infants requiring neonatal intensive care unit (NICU) admission. This influx of babies was difficult to accommodate with the existing capacity of Japanese NICUs in the early years of the twenty-first

century. The best solution to reduce the MPR was to transition to a single embryo transfer (SET) policy. Such a policy had originally been proposed by pioneers in northern European countries where comprehensive ART registries and social insurance already existed [16].

Web-Based Registry and Reimbursement for ART

In 2006, JSOG's Registry and Investigation Committee started to construct the totally new online web-based ART registry system because of the rapid progress of Internet availability everywhere. The new system enabled Japan to accumulate the details of each cycle automatically, accompanied by background and pregnancy outcome data. Each registered clinic was issued its own ID and password and was able to register data from its office at its own convenience. Each clinic can obtain its own generated summary data from the system and compare those with the average of all registered clinics nationwide. However, each clinic's own data are completely anonymous, and comparative data between clinics are not available.

Around the same time, in January 2005, following yearly discussions with ART specialists and patients' lobbying groups, and in response to a decreasing birth rate, the Japanese government introduced partial reimbursement for ART treatments. The government asked all registered clinics to report outcomes of individual reimbursed cycles to the JSOG registry if they wished to participate in the government reimbursement program. In practice, the patient couples who want to obtain the allowance from their local government need to request a specific certificate from their physician in charge that contains a specific number issued after online registration of the cycle in the JSOG registry. The reimbursement is received as a bank transfer after submission of their paperwork to the local government office. There were several requirements for submission, e.g. a limitation of annual income, but initially no age limit was set.

While the transition to SET was initiated by an urgent demand from a shortage of neonatal care in Japan, the timing synchronized with the preparation of a sophisticated ART registry and the governmental financial support for patients. Since SET became mandatory, under certain conditions, in 2007 by JSOG guidelines, MPR resulting from ART started to drop dramatically, and in recent years is less than 5% [17].

Amendment of the Registry

Since 2007, the Japanese ART registry has frequently incorporated small revisions. Current reporting is basically composed of two separate data input web pages [18]. The first page accommodates data from the point of intention to treat to pregnancy test. The required data for all cycles are as follows: age of wife and husband, height and body weight, gravidity and parity, indication for ART, method of ovarian stimulation, method of oocyte pickup (OPU), type of embryo(s) intended to use, type of treatment, method of sperm collection, semen characteristics and the name of local government for reimbursement. In cycles with fresh transfer, the numbers of retrieved eggs and fertilized eggs are also required. In the cycles with frozen-thawed embryos, the numbers of thawed embryos and viable embryos are required. In all transferred cycles, stage of embryos, number of transferred and frozen embryos, method of luteal support, side effects and pregnancy outcome are needed. The second page consists of data as follows: number of gestational sacs, number of fetuses, outcome of pregnancy, number of infants, method of delivery, obstetrical complications and detailed information on all infants including detected congenital anomalies at birth.

Ten years after implementation, the most recent revision of the reimbursement program occurred in 2015. For the first time, female age limitation of younger than 43 years was introduced and annual limitation of treatment cycles was lifted, although total reimbursement opportunities were reduced to six times. The main reason for this revision was to increase the number of younger couples who will have easier access to ART treatment, although it is not yet known what the actual impact will be.

Dissemination of ART Data

All clinics' combined summary data from the Japanese ART registry have been published annually since 1990, written in Japanese, as the annual report from the Registry and Investigating Committee. However, the committee decided to publish the same data in English as well as in Japanese starting in 2015. The most recent 2016 data included the reports from 603 out of 604 clinics (99.8%) containing 255, 828 cycles with intention to use fresh embryo and 191,962 cycles with intention to use frozen-thawed embryos. Live birth infants numbered 9,432 and 44,678, respectively. The detailed data are available in a summary report by Ishihara et al. [19].

Asian Regional Perspective

There has been no Asian regional ART registry established to date, unlike EIM (European IVF Monitoring Consortium) in the European region or REDLARA (Red Latinoamericana de Reproducción Asistida) in the Latin American region, one reason being that each of the three Asian countries described in this chapter has a huge number of ART cycles within its own registry. In other words, each national registry of these three countries could count annually as being primarily on the scale of a regional registry. However, several other Asian countries have also established their own national registries. Table 14.1 summarizes national registries in other Asian countries and the responses to the inquiry questionnaire sent by one of authors of this chapter (OI) to volunteer clinicians in various countries.

There are basically two types of operations regarding local ART registries already established in Asian countries. The first type is operated by local professional organizations, as in Korea, Taiwan and Japan. They can be independent from their government; however, the cost of the operation should be paid by the members of the professional organizations. This could cause financial problems, resulting in the unsustainability of the surveillance. The second ART registry type is operated by the government, as in governmental ART

Table 14.1 Summary of national ART registries in Asian countries

Country	Population (million)	Number of ART clinics	ART registry	Registry established (year)	ART data reporting	Registry operator	Source of registry financing	Data collection type	Est. coverage (% clinics)	Non-reporting penalty
China	1413	451	yes	1994	compulsory	government	taxpayers	cycle-based		
India	1351		yes	2000	voluntary	professional org	professional org	clinic-based		no
Indonesia	266		yes							
Japan	127	603	yes	1986	compulsory	professional org	professional org	cycle-based	99.3	no
Korea	51	188	yes	1995	voluntary	professional org	professional org	clinic-based	39.8	no
Malaysia	31	36	no							
Singapore	5.7	11	yes		compulsory	government	taxpayers	cycle-based	100	yes
Taiwan	23	83	yes	1998	compulsory	professional org	professional org	cycle-based	100	yes
Thailand	69		yes	2015	compulsory	government	doctors	cycle-based	100	yes
Vietnam	96	25	no							

registry systems established in Singapore and China. In these cases, the operational cost of the registry should be covered by their government; however, data accessibility is not always ideal.

Conclusion

In response to the rapid increase in the number of ART practices in many Asian countries, ART registries have been established. However, continuous efforts are still needed to improve registries to achieve safer and more efficient ART practices in these countries. The introduction of a national registry also is indispensable for safety and improvement of ART practices in countries without such a registry; however, a tolerant approach is necessary because of the sociocultural diversity of the Asian region.

References

1. Zhang L. *Clinical Reproductive Endocrinology and Infertility*, 2nd edn. Beijing: Science Press; 2006. pp.491–576.

2. Xu,Y, Zhuang G, Li M, et al. Detecting embryo sex by fluorescence in-situ hybridization in preimplantation genetic diagnosis. *Zhonghua Fu Chan Ke Za Zhi*. 2000;**35**(8):465–7. [In Chinese.]

3. Xie X, Gou W. *Obstetrics and Gynecology*, 8th edn. Beijing: People's Medical Publishing House; 2013.

4. Qiao J. Current situation and prospect of associated reproductive technology in China. *Zhonghua Fu Chan Ke Za Zhi*. 2013;**48**(4):284–6. [In Chinese.]

5. Policy compilation of ART management. Women and Children's Department, National Health Commission. 2013.

6. Yu X. *Ethics and Management of Assisted Reproductive Technology*. Beijing: People's Medical Publishing House; 2014.

7. Rowe PJ, Farley TMM. The standardized investigation of infertile couples. In PJ Rowe, EV Vikhlyaeva (eds.), *Diagnosis and Treatment of Infertility*. Geneva: WHO, Hans Huber Publishers; 1988.

8. Mukherjee S, Mukherjee S, Bhattacharya SK. The feasibility of long term cryogenic freezing of viable human embryos – a brief pilot study report. *Indian J Cryog*. 1978;**3**(1):80.

9. Sullivan EA, Zegers-Hochschild F, Mansour R, Ishihara O, de Mouzon J, Nygren KG, et al. International Committee for Monitoring Assisted Reproductive Technologies (ICMART) world report: assisted reproductive technology, 2004. *Hum Reprod*. 2013;**28**:1375–90.

10. Sharma RS, Bhargava PM, Chandhiok N, Saxena NC. *National Guidelines for Accreditation, Supervision & Regulation of ART Clinics in India*. New Delhi: Indian Council of Medical Research – Ministry of Health & Family Welfare, Government of India; 2005.

11. Department of Health Research: Assisted Reproductive Technology (Regulation) Bill-2017 [India].

12. Japan Society of Obstetrics and Gynecology. IVF-ET guideline. *Acta Obstet Gynaecol Jpn*. 1983;**35**(10):7. [In Japanese.]

13. Japan Society of Obstetrics and Gynecology. IVF-ET registry guideline. *Acta Obstet Gynaecol Jpn*. 1986;**38**(3):8. [In Japanese.]

14. Japan Society of Obstetrics and Gynecology. Committee report on the reproductive medicine registry. *Acta Obstet Gynaecol Jpn*. 1990;**42**(4):393–7. [In Japanese.]

15. Japan Society of Obstetrics and Gynecology. ART annual report. *Acta Obstet Gynaecol Jpn*. 1992;**44**(4):499–511. [In Japanese.]

16. Thurin-Kjellberg A, Olivius C, Bergh C. Cumulative live-birth rates in a trial of single-embryo or double-embryo transfer. *N Engl J Med*. 2009;**361**(18):1812–13.

17. Japan Society of Obstetrics and Gynecology. 2015 ART annual report. *Acta Obstet Gynaecol Jpn*. 2017;**69**(9):1841–915. [In Japanese.]

18. On-line registry of ART operated by JSOG. [In Japanese.] Available at: http://plaza.umin.ac.jp/~jsog-art/.

19. Ishihara O, Jwa SC, Kuwahara A, Ishikawa T, Kugu K, Sawa R, et al. Assisted reproductive technology in Japan: a summary report for 2016 by the Ethics Committee of the Japan Society of Obstetrics and Gynecology. *Reprod Med Biol*. 2018;**18**:1–10.

Chapter

15

ART Surveillance in Australia and New Zealand

Georgina M. Chambers, Paul Lancaster and Peter Illingworth

History of ART in Australia and New Zealand

Australia has a proud history of achieving many of the early scientific and clinical breakthroughs in assisted reproductive technology (ART) treatment, largely through the collaborative efforts of teams at the Royal Women's Hospital (Melbourne IVF) and Queen Victoria Hospital (Monash IVF) in Melbourne. Australia's first in vitro fertilization (IVF) baby, Candice Reed, was born at Melbourne's Royal Women's Hospital in 1980 from a natural cycle. This was also the first IVF pregnancy in Australia, although two biochemical pregnancies lasting less than a week were reported in Melbourne in 1973. The first baby born from a donor egg was achieved by Monash IVF in 1983, and the first baby born from a frozen-thawed embryo was also achieved by Monash IVF one year later. The first open international workshop on IVF was convened by Monash IVF in 1982 [1]. New Zealand's first IVF baby, Amelia Bell, was born in 1983 [2].

The Australian national IVF patient support and advocacy organization, Access, was established in 1987 and has played a key role in improving access to and affordability of ART treatments, working in close collaboration with fertility clinicians and the Fertility Society of Australia (FSA) to achieve many gains for patients (see Chapter 10, Use of ART Surveillance by People Experiencing Infertility).

Since the birth of Candice Reed in 1980, more than 230,000 babies are estimated to have been born following ART treatment in Australia (Fig. 15.1). In 2015, 71,479 ART treatment cycles were performed in Australian clinics, representing 14.4 cycles per 1,000 women of reproductive age (15–44 years) and 4.3% of all women who gave birth in Australia. This is compared with 6,242 cycles performed in New Zealand clinics, representing 6.5 cycles per 1,000 women of reproductive age in New Zealand [3].

The more than double utilization rate in Australia compared with that of New Zealand is largely due to New Zealand's more limited funding environment [4]. In 2015, in Australia and New Zealand, women used their own eggs (autologous ART) in 95% of ART cycles, and 38% of cycles involved the thawing of cryopreserved embryos.

There have been significant changes in the uptake, treatment approaches and multiple birth rates over the past decade or more, as shown in the Australian treatment data presented in Figures 15.2 and 15.3. There was a 130% increase in the number of initiated autologous ART cycles undertaken in Australia between 2002 and 2015. The total live birth rate per embryo transfer cycle increased from 19% in 2002 to 25% in 2015. This occurred despite a trend of older women seeking ART treatment and a 3-fold increase in single embryo transfer (SET) cycles to 85% of embryo transfers in 2015. The multiple birth rate was 4.4% in 2015, one of the lowest in the world. Treatment trends have also shown a marked shift towards blastocyst culture and intracytoplasmic sperm injection (ICSI), although the latter appears to have plateaued in more recent years [3, 5]. Furthermore, the cryopreservation of all oocytes or embryos for potential future use (freeze-all cycles) has risen rapidly in recent years, from 5% of all egg collection cycles in 2011 to 17.2% in 2015 [3].

Governance of ART and ART Surveillance

ART in Australia is regulated by a combination of ART ethical guidelines, which are prepared by the National Health and Medical Research Council (NHMRC), federal and state/territory legislation and accreditation by the Reproductive Technology Accreditation Committee (RTAC) of the FSA.

The history of ART governance in Australia dates back to 1981 when the NHMRC formed a working party

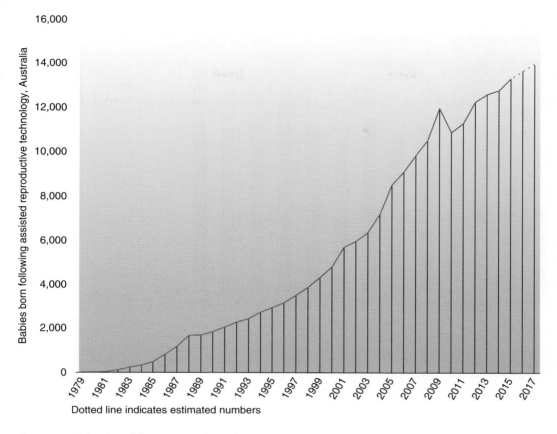

Dotted line indicates estimated numbers

Figure 15.1 Babies born following assisted reproductive technology treatments performed in Australia, 1979–2017.

to review the ethical guidelines for all programs in medical research receiving NHMRC grants and, in particular, guidelines for IVF research. These guidelines were published in 1983 and were the first national ethical guidelines on IVF procedures published in the world. The state of Victoria's Infertility (Medical Procedures) Act 1984 [6], which followed a report of a committee chaired by Professor Louis Waller [7], was enacted in 1988 and set out requirements in relation to counselling, a Central Registry, artificial insemination and donor expenses. This was the first legislation worldwide to regulate IVF and associated human embryo research.

Since the enactment of the National Health and Medical Research Council Act 1992, the Australian Health Ethics Committee (AHEC) has been responsible for the development and revision of ethical guidelines related to clinical practice and research in ART. The first set of guidelines from AHEC was published in 1996 [8], with the most recent revision of the guidelines issued in 2017 [9]. The NHMRC

ART ethical guidelines provide a set of standards for use by fertility clinicians, scientists, embryologists, counsellors, administrators, researchers, Human Research Ethics committees and governments.

The principal legislation that governs research in ART are the two national Acts that were enacted in 2002, the Research Involving Human Embryos Act 2002 and the Prohibition of Human Cloning for Reproduction Act 2002. These Acts and their state equivalents regulate research in ART. However, there is currently no national legislation covering the clinical practice of ART or ART registries, as the legislation in health care practice is the constitutional responsibility of state and territory governments. At the time of writing in 2017, four Australian states have enacted specific legislation to regulate ART:

- Victoria – Assisted Reproductive Treatment Act 2008 [10]
- New South Wales – Assisted Reproductive Technology Act 2007 [11]

143

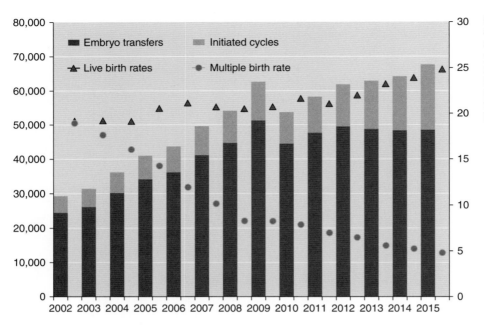

Figure 15.2 Trends in autologous ART treatment, Australia, 2002–2015.

Source: Australian and New Zealand Assisted Reproduction Database (ANZARD). A colour version of this figure is provided in the plate section.

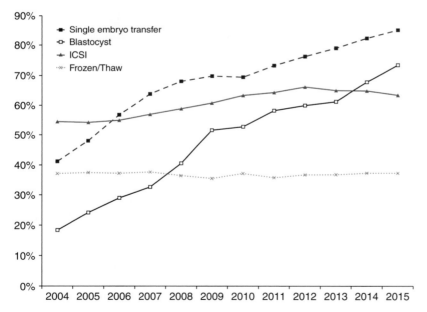

Figure 15.3 Trends in the proportion of embryo transfer cycles utilizing different ART techniques.

Source: Australian and New Zealand Assisted Reproduction Database (ANZARD)

- Western Australia – Human Reproductive Technology Act 1991 [12]
- South Australia – Assisted Reproductive Treatment Act 1988 [13]

National accreditation of fertility clinics is performed by the RTAC of the FSA. Under the 2002 Research Involving Human Embryos Act, RTAC accreditation is a legal requirement for all facilities that provide clinical services involving human embryos in Australia. In addition, the prescription of medications supporting ART services is only available to RTAC-accredited clinics. As a consequence, all ART clinics in Australia are subject to RTAC accreditation. The RTAC accreditation system is based on the NHMRC ethical guidelines and provides the basis of a nationally consistent approach for overseeing ART clinical practice [14].

In New Zealand, the Human Assisted Reproductive Technology Act 2004 (HART Act) provides for the regulation of procedures that assist with human reproduction [15].

History of ART Surveillance in Australia and New Zealand

The Early Days: The Assisted Conception Data Collection

Australia was the first country to establish a data registry to collate and report on birth outcomes for ART treatment. The registry, called the Assisted Conception Data Collection (ACDC), was a cooperative venture between the FSA and the National Perinatal Statistics Unit (NPSU) at the University of Sydney. The national voluntary registry was established after a request from the FSA, made on its behalf by Associate Professor Douglas Saunders from Sydney's Royal North Shore Hospital, and another from the NHMRC to Dr Paul Lancaster, director of the NPSU. Data collection commenced in 1983 when just over 200 IVF pregnancies had been conceived in the 8 existing fertility clinics in Australia. The NPSU had begun a national monitoring system for birth defects several years previously and was regarded as being suitably independent from the fertility clinics. While possible risks of birth defects were the initial concern, it was agreed that other information would also be included in the notification forms provided to the NPSU after each pregnancy was completed.

The IVF registry aimed to describe the characteristics of infertile couples and the management of IVF pregnancies, and to determine the incidence of pregnancy losses and major congenital malformations [16]. The Fourth World Congress on In Vitro Fertilization was held in Melbourne in November 1985. This provided an excellent opportunity to publicize the national IVF registry, leading to similar registries being set up in other countries and later to international collaboration in reporting results of treatment in many countries [17]. Data items on forms used to notify IVF pregnancies included the following: parental ages and the number of previous pregnancies; the causes and duration of infertility; the drugs used to induce

ovulation, the laparoscopy cycle in which pregnancy occurred and the number of oocytes collected; the use of donor sperm, oocytes and embryos and whether embryos had been frozen; the number of embryos replaced in the uterus after in vitro fertilization; the date of fertilization; any drugs used during the luteal phase; and the number of gestational sacs seen at the initial ultrasound examination. The outcomes recorded were the following: biochemical pregnancies (preclinical abortions); ectopic pregnancies; spontaneous abortions; stillbirths and live births; multiple pregnancies; and the infants' date of birth, sex, birth weight and method of delivery, as well as the presence of any congenital malformations. As confidentiality of infertile couples was essential, no identifying data about families were held in the registry; instead, a fertility clinic number for each couple enabled exchange of information between IVF units and the NPSU. Forms were manually completed by staff in the fertility clinics, using their records and follow-up information from referring doctors. The completeness and accuracy of data were maintained by requesting additional information if data were missing or ambiguous and by returning computer printouts summarizing the notified pregnancies to each fertility clinic for checking. Any corrections were subsequently sent to the NPSU.

The initial reports from the registry were published jointly by the NPSU and the FSA. On the suggestion of the NPSU director, Dr Paul Lancaster, the Australian In Vitro Fertilization Collaborative Group was formed with the purpose of using ART surveillance data for research. The initial members of the collaborative group were Dr W.I.H. Johnston (Reproductive Biology Unit, Royal Women's Hospital, Melbourne); Professor C. Wood (Queen Victoria Medical Centre, Melbourne); Associate Professor D.M. Saunders (Royal North Shore Hospital, Sydney); Professor W.R. Jones (Flinders Medical Centre, Adelaide); Dr J.F. Kerin (Queen Elizabeth Hospital, Adelaide); Dr J.L. Yovich (PIVET Laboratory and University of Western Australia); Dr J.F. Hennessey (Queensland Fertility Group, Brisbane); Professor J.F. Correy (Queen Alexandra Hospital, Hobart). Dr P. Lancaster prepared the articles for publication. At this early stage in the 1980s, IVF fertility clinics had been established in all six states and there were two clinics in Victoria and South Australia. As clinical services for treating infertile couples expanded rapidly in later decades, there were numerous fertility clinics established in capital cities and regional centres, some as satellite units of existing fertility clinics and others working independently. Following discussions with Dr Lancaster and Professor Dennis Bonham (National Women's Hospital in Auckland), soon after the first IVF birth in New Zealand in 1984, the fertility clinics in New Zealand also contributed data to the registry.

Collaboration and frequent communication with the directors and staff of fertility clinics came about by annual visits of the NPSU director to each unit, by meetings with fertility clinic directors and informal discussions with their staff at annual conferences of the FSA, and less frequently at international conferences. Such meetings were usually harmonious, but one IVF fertility clinic declined to contribute data for the first report published in 1984 [18]. Douglas Saunders, and later other fertility clinic directors, reviewed all NPSU reports before they were published.

It is unlikely that even the most enthusiastic pioneers of IVF would have predicted how rapidly the infertility services would develop (see Fig. 15.1). While infertile couples paid fees for their clinical care, supported partly by reimbursement from Medicare (Australia's universal health insurance scheme) and private health insurance policies, there was no funding in the early years for the work of developing the national registry and collecting and analyzing the data. Eventually it was agreed that individual fertility clinics would subsidize the NPSU work, with some assistance from major pharmaceutical companies.

Notifications of IVF pregnancies to the NPSU, and later data collection summarizing treatment cycles, were provided on paper forms for many years. New procedures such as gamete intrafallopian transfer (GIFT), intracytoplasmic sperm injection (ICSI) and numerous other variants of ART had to be reported separately. Difficulties arose because fertility clinics had their own, independent computing systems and programs and were initially reluctant to modify their systems to accommodate Australian and New Zealand Assisted Reproduction Database (ANZARD) reporting formats. After a time, individual clinic data were reported only in an anonymous format. Not surprisingly, the views of IVF directors on reporting varied according to how they perceived their results

compared with other units in an increasingly competitive field of clinical practice. Many in the wider community and representatives of patient groups were keen to know how individual fertility clinics were performing but often did not recognize how pregnancy rates might be influenced by considerable variation in underlying causes of infertility in different clinical settings for the fertility clinics. Australia continues not to report individual clinic success rates, and clinics are discouraged from publicly comparing themselves with the national ART annual reports. The approach of not publishing individual clinic results is widely debated in Australia and New Zealand. It has been argued that publication is important for consumer transparency. However, the decision not to publish recognizes the difficulty in adequately risk adjusting between the case mix of patients treated by different clinics. There is also a perceived need to avoid public reporting practices that incentivize strategies that artificially elevate success rates, such as the transfer of multiple embryos to maximize pregnancy rates and the refusal of treatment to women with relatively poorer prognoses due to factors such as obesity.

It is important to note that the first years of IVF and related research in the 1980s were often highly controversial. Religious and other community groups and individuals expressed opposition to many aspects of this work. Institutional ethics committees were established to oversee laboratory and clinical research, and legislation was gradually introduced in some states. In due course, the NPSU obtained data on laboratory procedures and the plight of embryos, often leading to discussion about the increasing number of cryopreserved embryos [19].

The initial report from the national registry was published in 1984 and included pregnancies completed by December 1983 [18]. Subsequent reports were all based on pregnancies conceived in individual years. In 1985, a fertilization cohort of 244 pregnancies resulting from IVF in eight fertility clinics showed that early pregnancy losses were high, with 5% tubal ectopic pregnancies and an incidence of spontaneous miscarriage of 27% [20]. Multiple pregnancies were common (22%) among pregnancies of at least 20 weeks' gestation, with 26 pairs of twins and four sets of triplets. The incidence of preterm births in singleton pregnancies was more than three times higher than in the general population. Preterm births and multiple pregnancies contributed to the high incidence of low birth weight. The initial data suggested that the sex ratio and the incidence of major congenital malformations were similar to those in naturally conceived pregnancies, although later research differed [21].

A second article from the Australian In-Vitro Fertilization Collaborative Group included data on 1,510 pregnancies from all 12 fertility clinics in Australia and one in New Zealand [22]. This confirmed the initial findings and also showed a high perinatal death rate of 47.5 deaths per 1,000 births, stillbirths accounting for three-quarters of these deaths. This study of population-based results from the registry emphasized the value of combining the data from the fertility clinics to analyze various risk factors and obtain information that could be used to counsel infertile couples.

In an era when multiple embryos were transferred in order to achieve optimal pregnancy rates, the incidence of multiple births remained at high levels for several decades, including quadruplet and the occasional quintuplet births [23]. While improvements in embryo culture were eventually the main reason that transfer of fewer embryos could be achieved, newspaper reports of these high-order multiple births, and media releases when each NPESU report was published, contributed to the efforts to reduce multiple pregnancies.

Analysis of data on 1,694 births and three terminations of pregnancy in the 1979–1986 fertilization cohort showed more infants than expected with two types of congenital malformation, spina bifida and transposition of the great vessels. In a subsequent analysis of a larger cohort of 2,543 IVF and 680 GIFT births and induced abortions, the overall incidence of major congenital malformations was not increased but there was a significant increase of spina bifida, oesophageal atresia and urogenital malformations. These findings stimulated epidemiologists in other countries to conduct more extensive studies [24, 25, 26].

Anecdotal reports to the NPSU of several children who had different types of cancer led to a brief published report [27]. This prompted a data linkage study in Victoria of a cohort of 5,249 children conceived in two clinics using IVF and related procedures. The data linkage study did not reveal a significantly increased incidence of cancer in comparison with the general population [28].

Within Australia, the highest treatment ratio was in Victoria. As these ratios were based on the states in

which the fertility clinics were located, comparisons between states could have been slightly affected by interstate movements of infertile women for treatment. In 1998, 47.8% of all treatment cycles in Australia were IVF, 43.0% were ICSI, 6.1% were GIFT and 3.1% were donor oocytes/embryos. In New Zealand, where the treatment ratio was much lower than in Australia, IVF accounted for a slightly higher proportion of all treatment cycles than in Australia [29].

The Later Years: Australian and New Zealand Assisted Reproduction Database (ANZARD)

From 2002, the Australian and New Zealand Assisted Reproduction Database (ANZARD) replaced the ACDC. ANZARD was commissioned by the FSA and implemented by the National Perinatal Epidemiology and Statistics Unit (NPESU), previously the NPSU, in recognition of the need for an expanded data collection that included consistent data definitions and a more robust and flexible data capture and storage framework. While the ACDC had been based on individual reports of each pregnancy, the other parameters of IVF activity were obtained from summative reports prepared and calculated by the clinics themselves and were therefore not able to be independently assessed or verified. It was generally agreed across the sector that a much more detailed and specifically electronic reporting system was urgently needed.

ANZARD was developed as a collaboration between the FSA, the NPESU and fertility clinics across Australia and New Zealand under the ANZARD committee chaired by Associate Professor Peter Illingworth. Unlike the ACDC, the fertility clinics provide the data to ANZARD on a per-cycle basis. ANZARD collects ART treatment data and data on artificial insemination using donor sperm from all fertility clinics in Australia and New Zealand. The comprehensive data collection is achieved because under RTAC accreditation, clinics are required to report all ART treatment to ANZARD as a condition of their licence to practise.

In 2009, as a further joint initiative of the NPESU and the FSA, ANZARD was upgraded to accommodate information on cryopreservation methods and duration of storage of oocytes and embryos, and to transform ANZARD from a cycle-based data collection to a woman-based data collection (ANZARD2.0). The upgrade to a woman-based data collection was achieved by introducing a statistical linkage key (SLK) that links successive treatment cycles undertaken by one woman. The SLK is a combination of the first two letters of a woman's first name, the first two letters of her surname and her date of birth [30]. This approach was developed to achieve a balance between having sufficient data to allow data linkages and still protecting individual privacy. The linkage of cycles performed across all Australian and New Zealand clinics allows the number of women undergoing treatment across time to be reported, as well as cumulative live birth rates to be tracked.

In addition to ANZARD, Victoria and Western Australia have state-based ART registries and donor registries, governed in part by their respective Assisted Reproductive Technology Acts [10, 12].

Variables Collected

ANZARD2.0 collects more than 90 data items on approximately 70,000 ART cycles and 13,000 babies each year, including patient demographics, treatment and outcome data. A list of data variables collected is provided in each annual ANZARD report and are summarized in Table 15.1. At the time of writing, the ANZARD data dictionary is being revised to include additional demographic and treatment data.

Assuring Data Quality

Each clinic submits its data to ANZARD on a calendar-year basis for validation checks before they are included in the database. The NPESU requests the annual data submission 12 months after the end of the treatment year; for example, 2016 treatment data were requested in early 2018. This allows the clinics to follow up all pregnancy outcome data before they are included in ANZARD. Generally, less than 3% of pregnancy outcomes cannot be ascertained by clinic staff, mostly due to women moving overseas following treatment.

Before 2017, data submission to the NPESU was via a spreadsheet template provided to the clinics. Upon receipt of the data, the ANZARD data managers would run the clinic data through a number of validation programs to check for logical errors and internal inconsistencies within cycles. A feedback report would be manually sent to the clinics that included

errors and inconsistencies to be corrected. This iterative process would continue until the data were suitable for uploading to ANZARD.

In 2017, the NPESU introduced a secure, automated, web-based data portal (ANZARD Data Capture Portal), which allows clinics to upload their data directly and receive automated validation reports. The advantages of the new data portal include secure and restricted upload of clinic data through a user-friendly, web-based interface; the ability to batch upload one or more clinic datasets or to enter single cycles; real-time validation of data with summary validation reports; and a flexible programming environment to allow the addition of new validation rules as required. In addition to the new ANZARD data portal, the underlying ANZARD database was transitioned in 2017 to an industry-standard SQL database server.

The validity of the ANZARD data is also assured by annual audits conducted by RTAC. A variety of checking mechanisms are used during the audits, including checking a random sample of cycle information provided in the annual submission to ANZARD, and auditing treatment and pregnancy outcome data.

Using ART Surveillance Data

ANZARD Annual Reports

The first ART surveillance report was prepared and published by the NPESU (previously the NPSU) in 1984, covering pregnancies completed in 1980–1983. Since then, an annual report has been produced each consecutive year. The thirty-third annual report was published in September 2018.

The ANZARD annual reports are widely accessed, with reports covering treatments performed since 1992 freely available on the NPESU website. Each annual report is traditionally released at the time of the FSA's annual scientific meeting in September (for example, ANZARD 2015 was released in September 2017) and is accompanied by a media release highlighting points of interest from the report. Each annual report is reviewed by a committee representing clinicians and scientists from a variety of fertility clinics across Australia and New Zealand. The ANZARD report is arguably the most comprehensive ART report in the world, with more than 80 tables produced each year. Each

Table 15.1 List of data variables collected by the Australian and New Zealand Assisted Reproduction Database (ANZARD2.0)

Patient demographics	Treatment	Outcome
Age	**Stimulation**	**Pregnancy**
Date of birth (female and partner)	First ART cycle FSH stimulation and date started Cancellation date	Number of fetal hearts Clinical pregnancy
Residential location	**Ovarian aspiration and fertilization**	**Adverse pregnancy outcomes**
Postcode of residential area	Aspiration date Number of eggs retrieved, treated with IVF/ICSI, fertilized	Ectopic pregnancy, Elective termination, Selective reduction, OHSS, Other maternal complications
Causes of infertility	**Cryopreserved eggs**	**Delivery**
Tubal disease, Endometriosis, Other female factors, Male factor, Unexplained	Cryopreservation date Slow frozen or vitrified Thawed or warmed	Vaginal or Caesarean
Parity	**Cryopreserved embryos**	**Baby outcomes**
Previous pregnancy ≥20 weeks	Cleavage or blastocyst Slow frozen or vitrified Thawed or warmed	Birth outcome (live born, stillborn, neonatal death), Plurality, Sex, Birth weight, Gestational age, Congenital anomalies
	Embryos transferred	
	Date of transfer Number of cleavage or blastocyst embryos Number of ICSI embryos	
	Additional procedures	
	PGT, Assisted hatching	
	Donor and surrogacy information	
	Donor age, Number of eggs/embryos donated or received, Surrogacy arrangements	

ART, assisted reproductive technology; FSH, follicle stimulating hormone; ICSI, intracytoplasmic sperm injection; IVF, in vitro fertilization; OHSS, ovarian hyperstimulation syndrome; PGT, preimplantation genetic testing

report typically receives between approximately 1,000 and 3,000 web views a year and attracts more than 100 citations in the academic literature.

Clinic Feedback

Unlike the ART treatment data collected by the Centers for Disease Control and Prevention (CDC) for US clinics and the Human Fertilisation and Embryology Authority (HFEA) for UK clinics, clinic success rates are not publicly available in Australia and New Zealand. The ANZARD annual report does include information about the relative performance of clinics, but in an anonymous format. The most recent ANZARD annual reports include a box-and-whisker plot providing a graphic representation of the median, quartiles and extremes of live birth rates per initiated fresh and thaw autologous and recipient cycles among fertility clinics [3].

However, the NPESU does provide each clinic with an annual detailed report showing its relative performance compared with the distribution of all other clinics. This includes success rates from fresh embryo transfers, frozen-thawed embryo transfers and recipient cycles.

The NPESU also produces crude and age/parity-adjusted funnel plots for quality assurance purposes. Clinics that fall below the expected range for critical parameters work with RTAC to develop quality improvements to improve their performance.

Research

The ANZARD data collection has been used widely by researchers to provide evidence relating to the safety and quality of ART, to inform public policy and to evaluate the clinical and cost-effectiveness of treatment strategies. In terms of safety and quality, the annual ANZARD reports provide ongoing surveillance of perinatal outcomes. However, a more detailed analysis of treatment effectiveness and outcomes of fresh versus cryopreserved embryos and single versus double embryo transfers has been presented in a series of publications [31, 32, 33, 34, 35].

ANZARD has also been used extensively in public policy research, particularly in providing evidence that supportive public funding incentivizes single embryo transfer, leading to better health outcomes for mothers and babies. Indeed, data from ANZARD have shown that providing supportive public funding not only reduces maternal and infant morbidity but also substantially reduces health care costs [34, 36, 37, 38, 39]. Furthermore, ANZARD data have been used in government reviews of the cost and cost-effectiveness of ART in Australia and to evaluate the impact of changes in public funding and legislative changes [40, 41, 42, 43]. Most recently, ANZARD data have been used to publish age-specific cumulative live birth rates that allow patients and clinicians to estimate the chance of a live birth after repeated ART cycles [44].

Successes, Challenges and Future Plans

ANZARD and the ACDC before it are examples of successful cooperation and collaboration between clinicians, fertility clinics, universities and regulators. Under their licensing agreement, all clinics must report to ANZARD, ensuring complete ascertainment is achieved. It is the oldest IVF registry in the world and was established with great foresight by the early IVF pioneers in Australia. The data from the registry have been publicly reported without interruption on an annual basis for more than 30 years and made widely available to consumers, policy makers and researchers. The NPESU and the FSA continue to have a strong and collaborative approach to ART surveillance, with the FSA funding the collection and the NPESU managing and independently preparing the annual reports.

One of ANZARD's important achievements has been in supporting the fertility sectors in Australia and New Zealand to reduce the multiple birth rate to become one of the lowest in the world. The reporting of aggregate multiple birth rates without identifying the results of individual clinics has incentivized the collective shift towards single embryo transfer. The identification of individual clinics' results

invariably leads to competition and creates perverse incentives for clinics to improve pregnancy rates at the expense of singleton live birth rates.

Future plans include developing a patient predictor tool that will allow patients to enter information, such as age, parity and number of previous cycles, into a web-based tool, which then generates individual success rate estimates. More interactive annual reports are also planned that will partially replace the paper-based reports and include more visual displays of descriptive statistics and user-driven menus. Finally, the ANZARD data dictionary is reviewed periodically, and it is anticipated that a number of changes will be introduced for treatments commencing in 2019 to reflect changing clinical and scientific practices and additional patient demographic and diagnostic information.

References
1. Leeton J. The early history of IVF in Australia and its contribution to the world (1970–1990). *Aust N Z J Obstet Gynaecol.* 2004;**44**:495–501.
2. Wilkinson J, Roberts SA, Showell M, Brison DR, Vail A. No common denominator: a review of outcome measures in IVF RCTs. *Hum Reprod.* 2016;**31**(12):2714–22.
3. Fitzgerald O, Harris K, Paul RC, Chambers GM. *Assisted Reproductive Technology in Australia and New Zealand 2015.* Sydney: National Perinatal Epidemiology and Statistics Unit, University of New South Wales Sydney; 2017. Report No. 978-0-7334-3655-0.
4. Farquhar CM, Wang YA, Sullivan EA. A comparative analysis of assisted reproductive technology cycles in Australia and New Zealand 2004–2007. *Hum Reprod.* 2010;**25**(9):2281–9.
5. Chambers GM, Wand H, Macaldowie A, Chapman MG, Farquhar CM, Bowman M, et al. Population trends and live birth rates associated with common ART treatment strategies. *Hum Reprod.* 2016;**31**(11):2632–41.
6. Infertility (Medical Procedures) Act 1984. No. 10163. (Victoria, Australia). Available at: http://www.austlii.edu.au/au/legis/vic/hist_act/ipa1984311.pdf, accessed April 2018.
7. The Committee to Consider the Social Ethical and Legal Issues Arising from In Vitro Fertilization. *Report of the Disposition of Embryos Produced by In Vitro Fertilisation.* Melbourne: F D Atkinson Government Printer; 1984.
8. National Health and Medical Research Council. *Ethical Guidelines on Assisted Reproductive Technology, 1996 (rescinded 16/09/2004).* Canberra: National Health and Medical Research Council; 1996.

9. National Health and Medical Research Council. *Ethical Guidelines on the Use of Assisted Reproductive Technology in Clinical Practice and Research*. Canberra: National Health and Medical Research Council; 2017.

10. Assisted Reproductive Treatment Act 2008. No. 76. (Victoria, Australia). Available at: http://www6 .austlii.edu.au/cgi-bin/viewdb/au/legis/vic/consol_act/ arta2008360/, accessed April 2018.

11. Assisted Reproductive Technology Act 2007. No 69. (New South Wales, Australia). Available at: http://www .health.nsw.gov.au/art/Pages/default.aspx, accessed April 2018.

12. Human Reproductive Technology Act 1991. (Australia, Western Australia). Available at: www .legislation.wa.gov.au/legislation/statutes.nsf/main_ mrtitle_435_homepage.html, accessed April 2018.

13. Assisted Reproductive Treatment Act 1988. (Australia, South Australia). Available at: www.legislation.sa.gov .au/LZ/C/A/Assisted%20Reproductive%20Treatment %20Act%201988.aspx, accessed April 2018.

14. Assisted Reproductive Technologies Review Committee. *Report of the Independent Review of Assisted Reproductive Technologies*; 2006. Report commissioned by the Australian Commonwealth Government. Available at: http://www.health.gov.au /internet/main/publishing.nsf/Content/ART-Report, accessed April 2018.

15. Human Assisted Reproductive Technology Act 2004. (New Zealand). Available at http://www.legislation .govt.nz/act/public/2004/0092/latest/whole.html, accessed April 2018.

16. Lancaster P. Health registers for congenital malformations and in vitro fertilization. *Clin Reprod Fertil*. 1986;4:27–37.

17. *Sydney Morning Herald*. An 'added risk' for in vitro babies. 20 November 1985.

18. National Perinatal Statistics Unit and Fertility Society of Australia. *In Vitro Fertilisation Pregnancies in Australia*. Sydney: University of Sydney; 1984.

19. Saunders D, Lancaster P. Frozen embryos – another population explosion? *Med J Aust*. 1992;157:148–9.

20. Australian In-Vitro Fertilization Collaborative Group. High incidence of preterm births and early losses in pregnancy after in-vitro fertilization. *BMJ*. 1985;291: 1160–3.

21. Dean J, Chapman M, Sullivan E. The effect on human sex ratio at birth by assisted reproductive technology (ART) procedures – an assessment of babies born following single embryo transfers, Australia and New Zealand, 2002–2006. *BJOG*. 2010;117:1628–33.

22. Australian In-vitro Fertilization Collaborative Group. In-vitro fertilization pregnancies in Australia and New Zealand, 1979–1985. *Med J Aust*. 1988;148(9):429–36.

23. *Canberra Times*. Multiple births in Perth through IVF. 20 January 1989.

24. Lancaster P. Congenital malformations after in-vitro fertilisation. *Lancet*. 1987;2(8572):1392–3.

25. Lancaster P. High incidence of selected congenital malformations after assisted conception. *Teratology*. 1989;40:288.

26. Lancaster PAL. Evaluation of birth defects after assisted conception. In P Mastroiacovo (ed.), *Proceedings of the 3rd ASM International Symposium on Birth Defects*. Rome: ICARO-ASM Press House; 1992. pp.225–33.

27. White L, Giri N, Vowels M, Lancaster P. Neuroectodermal tumours in children born after assisted conception. *Lancet*. 1990;336:1577.

28. Bruinsma F, Venn A, Lancaster P, Speirs A, Healy D. Incidence of cancer in children born after in-vitro fertilization. *Hum Reprod*. 2000;15:604–7.

29. Hurst T, Lancaster P. *Assisted Conception Australia and New Zealand 1998 and 1999*. Sydney: AIHW National Perinatal Statistics Unit; 2001. Assisted Conception Series No. 5.

30. Wang Y, Macaldowie A, Hayward I, Chambers G, Sullivan E. *Assisted Reproductive Technology in Australia and New Zealand 2009*. Canberra: AIHW; 2011. Assisted Reproduction Technology Series No. 15. Cat. No. PER 51. 2016/09/02/.

31. Chambers GM, Chughtai AA, Farquhar CM, Wang YA. Risk of preterm birth after blastocyst embryo transfer: A large population study using contemporary registry data from Australia and New Zealand. *Fertil Steril*. 2015;104(4):997–1003.

32. Wang YA, Chapman M, Costello M, Sullivan EA. Better perinatal outcomes following transfer of fresh blastocysts and blastocysts cultured from thawed cleavage embryos: a population-based study. *Hum Reprod*. 2010;25(6):1536–42.

33. Wang YA, Kovacs G, Sullivan EA. Transfer of a selected single blastocyst optimizes the chance of a healthy term baby: a retrospective population based study in Australia 2004–2007. *Hum Reprod*. 2010;25 (8):1996–2005.

34. Sullivan EA, Wang YA, Hayward I, Chambers GM, Illingworth P, McBain J, et al. Single embryo transfer reduces the risk of perinatal mortality, a population study. *Hum Reprod*. 2012;27(12):3609–15.

35. Wang YA, Sullivan EA, Healy DL, Black DA. Perinatal outcomes after assisted reproductive technology treatment in Australia and New Zealand: single versus double embryo transfer. *Med J Aust*. 2009;190(5):234–7.

36. Chambers GM, Hoang VP, Sullivan EA, Chapman MG, Ishihara O, Zegers-Hochschild F, et al. The impact of consumer affordability on access to

assisted reproductive technologies and embryo transfer practices: an international analysis. *Fertil Steril.* 2014;**101**(1):191–8.e4.

37. Chambers GM, Illingworth PJ, Sullivan EA. Assisted reproductive technology: public funding and the voluntary shift to single embryo transfer in Australia. *Med J Aust.* 2011;**195**(10):594–8.

38. Chambers GM, Sullivan EA, Ishihara O, Chapman MG, Adamson GD. The economic impact of assisted reproductive technology: a review of selected developed countries. *Fertil Steril.* 2009;**91**(6):2281–94.

39. Chambers GM, Wang YA, Chapman MG, Hoang VP, Sullivan EA, Abdalla HI, et al. What can we learn from a decade of promoting safe embryo transfer practices? A comparative analysis of policies and outcomes in the UK and Australia, 2001–2010. *Hum Reprod.* 2013;**28**(6):1679–86.

40. Chambers GM, Ho MT, Sullivan EA. Assisted reproductive technology treatment cost of a live birth: an age-stratified cost-outcome study of treatment in Australia. *Med J Aust.* 2006;**184**(4):155–8.

41. Griffiths A, Dyer SM, Lord SJ, Pardy C, Fraser IS, Eckermann S. A cost-effectiveness analysis of in-vitro fertilization by maternal age and number of treatment attempts. *Hum Reprod.* 2010;**25**(4):924–31.

42. Chambers GM, Hoang VP, Zhu R, Illingworth PJ. A reduction in public funding for fertility treatment – an econometric analysis of access to treatment and savings to government. *BMC Health Serv Res.* 2012;**12**(1).

43. Chambers GM, Hoang VP, Illingworth PJ. Socioeconomic disparities in access to ART treatment and the differential impact of a policy that increased consumer costs. *Hum Reprod.* 2013;**28**(11):3111–17.

44. Chambers GM, Paul RC, Harris K, Fitzgerald O, Boothroyd CV, Rombauts L, et al. Assisted reproductive technology in Australia and New Zealand: cumulative live birth rates as measures of success. *Med J Aust.* 2017;**207**(3):114–18.

Chapter

16

ART Surveillance in Europe

Christian De Geyter, Markus S. Kupka and Carlos Calhaz-Jorge

Introduction

Although the first treatment with assisted reproductive technology (ART) leading to the birth of a healthy girl was performed in Europe [1] and despite the highest numbers of treatment worldwide reported on this continent, systematic surveillance of ART took off in Europe rather late. Whereas national and regional reports on ART activities in both North and South America and in Australia–New Zealand were published between 1997 and 1999, the first European report containing datasets collected in 1997 appeared as late as 2001 [2].

Realizing the urgent need to embark on ART surveillance, in 1999 the European Society of Human Reproduction and Embryology (ESHRE) created the European IVF Monitoring (EIM) Consortium, which sent a first invitation to the national representatives of all European countries with an interest in national in vitro fertilization (IVF) data registries. In that letter, the goal of establishing a European-wide database was specifically expressed. The first meeting of 18 participating countries took place in June 1999. The European pioneers in ART surveillance were Karl G. Nygren (Sweden), Anders Nyboe Andersen (Denmark) and Jacques de Mouzon (France). Since 2001, a series of 17 subsequent reports has been published in the journal *Human Reproduction* covering the European activities in ART from 1997 to 2014 (Table 16.1). Recently, a comprehensive review of the first 15 years of EIM (from 1997 to 2011) was published [3].

According to the World Health Organization (WHO), surveillance in medicine is the "continuous systematic collection, analysis and interpretation of health-related data needed for the planning, implementation and evaluation of public health practice" (www.who.int). EIM has indeed managed to implement a continuous data collection system. However, Europe is made up of a diversity of countries with very different cultural, political and legal systems. The lack

of unifying structures and, often, the absence of any requirement for national data registration renders the undertaking of a systematic collection of data on ART particularly difficult. This task is further complicated by the high frequency of cross-border reproductive care in Europe [4], which naturally develops in countries with strict legislation neighbouring other countries with a more liberal legislation.

Notwithstanding these obstacles, EIM has successfully created an organizational structure with a 'bottom-up' type of data collection. Basically, EIM primarily consists of the national representatives of all participating European countries. Single devoted experts in ART have also been very dedicated to collecting data from their respective countries. All representatives meet once yearly. The meetings take place during the annual ESHRE congresses and have contributed much to mutual understanding. The annual meetings of all EIM members are always well attended and have become a platform for communication and dialogue among the national representatives. In addition to the annual meetings, targeted scientific workshops are organized regularly to discuss specific problems concerning the registry, to plan future developments and to develop interacting strategies to improve the national registries of countries with specific problems. EIM created the idea of a core dataset for countries without a functional registry, which is available on the ESHRE website (www.eshre.eu). All these activities are organized by ESHRE and could not be performed successfully without its support.

Participation of European Countries and ART-Providing Institutions in EIM and the Completeness of ART Surveillance in Europe

Since 1997, the number of participating countries has risen stepwise from 18 to 39 in 2014 (Fig. 16.1A).

Table 16.1 List of annual publications summarizing the European ART data, as collected and analyzed by EIM

C. De Geyter, C. Calhaz-Jorge, M.C. Wyns, S. Kupka, E. Mocanu, T. Motrenko, G. Scaravelli, J. Smeenk, V. Goossens, and the European IVF-monitoring (EIM) Consortium for the European Society of Human Reproduction and Embryology (ESHRE). Assisted reproductive technology in Europe, 2014: results generated from European registers by ESHRE. Hum. Reprod. (2018) submitted.

C. Calhaz-Jorge, C. De Geyter, M. S. Kupka, J. de Mouzon, K. Erb, E. Mocanu, T. Motrenko, G. Scaravelli, C. Wyns, V. Goossens, and the European IVF-monitoring (EIM) Consortium for the European Society of Human Reproduction and Embryology (ESHRE). Assisted reproductive technology in Europe, 2013: results generated from European registers by ESHRE. Hum. Reprod. (2017) 32:1957–1973.

C. Calhaz-Jorge, C. De Geyter, M.S. Kupka, J. de Mouzon, K. Erb, E. Mocanu, T. Motrenko, G. Scaravelli, C. Wyns, V. Goossens, and the European IVF-monitoring (EIM) Consortium for the European Society of Human Reproduction and Embryology (ESHRE). Assisted reproductive technology in Europe, 2012: results generated from European registers by ESHRE. First published online. Hum. Reprod. (2016) 31:1638–1652.

M.S. Kupka, T. D'Hooghe, A.P. Ferraretti, J. de Mouzon, K. Erb, J.A. Castilla, C. Calhaz-Jorge, C. De Geyter, V. Goossens, and the European IVF-monitoring (EIM) Consortium for the European Society of Human Reproduction and Embryology (ESHRE). Assisted reproductive technology in Europe, 2011: results generated from European registers by ESHRE. Hum. Reprod. (2016) 31:233–248.

M.S. Kupka, A.P. Ferraretti, J. de Mouzon, K. Erb, T. D'Hooghe, J.A. Castilla, C. Calhaz-Jorge, C. De Geyter, V. Goossens, and the European IVF-monitoring (EIM) Consortium for the European Society of Human Reproduction and Embryology (ESHRE). Assisted reproductive technology in Europe, 2010: results generated from European registers by ESHRE. Hum. Reprod. (2014) 29:2099–2113.

A.P. Ferraretti, V. Goossens, M. Kupka, S. Bhattacharya, J. de Mouzon, J.A. Castilla, K. Erb, V. Korsak, A. Nyboe Andersen, the European IVF-monitoring (EIM) Consortium, for the European Society of Human Reproduction and Embryology (ESHRE). Assisted reproductive technology in Europe, 2009: results generated from European registers by ESHRE. Hum. Reprod. (2013) 28:2318–2331.

A.P. Ferraretti, V. Goossens, J. de Mouzon, S. Bhattacharya, J.A. Castilla, V. Korsak, M. Kupka, K.G. Nygren, A. Nyboe Andersen, the European IVF-monitoring (EIM) Consortium, for the European Society of Human Reproduction and Embryology (ESHRE). Assisted reproductive technology in Europe, 2008: results generated from European registers by ESHRE. Hum. Reprod. (2012) 27:2571–2584.

J. de Mouzon, V. Goossens, S. Bhattacharya, J.A. Castilla, A.P. Ferraretti, V. Korsak, M. Kupka, K.G. Nygren, and A. Nyboe Andersen. Assisted reproductive technology in Europe, 2007: results generated from European registers by ESHRE. Hum. Reprod. (2012) 27:954–966.

J. de Mouzon, V. Goossens, S. Bhattacharya, J.A. Castilla, A.P. Ferraretti, V. Korsak, M. Kupka, K.G. Nygren, A. Nyboe Andersen, and the European IVF-monitoring (EIM) Consortium. Assisted reproductive technology in Europe, 2006: results generated from European registers by ESHRE. Hum. Reprod. (2010) 25:1851–1862.

A. Nyboe Andersen, V. Goossens, S. Bhattacharya, A.P. Ferraretti, M.S. Kupka, J. de Mouzon, K.G. Nygren, and the European IVF-monitoring (EIM) Consortium. Assisted reproductive technology and intrauterine inseminations in Europe, 2005: results generated from European registers by ESHRE. Hum. Reprod. (2009) 24:1267–1287.

A. Nyboe Andersen, V. Goossens, A.P. Ferraretti, S. Bhattacharya, R. Felberbaum, J. de Mouzon, K.G. Nygren, the European IVF-monitoring (EIM) Consortium. Assisted reproductive technology in Europe, 2004: results generated from European registers by ESHRE. Hum. Reprod. (2008) 23:756–771.

A. Nyboe Andersen, V. Goossens, L. Gianaroli, R. Felberbaum, J. de Mouzon and K.G. Nygren. Assisted reproductive technology in Europe, 2003: results generated from European registers by ESHRE. Hum. Reprod. (2007) 22:1513–1525.

A. Nyboe Andersen, L. Gianaroli, R. Felberbaum, J. de Mouzon and K.G. Nygren. Assisted reproductive technology in Europe, 2002: results generated from European registers by ESHRE. Hum. Reprod. (2006) 21:1680–1697.

A. Nyboe Andersen, L. Gianaroli, R. Felberbaum, J. de Mouzon and K.G. Nygren. Assisted reproductive technology in Europe, 2001: results generated from European Registers by ESHRE. Hum. Reprod. (2005) 20:1158–1176.

A. Nyboe Andersen, L. Gianaroli, and K.G. Nygren. Assisted reproductive technology in Europe, 2000: results generated from European Registers by ESHRE. Hum. Reprod. (2004) 19:490–503.

Assisted reproductive technology in Europe, 1999: results generated from European registers by ESHRE. Report prepared by K.G. Nygren and A. Nyboe Andersen. Hum. Reprod. (2002) 17:3260–3274.

Assisted reproductive technology in Europe, 1998: results generated from European registers by ESHRE. Report prepared by K.G. Nygren and A. Nyboe Andersen. Hum. Reprod. (2001) 16:2459–2471.

Assisted reproductive technology in Europe, 1997: results generated from European registers by ESHRE. Report prepared by K.G. Nygren and A. Nyboe Andersen. Hum. Reprod. (2001) 16:384–391.

Virtually all major European countries are now participating in the EIM Consortium. Among the 51 European countries, only 9 are not members of EIM, most of them small countries, usually without ART services.

Some countries provide full data coverage of all ART treatments, and the number of countries with full coverage has risen from 10 in 1997 to 17 in 2012 and decreased slightly to 14 in 2014. During the same time interval, the number of ART institutions

A

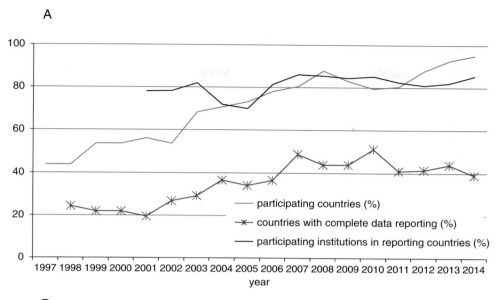

B

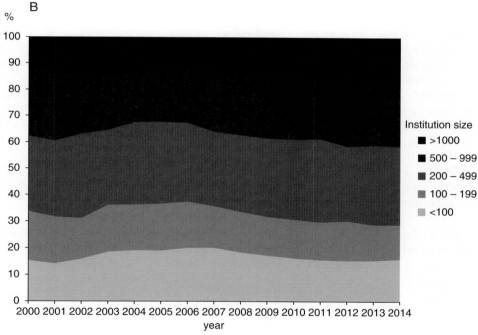

Figure 16.1 Participation of European countries and institutions offering ART services in EIM.
A. Since 1997, the number of participating countries has risen stepwise from 18 to 38 in 2014, now reaching 92.7% of all European countries, and 14 countries reported full data coverage in all participating institutions (39.0%). In addition, the number of reporting ART institutions rose from 482 in 1997 to 1,280, which represents 87.9% of all known ART clinics and institutions known to exist in Europe.
B. Since 2000, the distribution of different institutional sizes is given in the yearly reports (data given in %). The distribution of the different sizes of the active institutions has remained much the same over time. Only the larger institutions with more than 1,000 treatment cycles per year became substantially more prevalent over time.

Table 16.2 The effect of a shift from voluntary to compulsory data collection on data completeness, as exemplified by two European countries in 2012 and 2013

	Greece			Kazakhstan		
	2012	2013	Growth rate (%)	2012	2013	Growth rate (%)
Contributing centres	20	41	105.0	3	5	66.7
Cycles, IVF/ICSI	672	12,207	83.0	2,263	3,288	45.3
Cycles, FER	626	2,024	223.3	465	645	38.7
Pregnancies, IVF/ICSI	2,157	3,675	70.4	889	1,311	47.5
Pregnancies, FER	378	726	92.1	159	204	28.3
Deliveries, IVF/ICSI	1,083	1,684	55.5	593	947	59.7
Deliveries, FER	185	326	76.2	106	166	56.6

FER, frozen embryo replacement; ICSI, intracytoplasmic sperm injection; IVF, in vitro fertilization

providing data to their national registers and then to EIM has risen from 482 in 1997 to 1,280 in 2014 (90.1% of all known institutions offering ART services in Europe). Between 2000 and 2014, the proportion of large institutions (>1,000 treatment cycles per year) offering ART services has increased from 11.3 to 18.3% (together with more centres contributing to EIM), and this rise has substantially augmented the number of recorded cycles, while the proportion of smaller institutions has remained much the same (Fig. 16.1B). From 2000 to 2014, the large IVF units (>1,000 treatment cycles per year) increased their contribution to the EIM data collection from 31,411 to 142,023 cycles every year. Despite the preponderance of large institutions, the overall picture shows a continuing participation of all types of institutions.

Between 1997 and 2013, a total of 1,308,289 newborn children have been registered by EIM in Europe [5]. We are aware that there is an underreporting of these particular data, because in the first years of the EIM registry only countries with full coverage reported newborn children and a proportion of unknown outcomes of pregnancies still persists. Nevertheless, ART is having an increasing and significant impact on the overall numbers of children born in many European countries. In some European countries, such as Denmark, Iceland and Slovenia, the number of newborn children has risen progressively. Denmark has always been the leading country in the number of newborn children resulting from ART, and the percentage of all newborn children from ART in Denmark has risen from 3.5% in 1997 to 6.7% in 2013.

Despite the progress, a substantial number of institutions and registries still do not provide their data to EIM. One important factor contributing to better completeness of the reported datasets has been observed in countries with a shift from a voluntary to a compulsory data registration. From 2012 to 2013, two European countries, Greece and Kazakhstan, underwent such a process, and the compound growth rates were positive for all main reported parameters, including the clinical pregnancy and delivery rates (Table 16.2). A similar improvement in the quality of submitted data was observed in Spain from 2013 to 2014.

ART Results in Europe as Recorded by EIM

The data summarized in the 17 EIM reports are primarily given in absolute figures. For the purpose of this review chapter, we re-calculated all published data and expressed the results in percentage values. This way of presenting the data provides the opportunity to better appreciate ongoing trends and developments over time.

Since the early beginnings of ART surveillance in Europe, not only have increasing treatment numbers been recorded, but new treatment modalities have also been introduced (Fig. 16.2). Whereas IVF, intracytoplasmic sperm injection (ICSI) and frozen embryo replacement (FER) have been registered since 1997, the use of egg (oocyte) donation (ED) has been recorded since 1998, preimplantation genetic diagnosis (PGD) since 2002, in vitro maturation (IVM) since 2002 and frozen oocyte replacement

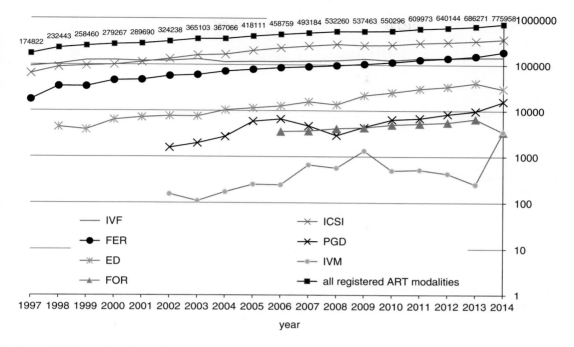

Figure 16.2 Since 1997, the overall number of treatment cycles (black line, with actual figures given) has constantly risen together with the diversity of treatment modalities: IVF, ICSI, FER (frozen embryo transfer), PGD (preimplantation genetic diagnosis), ED (egg donation), IVM (in vitro maturation) and FOR (frozen oocyte replacement). Except for IVM, which has declined since 2009, all treatment modalities are on the rise in Europe.

(FOR) since 2006. In 2014, the leading European countries with the largest treatment numbers were Spain (109,275 treatments), Russia (94,985), France (90,434) and Germany (81,177).

Ideally, the intention for treatment should be recorded together with all intermediate steps up to the final outcome, i.e. the birth of a healthy child. Although intention for treatment is one of the variables recorded by EIM, the number of initiated treatments is always lower than the number of reported oocyte collections, suggesting frequent underreporting of that variable. In addition, in several well-established national registries this parameter has not been recorded. The same holds true for thawing cycles. In contrast, oocyte collections, embryo transfers and thawings all seem to have been reported reliably. We therefore calculated treatment outcome variables with respect to these better registered ART landmarks.

Both in stimulated cycles (so-called fresh treatments) and in thawing cycles, the clinical pregnancy and delivery rates more or less rose steadily with time (Fig. 16.3). Taking the number of embryo

transfers as the comparator between fresh and thawing cycles, the clinical pregnancy rates improved from 26.2% in 1997 to 33.8% in 2014 (a rise of 7.6%; Fig. 16.3A), whereas the clinical pregnancy rates in thawing cycles improved during the same time interval, from 15.2% to 29.4% (a rise of 14.2%; Fig. 16.3B). Improvements in the cryopreservation technology (including vitrification) together with broader use of embryo cryopreservation (as in 'freeze-all' cycles for the prevention of ovarian hyperstimulation syndrome (OHSS)) are likely responsible. In the near future, the observed improvements in outcome data of thawing cycles may result in more children born after thawing cycles than after fresh treatments.

This trend is not without importance for ART surveillance in Europe and elsewhere, as traditional surveillance in ART has been carried out with cross-sectional datasets (e.g. data collected on a yearly basis, as given by the EIM reports). The ongoing trend towards more cryopreservation of embryos (FER) and oocytes implies that the concept of treatment segmentation in ART [6] is increasingly gaining

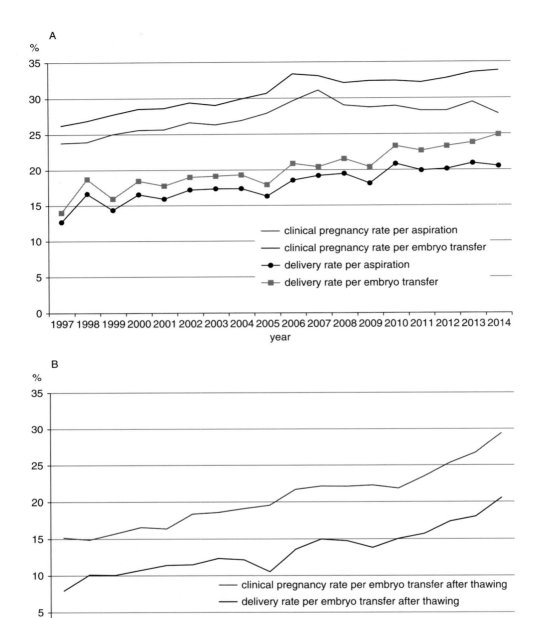

Figure 16.3 The reported clinical pregnancy and delivery rates (in %) per embryo transfer after IVF and ICSI (panel A) and in thawing cycles (panel B).

ground. Current cross-sectional ART surveillance will inevitably have to develop towards a cumulative type of data collection in the near future.

Complications of ART

Conventionally, most treatments with ART necessitate ovarian hyperstimulation for the growth and maturation of a supraphysiological number of follicles, the collection of mature oocytes through the more or less invasive aspiration of the contents of the grown follicles and the transfer of one or more embryos to secure the highest possible pregnancy rates. None of these activities is without risk for mother and offspring. The following complications have been recorded systematically in the EIM reports: multiple pregnancies and deliveries, fetal reduction, OHSS, haemorrhage and infections resulting from oocyte collection and maternal death.

Multiple pregnancies are often associated with premature delivery (defined by birth before week 37 of pregnancy) that may harm the newborn, occasionally with lifelong consequences. In order to prevent the complications of multiple gestation (including premature delivery) and supported by the increasing efficacy of cryopreservation, fewer embryos are being transferred today as compared with previous years. This trend is mirrored by a steady decline in the twin and triplet birth rates (Fig. 16.4A). Figure 16.4B plots the premature delivery rates of singleton, twin and triplet pregnancies per embryo transfer. Since the start of the registration of the numbers of premature deliveries in 2006, the number of premature deliveries has declined because fewer embryos are being replaced per cycle, leading to fewer multiple pregnancies. During the same time interval, however, the relative number of premature deliveries in singleton pregnancies per embryo transfer has risen from 0.9% of all embryo transfers in 2006 to 2.8% in 2014 (Fig. 16.4B). The descriptive nature of ART surveillance does not provide an immediate clue for this development.

The other complications of ART listed in the EIM reports are much rarer; although from 1997 to 2013 the incidences of maternal deaths, OHSS, haemorrhage and infection had increased or remained stable, considering the steep increase in treatment numbers resulting in a steady decrease in the relative incidence numbers (Fig. 16.4B). Underreporting is, however, likely to be responsible for a consistent underestimation of some of those risks. A Dutch survey has shown an incidence of maternal mortality of 6/100,000 directly related to ART and of 42.5/100,000 pregnancies resulting from ART, mainly in twin pregnancies [7].

The Future of ART Surveillance in Europe

Since its origin, the EIM data registry has been thriving as a 'bottom-up' endeavour of the national representatives of the participating European countries. The EIM reports published in the journal *Human Reproduction* rank among the most cited publications in that journal. The EIM also contributes to the dataset of the International Committee Monitoring Assisted Reproductive Technologies (ICMART), which regularly publishes global ART data [8]. Currently, 90.5% of all participating European countries, in which ART services are offered to infertile couples (41 countries), and 90.2% of all European institutions active in ART provide their results to EIM, but only 34.1% of participating countries provide full coverage data. As the level of completeness has been rising from the early beginnings of EIM, it can be expected that further improvements may still be achieved.

The face of ART is now changing rapidly. Traditionally, ART treatments were started with the clear-cut intention to obtain a positive pregnancy test as quickly as possible. This aim was to be achieved while often taking a number of complications into account, such as OHSS and multiple gestation. Today, with the improvements in cryopreservation [9], with the advent of human chorionic gonadotropin (hCG)-free ovarian hyperstimulation protocols [10] and with better embryo selection criteria allowing elective single embryo transfer (eSET), all of these complications can now be reduced significantly. The scope of most current ART protocols encompasses the initiation of the treatment including ovarian hyperstimulation, oocyte collection, fertilization and embryo culture. Depending on the individual situation of the treated patient, oocytes, zygotes or embryos may be stored frozen until a new thawing cycle is initiated. Such a segmentation of ART protocols in time allows the prevention of OHSS (through the avoidance of exposure to exogenous or endogenous hCG) and eSET.

Conventional surveillance in ART focused on the collection of oocytes and spermatozoa and the verification of the outcome of their fusion after embryo transfer up to a clinical pregnancy resulting in the delivery of a newborn child. Infertility treatment is increasingly going beyond the collection and storage of gametes, as ovarian tissue may be biopsied and stored frozen until retransplantation. There is a demand to record this

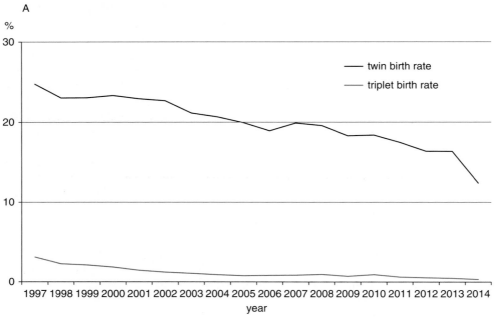

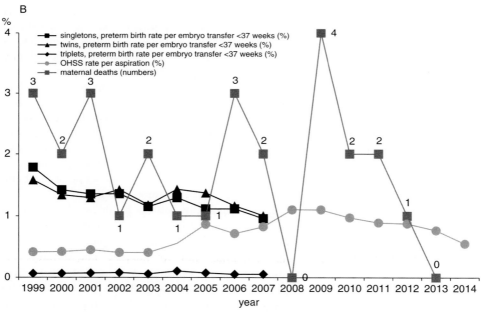

Figure 16.4 Complications in ART as given by the EIM Consortium. Panel A depicts the steady decline in the twin and triplet birth rates since 1997 as a result of the adoption of a strategy of replacing fewer embryos per treatment cycle. Lower multiple delivery rates (panel A) paralleled a similar drop in the incidence rates of premature delivery (<37 weeks) (panel B). Whereas the incidence rate of OHSS has fallen over time, maternal deaths continue to be recorded (numbers added).

type of intervention together with its outcome. This type of surveillance will also require a long-term follow-up, as retransplantation, pregnancy and eventual delivery may be observed many years later.

All these treatment modalities involve frequent storage of reproductive material from women at an age in which this material still has sufficient potential for successful procreation. As a result, the age of the woman at the time of storage of reproductive potential can now be separated effectively from the actual age of childbearing. This time interval can now be prolonged at will, but this poses serious problems with the current concepts of ART surveillance, which traditionally consist of cross-sectional surveys [11].

Ideally, the linkage of single separate therapeutic steps should be managed both in time (spanning time intervals exceeding single years) and in space (if the patient/the couple has her/their reproductive material transported from one institution to another or even across borders). Future surveillance in ART could develop towards analyzing data in a cumulative way and across regions and countries while linking the different segments of serial therapeutic steps together. Future surveillance of all infertility interventions may be carried out effectively only if the individuals (men and women) seeking reproductive assistance are registered by one unified European-wide coding system. A central office could be installed somewhere in Europe that would provide to all European institutions offering ART a code for each individual seeking reproductive care for the first time through easy-to-access software. The code should follow the individual or couple during the various steps of infertility care, even if the individual or the couples change the treatment unit or the country of residence. For data protection purposes, the identity of the individuals should not be given to the central office, but all local stakeholders should link the code to all reports. All reporting to the national ART registry should be accompanied by this individual code, and all treatment results should be labelled with the code, even after 10 or more years. The attribution of such a code could become an integral part of all early infertility care. With time, this code could be promoted as a quality label of infertility care. Ultimately, such a system will allow the construction of true cumulative outcome data.

The organization of such a centralized registration system will push the development of EIM from mere ART surveillance to real vigilance. The question of who will implement such a central office remains to be answered. Certainly, because of its expertise in what matters to modern reproduction and because of its access to the practitioners involved in ART, ESHRE should be the leading body in the organization of such a central office. But is the bottom-up structure of EIM sufficient to motivate all stakeholders in the process of attributing a single, unique European code to all new individuals seeking reproductive care?

Ideally, a partner with the power to install a 'top-down' compulsory data collection initiative should be involved. The European Commission (EC) has already been active in setting up a coding system for cells and tissues (Directive 2015/565/EC of 9 April 2015 that partially amended Directive 2006/86/EC of 24 October 2006), but the European Union (EU) does not represent the totality of all European states. Currently, 28 countries are EU members and almost all reliably provide data to the EIM. Eleven members of EIM are not members of the EU. Ideally, another strong partner should be sought beyond the EU. The Organisation for Economic Co-operation and Development (OECD) could be another international institution promoting ART surveillance in Europe. OECD has been involved in health politics, but not in infertility issues.

Conclusions

Surveillance of ART in Europe is carried out by the EIM Consortium and is a bottom-up organization of the representatives of national registries of nearly all European countries offering ART services. The first dataset of 1997 was published in 2001, and since then 17 reports have been published in the journal *Human Reproduction*. These reports are among the most cited publications from this journal. Reported treatment modalities are IVF, ICSI, frozen-thawed embryo and oocyte replacement, egg donation, preimplantation genetic diagnosis and in vitro maturation. Outcome data, such as clinical ongoing pregnancies and deliveries, are given for each participating country. Ongoing observed trends are the continuous rise in the number of (successful) treatments and a steady decline in the incidence of multiple deliveries and of ovarian hyperstimulation syndrome. Over the years high levels of completeness have been reached, but the current trend towards a higher diversity in treatment modalities demands changes in the setting of data collection. ART surveillance in Europe should now develop from cross-sectional data analysis towards prospective surveillance of cumulative data. In the very fragmented national and legal European landscape governing ART activities, this goal can be achieved only when an easy-to-access, centralized coding system is installed to tag and follow all newly recruited cases presenting with infertility.

References

1. Steptoe PC, Edwards RG. Birth after the reimplantation of a human embryo. *Lancet*. 1978;2:366.

2. Nygren KG, Nyboe Andersen A. Assisted reproductive technology in Europe, 1997. Results generated from European registers by ESHRE. *Hum Reprod*. 2001;16: 384–91.

3. Ferraretti AP, Nygren, K, Nyboe Andersen A, de Mouzon J, Kupka M, Calhaz-Jorge C, et al.; the European IVF-monitoring (EIM) Consortium for the European Society of Human Reproduction and Embryology (ESHRE). Trends over 15 years in ART in Europe: an analysis of 6 million cycles. *Hum Reprod*. 2017;2(12):hox012.

4. Shenfield F, de Mouzon J, Pennings G, Ferraretti AP, Andersen AN, de Wert G, et al.; ESHRE Taskforce on Cross Border Reproductive Care. Cross border reproductive care in six European countries. *Hum Reprod*. 2010;25:1361–8.

5. Calhaz-Jorge C, De Geyter MS, Kupka J, de Mouzon K, Erb E, Mocanu T et al.; the European IVF-monitoring (EIM) Consortium for the European Society of Human Reproduction and Embryology (ESHRE). Assisted reproductive technology in Europe, 2013: results generated from European registers by ESHRE. *Hum Reprod*. 2017;32:1957–73.

6. Devroey P, Polyzos NP, Blockeel C. An OHSS-free clinic by segmentation of IVF treatment. *Hum Reprod*. 2011;26:2593–7.

7. Braat DDN, Schutte JM, Bernardus RE, Mooij M, van Leeuwen FE. Maternal death related to IVF in the Netherlands 1984–2008. *Hum Reprod*. 2010;25:1782–6.

8. Dyer S, Chambers GM, de Mouzon J, Nygren KG, Zegers-Hochschild F, Mansour R, et al. International Committee for Monitoring Assisted Reproductive Technologies world report: assisted reproductive technology 2008, 2009 and 2010. *Hum Reprod*. 2016;31:1588–609.

9. Cobo A, Garrido N, Pellicer A, Remohí J. Six years' experience in ovum donation using vitrified oocytes: report of cumulative outcomes, impact of storage time, and development of a predictive model for oocyte survival rate. *Fertil Steril*. 2015;104:1426–34.

10. Humaidan P, Polyzos NP, Alsbjerg B, Erb K, Mikkelsen AL, Elbaek HO, et al. GnRHa trigger and individualized luteal phase hCG support according to ovarian response to stimulation: two prospective randomized controlled multi-centre studies in IVF patients. *Hum Reprod*. 2013;28:2511–21.

11. De Geyter Ch, Wyns C, Mocanu E, de Mouzon J, Calhaz-Jorge C. Data collection systems in ART must follow the pace of change in clinical practice. *Hum Reprod*. 2016;31:2160–3.

Chapter

17

ART Surveillance in the Middle East: Governance, Culture and Religion

Johnny Awwad, Dalia Khalife and Ragaa Mansour

History of ART and ART Surveillance in the Middle East

The Middle East (ME) is a region rich in history and tradition, with long-standing, ongoing economic and political struggles. It includes about 18 countries for the purposes of this chapter, with a prevalence of infertility affecting 10 to 15% of couples [1, 2, 3]. In this chapter, the authors highlight the interconnectivity between regulation, culture and religion in the Middle East in relation to reproductive practices and assisted reproductive technology (ART) surveillance. While this aspect of the discussion appears to be unique to Islamic countries, it may not apply to other regional countries, such as Israel. Because the relationship between the state and religion in Israel follows different dynamics, the authors will not be discussing the case of ART surveillance in this particular country.

Although male factor infertility is believed to account for a significant proportion of cases in the region, culturally the major blame lies with women [4, 5]. The Middle East has observed a significant proliferation of ART services over the past few decades [6]. The first in vitro fertilization (IVF) clinics in the region were established in 1986 in Egypt, Jordan and Saudi Arabia [7].

Today, the Middle East claims some of the busiest programs in the world. The number of IVF clinics in the area, reportedly, has been rapidly proliferating: by 2010, there were about 55 centres in Egypt, 40 in Saudi Arabia and 20 in Lebanon [8]. This rapid spread of ART technology is not surprising given the fact that childbearing is highly esteemed, culturally and religiously, in this part of the world. In the ME, a marriage is valued by the number of children it produces. Being pronatalist, Muslim societies expect all adults to marry and reproduce [9, 10]. For this reason, childless Muslim women are haunted by the fear of divorce, and Islamic personal status laws

consider infertility as an acceptable ground for divorce and/or second marriage.

Although assisted reproductive technologies are well established in the Islamic countries of the Middle East, no country besides Egypt monitors IVF practice by reporting it to a registry.

National ART Surveillance in Egypt. In view of the rapid spread of ART clinics across Egypt, reaching about 100 centres today, the need for a national registry became evident. In 2001, the Egyptian IVF Registry was formed by a non-governmental group independent of any current organization or society, with the purpose of gathering and disseminating information on the benefits, risks and success rates of assisted reproduction in the country. The Egyptian Medical Syndicate and the Egyptian Ministry of Health, both of which regulate the practice of ART in Egypt, provide no specific guidelines for the reporting of data to a national registry.

Because of the noncompulsory nature of the Egyptian registry, the process of data collection has proved to be a real challenge. In an effort to gather IVF data, the registry routinely contacts all IVF centres in the country through emails, faxes, phone calls and personal contacts, inviting them to participate. The world report on ART forms, prepared by the International Committee Monitoring Assisted Reproductive Technologies (ICMART), is usually distributed along with a cover letter setting a date for a meeting to collect the completed anonymous forms. In 2003, the first and second reports of the Egyptian IVF Registry were collectively published for cycles beginning in 1999 and 2000 [1].

Regional ART Surveillance Efforts by the Middle East Fertility Society. A regional registry is currently in the planning and development phases by the Middle East Fertility Society (MEFS), which is seeking close collaboration with ICMART and the Society for Assisted Technology (SART) for technical and advisory support. During its twenty-second annual scientific meeting at Sharm El Sheikh in 2016, MEFS invited its members to an open forum to discuss perceptions and attitudes towards the establishment of a regional ART registry. Representatives from more than 30 IVF centres attended and shared opinions and concerns.

Participants voiced concerns about confidentiality of centre-specific success rates. Misconceptions were also displayed in relation to the perceived role of the registry as a means of 'spying' on the success rate of centres and monitoring their activities. Publication of the data, potentially leading to the ranking of IVF centres by success rates, was another point of major concern.

Global ART Surveillance in the Middle East. The International Committee Monitoring Assisted Reproductive Technologies (ICMART), an independent, global, non-profit organization, has taken a leading role in the collection of data on ART in the ME. Individual IVF centres in the region have been solicited yearly since 2001 to share their data by filling in the world report on ART forms distributed through email.

Oversight

The Middle East lacks IVF laws and directives in most of its nations, despite the existence of well-established regulatory bodies in a few countries [11]. While ART practice is managed by laws in Saudi Arabia and Tunisia, it is regulated by guidelines in Egypt by the medical syndicate and Ministry of Health. In most other communities, neither guidelines nor regulations exist regarding the practice [12].

It should be noted that in the Middle East, ART practice is highly dominated by religion, namely, the major religious denomination of Islam [13]. In the quasi-absence of governmental oversight in many Middle Eastern countries, it is important to review religious morality for its strong influence on political life and day-to-day decisions. In Muslim-dominated countries, nonbinding but authoritative Islamic religious proclamations (*fatwas*) significantly influence the practice of IVF in ways that are not commonly seen in the United States (US) and Europe [14].

Sunni Religious Influence. In Islam, ART treatment is allowed within the frame of marriage and is permitted during the validity of the marriage contract. The supreme Sunni authority Al Azhar issued a *fatwa*

in 1980 regulating the practice of ART [15]. This was supported in 1997 by a landmark five-point bioethical declaration presented at the ninth Islamic law and medicine conference, convened by the Islamic Organization for Medical Sciences (IOMS) in Casablanca [16]. For Sunni Muslims, in vitro fertilization is allowed as long as it involves gametes from the husband and wife [17, 18, 19]. Sharia law teachings and directions, however, are against any mixing of genes, as in the case of gamete donation [20, 21]. As Islam mandates biological inheritance, the donation of gametes undermines kinship, descent and inheritance. Reproductive third parties are not admissible into the marital function of procreation, including all forms of gamete/embryo donations and surrogacies [5], under threat of treating the products of such practices as illegitimate children under inheritance laws [6]. Cryopreservation of supernumerary embryos is permissible, and preserved embryos are the sole property of the married couple [8]. Multifetal selective reduction may be allowed in the exceptional case in which the well-being of the mother and/or pregnancy is believed to be under serious threat [15].

Shiite Religious Influence. While Sunni Muslim religious thinking is literarily based on the scripture with unwavering rigidity, Shiite scholars favour some forms of individual intellectual reasoning, which introduces a wide range of pragmatism in the interpretation of the religious literature [22]. As a result, a great deal of heterogeneity of practices has emerged across the Shiite community, leaving many clerics divided on many sensitive topics in ART. In 1999, for example, a *fatwa* from the Supreme Jurisprudent of the Iranian Shiite Islam, Ayatollah Ali Hussein Khamenei, permitted the use of male and female donor gametes and surrogacy under certain regulations [15]. According to the religious codes on parenting, the child born out of a donation process would follow the name of the infertile parent, but that child can inherit only from the biological parent. In contrast, another eminent Shiite religious authority based in Lebanon, Ayatollah Muhammad Hussein Fadlallah, did not allow the use of donor male gametes, but proposed a legal way around it. The wife has to divorce her infertile husband and marry the sperm donor throughout the whole duration of gestation and until her delivery, at which time she will be allowed to return to her initial husband.

Infertile couples very often find themselves with little choice but to move between religious denominations in order to accommodate their reproductive needs. Sunni Muslim couples, for instance, may seek cross-border medical tourism to countries with religious diversity, such as Lebanon.

Oversight in Lebanon. Lebanon is just one example of a Middle Eastern country in which a lack of any ART governmental legal oversight and/or professional regulatory system exists [19]. There is also no national ART registry to report on quantitative statistics and qualitative outcome measures.

Attempts to introduce legislation on regulating ART practice in Lebanon repeatedly failed because of multisectarian resistance. The necessity of gaining consensus between diverse religious communities frequently paralyzed proposed legislature on ART regulation, primarily because religious opinions on this matter remained far from being reconciled. As a result, ART practice in Lebanon has remained largely guided by the personal judgement of IVF physicians and their bioethical convictions [15].

It is not uncommon, therefore, to observe practices which are not compliant with standard guidelines proposed by international professional societies. Some of these practices support unsafe medical behaviours, such as the use of fresh sperm for donation and the absence of genetic screening for donors and recipients. Other practices do not comply with specific ethical codes, such as the selection of egg donors among financially underprivileged refugees.

The implementation of an ART registry in similar countries, although of unparalleled benefits in highlighting abuse and setting the ground for corrective measures, may be out of reach in these communities with lack of oversight.

The case may be different in countries with more homogeneous religious views such as Egypt. Here, despite the development of bioethical and professional codes, IVF physicians exert a great deal of self-restraint on particular controversial practice matters, more on the basis of Islamic morality than on laws and regulations.

Process of Data Collection

ICMART monitors ART cycles performed in the Middle East annually through the collection of aggregate data on standardized forms provided by individual clinics and by the Egyptian national registry. The data obtained annually through the world report on ART forms provide an overview of outcomes at the national and regional levels [23]. The data are then transferred to the Uppsala Clinical Research Center in Sweden for analysis and generation of reports [24, 25]. Surveys provide information on availability, effectiveness, safety and perinatal outcomes of ART procedures performed in each contributing country (see Chapter 11, Global ART Surveillance: The International Committee Monitoring Assisted Reproductive Technologies (ICMART)).

Because of the voluntary nature of reporting, the number of clinics reporting to ICMART from the Middle East has declined steadily over the past few years. While the estimated rate of participation in 2008 was 22.2%, it declined to 7.5% in 2010. Declining compliance may be multifactorial and could be attributed to the lack of governance [26], as well as the political turmoil and unrest that affected the region in the second decade of the twenty-first century.

At a country level, Egypt accounts for almost all participating clinics [25, 27, 28]. Data collected include numbers and outcomes of intrauterine insemination (IUI), intracytoplasmic sperm injection (ICSI) and frozen embryo transfer (FET).

This type of retrospective reporting is often flawed because of incomplete information and missing entries; not infrequently, rough estimations are made to account for these omissions. In view of all these hurdles to proper reporting, a workshop was conducted in Egypt in 2003 with the aim of developing an action plan to lay the foundations for a Middle East IVF registry. The project aimed to entice and assist physicians to develop national registries in their own countries [23]. Beside Egypt, unfortunately, no other regional country succeeded in establishing registries to report ART practice on a periodic basis.

Data Collected

According to ICMART, the total number of ART activities reported from the Middle East in 2001 was 16,293 cycles. Unfortunately, these figures were calculated on the basis of information provided by only 30 participating centres [23]. It is interesting to observe how the total number of cycles reported to ICMART decreased to 9,732 in 2010 [24]. It should be noted that Egypt conducted most of these interventions, and therefore these numbers cannot be used to estimate quantitatively the total ART activity load in the whole region.

One main limitation of the ICMART database, in relation to the number of cycles reported from the Middle East, is actually underreporting. Many centres in the region find no vested interest in contributing to this 'out-of-the-borders' initiative. Others suffer internal logistic hurdles related to limited human and technological resources. Many centres have no dedicated IVF software to facilitate the reporting task and rely solely on paper documentation. It is therefore obvious that reported figures represent a significant misrepresentation of the actual number of cycles performed in the region for any given year. Taken together, ICMART data ought to be interpreted with great caution, as they underestimate actual quantity. The real value of the information provided rather lies in the qualitative interpretation of practices and their changing trends over time.

As an example, the reports of the Egyptian IVF registry in collaboration with ICMART indicate that male factor infertility alone, or in combination with other factors, represented the largest indication for undergoing assisted reproductive technologies in the region. As many as 73.6% of ART treatment cycles in 2001 were for male infertility, and only 25.8% were for anovulation, tubal disease and unexplained aetiologies [23]. On this topic, registry data provided valuable qualitative information by pointing out the fact that spermatogenic defects represented a larger proportion of ART indications than previously estimated. Such information may prove to be of great value in guiding research on the underlying pathophysiological mechanisms of male infertility in this part of the world. It may also influence the way reproductive medicine is practised in the area by putting more focus on male reproductive disorders, thus far considered taboo because male fertility is traditionally linked to pride and manhood.

ICMART reports have also pointed out a high utilization rate of the ICSI procedure in the Middle East compared with conventional IVF: 90.7% of all ART cycles reported in 2001 were ICSI procedures. This ratio increased gradually to 94.0% in 2005 and 98.3% in 2010 [23, 25, 28]. Compared with ICSI utilization rates of 60 to 65% in Europe and the US, these figures are alarming and may warrant investigation. Although they may be partially influenced by the higher prevalence of male infertility presenting for ART, they do not provide a complete explanation for the rising trend in utilization rates over the following years. It seems evident, however, that the routine practice of 'ICSI-for-all' is gaining popularity over conventional IVF in this part of the world. It is not clear to what extent this growing tendency is socially

and/or financially driven. One study argued that it may be the result of a combination of factors, including limited financial resources, mislabelling and elevated patient expectations [29]. Unfortunately, attitudes and perceptions of patients and physicians concerning this subject have never been fully probed. Much research is therefore needed to understand the socio-economic drivers behind certain ART practices in particular regional communities.

ICMART data indicate that very few centres volunteered information on the outcome of their cryopreservation programs and/or techniques utilized [23, 30]. It is very likely that many centres do not feel comfortable sharing data they deem less satisfactory compared with the outcome of fresh cycles. These findings once more underscore a potential field of weakness in ART practice in the Middle East. Developing training programs for embryologists targeting cryopreservation techniques may be an option to improve the laboratory performance and serve the best interests of the infertile patient population.

In many countries of the Middle East, transferring too many embryos is still common practice [23, 24, 30, 31]. The ICMART registry demonstrated that the average number of embryos transferred in a fresh cycle dropped from 2.95 in 2008 to 2.48 in 2010, whereas the rate of elective single embryo transfer increased from 6.6% in 2008 to 17.2% in 2010 [24]. In parallel, the rate of multiple births continued to rise from 11.4% in 2008 to 22.0% in 2010. No guidelines exist to regulate and monitor the number of embryos transferred. Although individual policies have been developed internally by some ART centres, such endeavours remain largely isolated and are left to the discretion of individual physicians. In general, many centres are under pressure to achieve pregnancies punctually as part of their reported successes, irrespective of the outcome of multiple births order. This driver appears to have two components. First, physicians are known by the achievement of a pregnancy irrespective of the order of multiple pregnancies. A physician's success is all too often judged on the basis of pregnancy successes irrespective of healthy births. Second, patients are looking for a quick conception notwithstanding the risks of long-term complications. Patients in many instances seek financial support from immediate family members and are under pressure to achieve success as soon as possible, because they understand that another opportunity may not be feasible.

One major advantage of the ICMART registry is that it sheds light on actual complications of ART practice in the region. Treatment complications such as ovarian hyperstimulation syndrome (OHSS), bleeding and infection are all reported. The 2001 world report showed that clinically significant OHSS complicated 1.82% of cycles, while post-ovum pickup bleeding and infection occurred in 0.21% and 0.06% of all follicle aspirations, respectively [23]. The country which reported the highest rate of adverse effects was Bahrain, where 2.26% of all cycles performed during 2001 were complicated with clinically significant OHSS [32]. These figures compare with an overall OHSS incidence of 1.0% in the European registry [33].

In 2005, ICMART Middle East reported an overall perinatal death rate of 47.3 per thousand births after fresh embryo transfers and 64.7 per thousand births after frozen-thawed transfer cycles [25]. The overall rate of preterm deliveries was 34.2% for fresh transfer pregnancies and 19.0% for FET pregnancies. This information, however, was reported by only a handful of centres and may not be representative of the whole population of the Middle East; therefore, the data should be interpreted with great caution. It should be noted that no data on the risk of congenital malformations after ART are available. Unfortunately, most ART centres in the region do not have a well-defined traceability policy for obstetrical and/or postnatal complications after ART. Once pregnant, women often move away to their obstetricians with no way to trace or track them. The medical information regarding the process of conception is carefully concealed for the purpose of safeguarding confidentiality and for fear of compromising third-party coverage of obstetrical expenses.

It should be noted that, except for Lebanon, no gamete donation was reported from the Middle East. The practice of maternal surrogacy in the area is forbidden by most religions, although a few religious authorities permit it in the context of maintaining the integrity of the family. This view, however, is highly contested and not universally approved. In addition, there is the legislative complication at the time of delivery. The laws in most Arab countries have not been adapted to deal with gestational carriers and surrogacy, so the birth certificate would be issued with the name of the carrier as mother. Any change in the civil state will consider the infant as adopted and the biological mother as the stepmother.

Surrogacy is therefore not practised in the Middle East because it contradicts religious beliefs and legalities.

Assuring Data Quality

With the current method of data collection, it may be difficult to measure accurately the success of ART cycles in the Middle East. According to ICMART, the pregnancy rates (PRs) and delivery rates (DRs) per follicle aspiration have been reported as 34.5% and 25.6%, respectively, for fresh embryos in 2004, and remained practically unchanged through 2010 [24, 25, 28]. Similarly, the PRs and DRs from frozen-thawed embryos were 22.1% and 13.7%, respectively, in 2004 and showed no change until 2010 [24, 25, 28]. When considering fresh and frozen embryo transfers, the cumulative DR per follicle aspiration ranged from 32.2% in 2005 to 37.5% in 2010 [24, 25].

It is generally agreed that the preferred method of data collection which ensures high-quality data validity and transparency is the mandatory, prospective cycle-by-cycle reporting registry system established at the national level. In countries in which no governance of ART exists, however, the voluntary collection of aggregate data is deemed more convenient. This is largely the case in Middle Eastern countries, which report their data inconsistently to the ICMART registry.

Limitations inherent in voluntary registries nonetheless include reporting biases. Differences in clinical practice among clinics may lead some to abstain from sharing parts of their data. This may be related to clinics that do not follow standard norms and policies, such as capping the number of replaced embryos. Centres that offer significant levels of cross-border reproductive care, namely, gamete donation, may also feel uncomfortable reporting their data for privacy reasons and for fear of being labelled. It should be noted that full practice visibility may also mean taxation vulnerability, as some centres refuse participation for fear of having to follow proper tax reporting procedures. Taken together, the validity of noncompulsory registries has been called into question, as some contributing centres do not feel comfortable sharing genuine data. Because clinics that declare their data are often those with better clinical practice, a trend towards an overestimation of good outcomes is to be expected [34]. Without on-site data monitoring, the accuracy of these data will remain questionable.

Limitations of aggregate data collection also include the inability to establish record linkage between various registries, namely, birth, congenital malformation, hospital discharge and death registries. Record-linking health data registries may be the best means of establishing long-term health risks in the progeny of IVF technologies, namely, the outcome of certain practices.

Despite inherent limitations, aggregate data analyses offer several advantages. They may be preferred in environments in which integrity about information misuse and data confidentiality is of high concern. Aggregate data may also constitute valuable material for research, namely, when it is not possible to conduct large-scale studies for financial and economic reasons. From that perspective, registry-based studies have proved to be very cost-effective, as they entail data which have already been collected a priori as long as they are properly interpreted. On the other hand, aggregate data may be valued for their qualitative rather than quantitative data interpretation, referred to as 'ecological studies' [35]. In this case, the group demonstrating common collective characteristics becomes the entity of observation and analysis. Although ecological studies describe group-level conditions while failing to establish causal inferences at individual levels, useful correlations between group data are achievable and may constitute grounds for valuable hypothesis generation.

Challenges and Strategies

Challenges. The ART surveillance system in the Middle East lacks consistency, quality and completeness, as ICMART-collected information includes only voluntary aggregate data, having many gaps and being collected in a retroactive manner. Because the practice is not regulated by legislation or laws, not all centres are expected to be compliant with data reporting.

As discussed earlier, this form of retrospective aggregate data collection cannot estimate utilization rates of ART and access to fertility care. It may nevertheless determine practice variations and trends by governorates within the same country and/or between countries of the region. It may also provide information on ART practices in relation to local rules and regulations as well as to variation in insurance coverages [36].

Nation-based compulsory prospective data collection remains the most beneficial type of IVF registry. In the Middle East, such registries may face significant challenges in relation to continuity and sustainability.

They should be managed by a competent multidisciplinary scientific team including epidemiologists, statisticians, physicians, computer scientists and information technology (IT) technicians. Secure and sustained funding is all too often difficult to acquire but is essential for the support of clerical functions as well as statistical and research scientific activities. While some direct or indirect personal identifiers are usually required in individual-based registries, such a requirement may pose serious confidentiality concerns among Middle Eastern communities as a result of administrative corruption and mistrust of governmental organizations. Because infertility is a taboo subject, especially when it comes to male factor infertility, to safeguard their privacy couples may shy away from centres that report to registries.

Strategies. A successful implementation of a voluntary registry may require a more active engagement than a simple impersonal solicitation through an electronic data sheet. It may involve methods such as educational meetings, local consensus processes and the employment of local opinion leaders [37]. The value of the registry for both clinics and physicians could be enhanced by publishing the data collected. An internal, personally driven commitment remains, nonetheless, the main driver of a firm involvement in these types of registries.

Several strategies to facilitate compliance with a voluntary registry have been proposed:

(a) *Pilot phase.* An initial small-scale launch is invariably favoured during which the levels of participants' adherence are identified [38] and operational details sorted, notwithstanding the fact that data reporting is largely dependent on 'buy in' strategies. It should also be noted that higher coverage should not be sought at the expense of high accuracy in data reporting.

(b) *Pruning of data entries.* Reduced data fields may be adopted for start-up registries. Failure to prune data entries to a minimum may lead to poor adherence by demotivated centres, particularly when no funding for data collection is offered.

(c) *Timely feedback.* Prompt feedback on the quality of data received within a short time frame may serve to enhance the level of compliance, allowing contributing centres to make the requested adjustments to the data within reasonable working memory [38, 39].

(d) *Introducing a competitive element.* Awarding a prestigious status to data supply centres on the basis of data quality has been shown to instigate a competitive spirit and enhance overall compliance [39]. While the public awarding of gold certificates to highly compliant centres was shown to bolster their commitment to excellence, the award of bronze certificates in sealed envelopes could encourage less compliant ones to make the necessary improvements to attain the gold status by the next reporting deadline [39].

(e) *Maintaining confidentiality.* Registries that collect IVF data are subject to serious pressure for ensuring that the confidentiality of individual health data is tightly secured. Although a universal concern, proper disposal of health information is particularly important in societies such as the Middle East in which infertility is a taboo subject and in which administrative and social corruption is often prevalent. Seeking a trusted third party that owns the exclusive access to the de-identified personal data and that can guarantee their anonymity may be considered. The designation of such an authorized guardian may be a particularly challenging task in societies with a great deal of mistrust of their government leaders. Proper patient consent should clearly designate the trusted party and state the circumstances in which access to personal health data is granted [38, 39].

(f) *Financial sustainability.* Adequate and sustainable financial resources are necessary for the proper support of good registry practices. Unfortunately, it is not uncommon to witness restricted funding eroding the overall performance of registries, which all too often may find themselves struggling to gain support from government establishments, non-government organizations and industry.

(g) *Open access for research.* One important buy-in policy is data usefulness to contributing members of the registry. The proper design of the data collection scheme will facilitate the execution of approved research inquiries and will ultimately boost the value of the data collected. Obtaining data of low quality could erode confidence and commitment [39].

Conclusion

The assisted reproductive technology industry is blossoming in the Middle East [11]. Infertility treatment services are spread widely across the region as additional IVF clinics are founded every year. Despite the financial, psychological and religious dilemmas, ART

has been embraced by Middle Eastern cultures because the final point is procreation [5].

In the quasi-absence of governmental legislative control and professional society regulations, ART surveillance systems are critically needed to provide missing information about IVF practices and outcomes in each country of the region. Collected data may constitute a valuable platform on the basis of which future regulations may be established. An effective monitoring of ART practice is critical to determine the effectiveness and safety of treatment and identify the level of access to fertility services as well as high-risk behaviours.

The most suitable form of ART surveillance systems remains to be determined, considering the lack of governance and the unique qualities of Middle Eastern culture. Although nation-based, prospective, compulsory registries are highly valued and ultimately sought, a regional retrospective and voluntary surveillance system may be a more realistic project. Well-designed and comprehensive strategies should be installed to ensure the long-term sustainability of such a system. Transparent processes to ensure the anonymity of participants and confidentiality of health information should also be employed.

References

1. Boivin J, Bunting L, Collins, JA, Nygren, KG. International estimates of infertility prevalence and treatment-seeking: potential need and demand for infertility medical care. *Hum Reprod.* 2007;**22**(6): 1506–12.

2. Serour GI. Medical and socio-cultural aspects of infertility in the Middle East. *ESHRE Monographs.* 2008;**1**:34–41.

3. Egyptian Fertility Care Society. *Community-Based Study of the Prevalence of Infertility and Its Etiological Factors in Egypt: The Population-Based Study.* Cairo: The Egyptian Care Society; 1995.

4. Inhorn M, Van Balen F (eds.). *Infertility around the Globe: New Thinking on Childlessness, Gender, and Reproductive Technologies.* Berkeley: University of California Press; 2002.

5. Gürtin ZB, Inhorn MC, Tremayne S. Islam and assisted reproduction in the Middle East: comparing the Sunni Arab World, Shia Iran and secular Turkey. In *The Changing World Religion Map.* Dordrecht: Springer; 2015. pp.3137–53.

6. Inhorn MC, Tremayne S (eds.). *Islam and Assisted Reproductive Technologies: Sunni and Shia Perspectives.* New York: Berghahn Books; 2012.

7. Inhorn MC. *Local Babies, Global Science: Gender, Religion, and In Vitro Fertilization in Egypt.* London: Psychology Press; 2003.

8. Inhorn MC, Patrizio P. Infertility around the globe: new thinking on gender, reproductive technologies and global movements in the 21st century. *Hum Reprod Update.* 2015;21(4):411–26.

9. Zuhur S. *Revealing Reveiling: Islamist Gender Ideology in Contemporary Egypt.* Albany, NY: SUNY Press; 1992.

10. Inhorn MC. *Infertility and Patriarchy: The Cultural Politics of Gender and Family Life in Egypt.* Philadelphia: University of Pennsylvania Press; 1996.

11. Bento F, Esteves, S, Agarwal, A. *Gulf Countries.* New York: Springer; 2013.

12. Cohen J, Jones HW. *Worldwide Legislation. Textbook of Assisted Reproductive Techniques, Laboratory and Clinical Perspectives.* London: Martin Dunitz; 2001. pp.731–51.

13. Serour GI. Ethical considerations of assisted reproductive technologies: a Middle Eastern perspective. *Middle East Fertil Soc J.* 2000;5:13–18.

14. Inhorn M, Tremayne S (eds.). *Islam Assisted Reproductive Technologies: Sunni and Shia Perspectives.* New York: Berghahn Books; 2012.

15. Inhorn, MC. Islam, assisted reproductive technologies, and the Middle Eastern state. *Babylon.* 2008;6(1):32–43.

16. Moosa E. Human cloning in Muslim ethics. *Voices across Boundaries.* 2003;2003:23–6.

17. Serour, GI. Traditional sexual practices in the Islamic world and their evolution. *Global Bioethics.* 1995;8(1–3):61–9.

18. Serour, GI. Attitudes and cultural perspectives on infertility and its alleviation in the Middle East area. In E Vayenna (ed.), *Current Practices and Controversies in Assisted Reproduction.* Geneva: WHO; 2002. p.41.

19. Aboulghar M, Serour GI, Mansour RT. Ethical aspects and regulation of assisted reproduction in the Arabic-speaking world. *Reprod BioMed Online.* 2007;14:143–6.

20. Serour GI, Omran AR. *Ethical Guidelines for Human Reproduction Research in the Muslim World.* Cairo: International Islamic Center for Bioethics, Population Studies and Research; 1992. pp. 29–31.

21. Serour GI, Aboulghar MA, Mansour RT. Bioethics in medically assisted conception in the Muslim world. *J Assist Reprod Genet.* 1995;12(9):559–65.

22. Cole JR, Kandiyoti D. Nationalism and the colonial legacy in the Middle East and Central Asia: introduction. *Int J Middle East Stud.* 2002;34(2):189–203.

23. Mansour RT, Abou-Setta AM. Results of assisted reproductive technology in 2001 generated from the Middle East IVF registry. *Middle East Fertil Soc J.* 2006;11(3):145–51.

24. Dyer S, Chambers GM, De Mouzon J, Nygren KG, Zegers-Hochschild F, Mansour R, et al. International Committee for Monitoring Assisted Reproductive Technologies world report: assisted reproductive technology 2008, 2009 and 2010. *Hum Reprod.* 2016;31(7):1588–609.

25. Zegers-Hochschild F, Mansour R, Ishihara O, Adamson GD, de Mouzon J, Nygren KG, et al. International Committee for Monitoring Assisted Reproductive Technology: world report on assisted reproductive technology, 2005. *Fertil Steril.* 2014;101(2):366–78.

26. Zegers-Hochschild F, Nygren K, Ishihara O. The impact of legislation and socioeconomics factors in the access to and global practice of assisted reproductive technology (ART). In *Textbook of Assisted Reproductive Techniques.* London: Informa Healthcare; 2011. pp.441–50.

27. Nygren KG, Sullivan E, Zegers-Hochschild F, Mansour R, Ishihara O, Adamson GD, et al. International Committee for Monitoring Assisted Reproductive Technology (ICMART) world report: assisted reproductive technology 2003. *Fertil Steril.* 2011;95(7):2209–22.

28. Sullivan EA, Zegers-Hochschild F, Mansour R, Ishihara O, de Mouzon J, Nygren KG, et al. International Committee for Monitoring Assisted Reproductive Technologies (ICMART) world report: assisted reproductive technology 2004. *Hum Reprod.* 2013;28(5):1375–90.

29. Grimstad FW, Nangia AK, Luke B, Stern JE, Mak W. Use of ICSI in IVF cycles in women with tubal ligation does not improve pregnancy or live birth rates. *Hum Reprod.* 2016;3:1–6.

30. Mansour R. The Middle East IVF registry for the year 2000. *Middle East Fertil Soc J.* 2004;9(3):181–6.

31. Aboulghar MA. Perinatal complications of assisted reproduction. *Croat Med J.* 2005;46(5).

32. Eskandarani HA. A Bahraini registry of assisted reproductive technology for period of 2000–2006: hoping to stave off reporting stalemate. *J Reprod Contracept.* 2010;21(2):101–10.

33. Nyboe Andersen A, Gianaroli L, Nygren KG. Assisted reproductive technology in Europe, 2000. Results generated from European registers by ESHRE. *Hum Reprod.* 2004;19(3):490–503.

34. Bosser R, Gispert R, Torné M, Calaf J. Status of human assisted reproduction in Spain: results from the new

registry of Catalonia. *Reprod Biomed Online.* 2009;**19**:727–33.

35. Robinson WS. Ecological correlations and the behavior of individuals. *Am Sociol Rev.* 1950;**15**:51–7.

36. Jain T, Hornstein MD. Disparities in access to infertility services in a state with mandated insurance coverage. *Fertil Steril.* 2005;**84**(1):221–3.

37. Luceno F, Castilla JA, Gomez-Palomares JL, Cabello Y, Hernandez J, Marqueta J, et al. Comparison of IVF cycles reported in a voluntary ART registry with a mandatory registry. *Reproduction.* 2010;**25**(12): 3066–71.

38. Mehta G, Sims EJ, Culross F, McCormick JD, Mehta A. Potential benefits of the UK Cystic Fibrosis Database. *J R Soc Med.* 2004;**97**(Suppl 44): 60–71.

39. Mehta A. The how (and why) of disease registers. *Early Hum Dev.* 2010;**86**(11):723–8.

Chapter

18

ART Surveillance in North America

James Patrick Toner, Andrea Lanes and Dmitry M. Kissin

The findings and conclusions in this report are those of the authors and do not necessarily represent the official position of the Centers for Disease Control and Prevention.

ART Surveillance in the United States

History of ART Surveillance in the US

After years of diligent work on in vitro fertilization (IVF) by the pioneering British team of Robert Edwards and Patrick Steptoe, Louise Brown was born in England on 25 July 1978 [1]. Scientists and clinicians around the world understood the significance of this event and clamoured to reproduce it. In the United States (US), several teams undertook the challenge, and Drs Howard and Georgeanna Jones were the first to be rewarded for their efforts with the birth of Elizabeth Carr on 28 December 1981 [2]. Success by other US teams soon followed.

Shortly after the birth of Elizabeth Carr in the US, Dr Howard Jones gathered the leading practitioners of the five existing US IVF programs (Norfolk, Vanderbilt, the University of Texas at Houston, University of Southern California and Yale) to discuss establishing a national registry of IVF attempts and outcomes. Two years later, in 1985, Drs Alan DeCherney and Richard Marrs founded the Society for Assisted Reproductive Technology (SART) as a special interest group in the American Fertility Society (now the American Society for Reproductive Medicine (ASRM)) [3]. This reporting was entirely voluntary, but participation was at a high level. SART has coordinated an annual tabulation report since 1985. Annual reports tabulating the clinical assisted reproductive technology (ART) activity in the US from 1985 to 1999 are published in *Fertility and Sterility* [4].

Federal Oversight

In 1992, reporting became federally mandated with the passage of the Fertility Clinic Success Rate and Certification Act (FCSRCA) (Public Law No. 102–493, 1992) [3, 5, 6]. FCSRCA mandated that all clinics performing ART annually provide data for all procedures performed in a standardized manner to the Centers for Disease Control and Prevention (CDC), the nation's public health agency. The same mandate required the CDC to publish clinic-specific success rates and certification of embryo laboratories. The first publication required by this law tabulated ART cycles performed in 1995 [7]. Since that time, ART surveillance in the US is unique in having two relatively independent data collection systems: one operated by the government and the other operated by the professional society. To avoid duplicate reporting, SART reports ART data to the CDC on behalf of SART-member clinics. Non-SART clinics report directly to the CDC. A comparison of current features of the two data collection systems is shown in Table 18.1.

Manner of Data Collection

Before FCSRCA, the data were tabulated at the clinic level and reported at the national level. National reports were made public by way of annual publications in *Fertility and Sterility*. Subsequent modifications to reporting included a transition to both cycle-specific reporting and public reporting of outcomes at the individual clinic level, as required by the FCSRCA.

The reports of ART cycles performed from 1985 to 1990 were based on data collected by the special interest group for IVF within the then AFS (through a contract with Medical Research International). This reporting required cycle-specific information and was deemed cumbersome. The reports for the activity in 1991 to 1993 were managed directly by the Registry Committee of the newly named Society for Assisted Reproductive Technology (SART) through simplified Summary Sheets, which captured some general outcome data but no cycle-specific information. The report for 1994 cycles was based on data collected under a contract with a national accounting firm (KPMG). This process collected cycle-specific information, but was extremely time-consuming for the clinics, expensive for the

American Fertility Society (now the American Society for Reproductive Medicine (ASRM)), unwieldy for the Registry Committee and consequently untenable for future collections.

Since 1995, the Registry Committee has collected data via its own Clinical Outcomes Reporting System (CORS). This computer program was developed to collect the minimum cycle-specific information judged to be needed by the SART, ASRM and CDC.

In 2004, the CDC developed a reporting system independent of SART, the National ART Surveillance System (NASS). The CDC reporting system is currently administered by contract with Westat, Inc. On an annual basis, SART collects data from SART-

Table 18.1 The comparison of two assisted reproductive technology data collection systems in the US

Characteristics	US National ART Surveillance System (NASS, CDC)	Clinical Outcomes Reporting System (SART CORS, SART)
Reporting Requirements, Coverage and Data Validation		
Reporting requirements	All ART clinics	SART member clinics
Legal requirements	FCSRCA	SART by-laws
Reporting clinics	94% of all clinics	78% of all clinics
Reported cycles	~98% of all cycles	~90% of all cycles
Data validation	Random validation to assess discrepancy rates for key variables (approximately 35 clinics annually)	Targeted validation to detect systematic reporting errors (approximately 10 clinics annually)
Data cleaning	Basic data cleaning and reconciliation prior to publication	Publication as is with option to correct the data
Using ART Data for ART Reports and Clinical Practice		
Reporting clinic-specific data	ART Success Rates Report online at www.cdc.gov/ART	Clinic Tables online at www.sart.org
Reporting national data	National ART success rates data and ART National Summary Report	National ART success rates data
Reporting state-level data	State-specific ART Surveillance Summary	None
Using data for clinical guidelines / recommendations	Through peer-reviewed publications informing practice guidelines	Through peer-reviewed publications, practice guidelines, committee opinions
Primary research focus	Infant health outcomes (multiple births, preterm births, low birth weight, long-term outcomes), maternal health outcomes (pregnancy and birth complications, long-term outcomes), access to fertility treatments	ART effectiveness (laboratory quality, effectiveness of various ART methods), ART safety (multiple births, preterm births)
Using data to improve clinical care	Patient and provider education, prevention of multiple births (CDC/SART joint projects)	Patient and provider education, prevention of multiple births (CDC/SART joint projects), quality assurance activities
Using ART Data for Research and Data Linkages		
Data users	Any researcher with strong research proposal	SART member or individuals approved by the SART Executive Council
Data access	Onsite at the Division of Reproductive Health (CDC)	De-identified dataset provided to approved researcher
Confidentiality protection	Assurance of Confidentiality; public health surveillance does not require patient informed consent	Health Insurance Portability and Accountability Act of 1996 (HIPAA) requirement; patient informed consent may be required

Table 18.1 (cont.)

Characteristics	US National ART Surveillance System (NASS, CDC)	Clinical Outcomes Reporting System (SART CORS, SART)
State-based linkages	States Monitoring ART (SMART) Collaborative with Massachusetts, Michigan, Florida and Connecticut; other research projects with linked data	Massachusetts Outcomes Study of ART (MOSART) with Massachusetts; other research projects with linked data
National linkages	Linkage with National Vital Statistics System (all live births in the US)	Not applicable
Linkage methods	Probabilistic linkage (using indirect identifiers)	Deterministic linkages (using direct identifiers)
Linkage rates	Above 90%	Above 90%
Current statistics		
Number of cycles in the database (to 2016)	2,995,822	2,073,692
Number of infants in the database (to 2016)	1,087,546	762,513
Years of data collection	1996 to 2016	2003 to 2016

ART, assisted reproductive technology; CDC, Centers for Disease Control and Prevention; FCSRCA, Fertility Clinic Success Rate and Certification Act; NASS, National ART Surveillance System; SART CORS, Society for Assisted Reproductive Technology Clinical Outcomes Reporting System

member clinics and sends the data required to Westat for upload into the NASS. Clinics that are not members of SART report directly to the CDC via Westat.

Data Collected

The following information is currently being collected: patient demographics (age, race/ethnicity, residency), patient obstetrical and medical history (prior pregnancies and their outcomes, prior use of ART), reasons for ART (infertility diagnosis), detailed clinical parameters of the ART procedure (source of gametes, details about stimulation, details about oocyte retrieval, micromanipulations involving oocytes or embryos, information about the embryo(s), details about embryo transfer) and finally cycle outcome (information about pregnancies, births and infants, as well cycle cancellations or complications). See Appendix A for more details.

Because the method of collecting data and clinical practice have changed over time, the annual reports contain some changes that are pertinent when interpreting trends in practice and outcome. ART is a rapidly developing field, and one of the challenges of ART surveillance is to constantly adjust data collection systems to incorporate new methods of treatment or risk factors. While

changes to data collection are made on a regular basis, SART and the CDC have coordinated two major upgrades of the data collection system to reflect evolving clinical practice, once in 2000 and again in 2016.

The first published report of gamete intrafallopian transfer (GIFT) appeared in 1984 [8], and SART started collecting this information the following reporting year. Zygote intrafallopian transfer (ZIFT) was first described in 1986 [9] and was added to the ART registry in 1988. Micromanipulation of eggs to improve fertilization was first reported in 1992. The first techniques were reported about 1990 – partial zona dissection in 1989 [10] and subzonal insertion in 1990 [11] – but neither proved particularly effective. A more effective form of micromanipulation, intracytoplasmic sperm injection (ICSI), was first described in 1988 [12], but was not shown to be highly effective until 1992 [13]. It was singled out in the 1995 ART report, at which time other forms of micromanipulation were dropped.

Beginning with the 1985 reporting year, ART reports have been published annually [4]. ART cycles from programs in the US and Canada were reported together from 1991 to 1995, but not before or since. Female age, an important factor known from early on, has been collected since the ART registry's

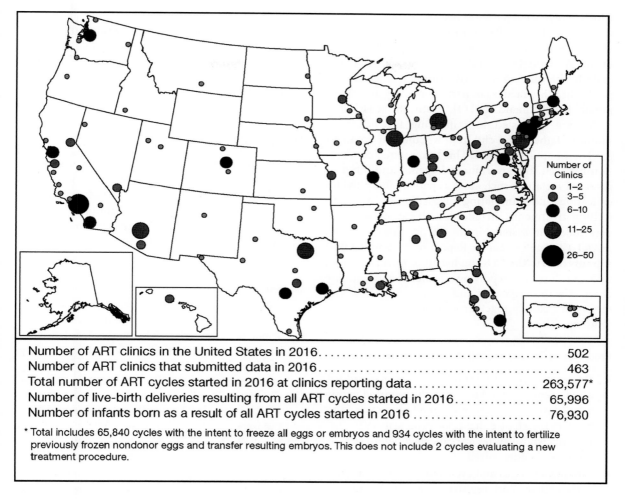

Number of Clinics

- 1–2
- 3–5
- 6–10
- 11–25
- 26–50

Number of ART clinics in the United States in 2016. 502
Number of ART clinics that submitted data in 2016. 463
Total number of ART cycles started in 2016 at clinics reporting data 263,577*
Number of live-birth deliveries resulting from all ART cycles started in 2016. 65,996
Number of infants born as a result of all ART cycles started in 2016 76,930

* Total includes 65,840 cycles with the intent to freeze all eggs or embryos and 934 cycles with the intent to fertilize
previously frozen nondonor eggs and transfer resulting embryos. This does not include 2 cycles evaluating a new
treatment procedure.

Figure 18.1 Locations of ART Clinics in the US and Puerto Rico, 2016.
Source: Centers for Disease Control and Prevention, American Society for Reproductive Medicine, Society for Assisted Reproductive
Technology. *2016 Assisted Reproductive Technology National Summary Report*. Atlanta, GA: US Department of Health and Human Services; 2018.
A colour version of the figure is provided in the plate section.

inception. Given that female age is one of the main predictors of ART outcomes, annual ART reports stratified ART success measures by age. But the reports used different female age groups over the years, as our understanding of this dimension has improved. From 1988 to 1990, female age was reported as <25, 25 to 29, 30 to 34, 35 to 39 and 40+ years. The years 1991 to 1994 divided age only into two categories: <40 and 40+ years. In 1995 and 1996, three categories were used: <35, 35 to 39 and 40+ years. In 1997 and 1998, four categories were reported: <35, 35 to 37, 38 to 40 and 41+ years. In 1999, the last age category was further divided into 41 to 42, and 43+ years.

Successes, Challenges and Future Plans

In the 2016 reporting year, more than 500 fertility clinics were operating in the US. The locations of these clinics throughout the country are shown in Figure 18.1. Although having two data collection systems in the US may seem redundant, each system plays an important role. SART is the primary organization of ART professionals, representing the majority of the ART clinics in the US. SART uses ART data to establish and maintain standards for ART practice through guidelines and committee opinions and to ensure that patients receive the highest possible level of care. The CDC is the nation's public health agency, which protects people from health threats. The CDC is using ART surveillance to calculate standardized, clinic-specific success rates as required by the FCSRCA mandate [5] and to improve maternal and child health outcomes of ART through research and public health practice as part of the organization's public health mandate [14]. Both the CDC and SART are interested in improving the health of mothers, fathers and children, whether on a patient level or a population level. This has fostered cooperation between the governmental agency and the professional society in such areas as patient and provider education and eliminating disparities in access to fertility treatments. In addition, because two ART data collection systems in the US are closely aligned (SART Clinical Outcomes Reporting System (CORS) submits data to the CDC on behalf of member clinics to avoid duplicate reporting), professionals who are charged with developing and maintaining these systems work closely together on many aspects of systems' operation.

Processes to Reduce Inaccurate Reporting by Clinics

- Prospective reporting. Both registries have added a requirement that ART cycles be reported within a few days of the start of the treatment cycle. This reduces the chance that poor prognosis IVF patients whose cycles are cancelled before egg retrieval go unreported.
- Linking all cycles and cycle components for the same patient. Both registries now capture all treatment cycles and link them back to the cycle from which the eggs were obtained. This permits calculation of the 'total reproductive potential' of a stimulation cycle by adding the outcomes of all the transfers stemming from one retrieval to calculate the value of one initiated cycle. This approach also allows accurate calculation of success rates if clinics are practising an embryo accumulation strategy. With the increased utilization of preimplantation genetic testing (PGT) and embryo accumulation, the outcome of an embryo transfer is based on the number of prior stimulation cycles that occurred before that transfer. For example, if a clinic accumulated eggs from three cycles and then transferred the best embryo, the 'per-cycle' rate would use a denominator of three, not one.
- Data validation. Assuring the accuracy of the reported data is an essential process in any

registry. At this time, the CDC does random validation to assess discrepancy rates for key variables (e.g. infertility diagnosis, number of embryos transferred, cycle outcome), and SART does targeted validation to detect systematic reporting errors. Each organization has a role in assuring accurate reporting.

Successes of ART Monitoring

- Public reporting. Allowing patients to see both national and clinic-specific pregnancy outcomes is helpful to guide their choices and expectations.
- Reducing multiple births. By examining the data, guidelines have been developed. The most important of these pertains to the maximum number of embryos to transfer by patient prognosis. This guidance has helped to drastically reduce the incidence of multiple pregnancies, especially high-order multiple pregnancies [15].
- Data linkage studies. Given the information available in the SART CORS and NASS datasets, it has been possible to do linkage studies regarding childhood cancer, autism and birth defects using other registries that collect that information. See Chapter 9, Monitoring Long-Term Outcomes of ART: Linking ART Surveillance Data with Other Datasets.
- Research. Because both ART data collection systems in the US are collecting cycle-level data, they were used for epidemiological and clinical research addressing safety and effectiveness of ART. More than 200 articles have been published using data from these databases. See Chapter 6, Using ART Surveillance Data in Clinical Research.

Future of ART Surveillance in the US

- ART data collection systems in the US and reporting of clinical outcomes of ART will continue to evolve to reflect current clinical practice [16].
- The CDC, SART and other governmental and non-governmental partners and consumer groups will continue their efforts to improve access to effective fertility treatments in the US and to further improve ART outcomes [17, 18].
- Real-time quality assurance dashboard. SART is developing a tool that clinics can use to benchmark certain performance metrics 'in house'

over time and to the current national averages of other clinics reporting prospectively.

ART Surveillance in Canada

History of ART Surveillance in Canada

In 1983, the first IVF baby was conceived and born in Canada. From 1999 to 2012, Canadian ART data were collected in the Canadian Assisted Reproductive Technologies Register (CARTR). This was the first documented nationally representative ART registry in Canada. All data contained in CARTR were owned by the Canadian IVF Medical Directors and were voluntary. These data were manually collected each year and used to inform an annual report on national population-level trends. Reports on these data were published in *Fertility and Sterility* [19, 20]. Data from CARTR were used to inform a number of Canadian clinical practice guidelines including Guidelines on the Number of Embryos Transferred [21] and the Canadian Framework for the Prevention of Multiple Births associated with Infertility [22]. These guidelines, along with other initiatives, were strengthened by the use of nationally representative data to produce evidence-based rationales for changing clinical practice.

In 2011, the medical directors of the fertility clinics in the province of Ontario and the Better Outcomes Registry & Network (BORN) Ontario (Ontario's birth registry) began to develop a more comprehensive national ART registry. BORN Ontario contains detailed information on maternal demographic characteristics, prenatal screening, congenital anomalies, pregnancy and birth outcomes and newborn screening. Both BORN Ontario and the IVF Medical Directors recognized the value of this partnership and a new data entry and repository platform was designed (CARTR Plus). This ART registry is able to provide near real-time information. ART treatment cycle information and birth outcome information is entered by fertility clinics in each province. However, in Ontario the partnership with BORN Ontario has enabled the linkage to birth outcomes data in the province (births ≥20 weeks' gestation). In 2014, there were 140,181 births in Ontario (36.5% of Canada's live births) [23]. Similarly, in 2015 Ontario was responsible for 37.6% of births (live births and stillbirths) from ART treatment cycles. This linkage allows for greater information to be obtained for these ART cycles without the need for manual follow-up with patients.

CARTR Plus was designed to improve quantity and quality of fertility treatment data captured in Canada, as well as to increase the use of these data for clinical practice, research and the development of health policies. CARTR Plus was planned with advice from four essential committees (CARTR Plus Steering Committee, Data Collection Subcommittee, Reporting and Outcomes Subcommittee and the Technical Subcommittee) to create a concept and design that would benefit Canadian ART clinics. Additionally, CARTR Plus was developed to be comparable to other international ART databases.

CARTR Plus Data Collection Process and Variables Collected

CARTR Plus started collecting information on Canadian fertility treatment cycles on 1 January 2013. Contributing to CARTR Plus is voluntary. In 2017, all but one fertility clinic contributed to the database. Data are entered into CARTR Plus either through a manual entry process in a secure web-based application or through a direct upload from a fertility clinic's electronic medical record system. The main electronic medical record systems used in CARTR Plus are BabySentry, IDEAS and eIVF. The fertility clinic must produce an extract file from its electronic medical record, which is then uploaded and processed through the secure web-based application.

CARTR Plus collects information from the initiation of the fertility treatment cycle through the documented birth outcomes. CARTR Plus captures in vitro fertilization (IVF), frozen embryo transfer (FET), frozen oocyte IVF, in vitro maturation (IVM) and oocyte banking cycles. It contains the socio-demographic information on the patients, detailed information about the treatment cycles (i.e. reason for treatment, stimulation protocol used, number of follicles, endometrial thickness, day of transfer, embryo cryopreservation method and number of embryos transferred), treatment success rates (i.e. clinical pregnancy, ongoing clinical pregnancy (clinical pregnancy with ≥1 fetal heart beat on ultrasound) and multiple pregnancy (ongoing clinical pregnancy with >1 fetal heart beat on ultrasound)) and birth outcomes (i.e. live birth, stillbirth, pregnancy loss, multiple live birth). It also contains information on the use of autologous or donor gametes, as well as the use of gestational carriers. (A comprehensive list of variables can be found at http://datadictionary.bornontario.ca/encounters-and-alphabetical-lists/fertility-cartr-plus/.)

CARTR Plus: Current Results

As of 31 December 2016, there were 114,227 fertility treatment cycles in CARTR Plus. The number of cycles performed by each clinic varies. There are clinics that perform fewer than 200 fertility treatment cycles annually and clinics that perform more than 1,000 fertility treatment cycles. In Canada, IVF and FET treatment cycles have been the most prevalent type of treatment. The rate of FET cycles has been steadily increasing with the practice change towards *freeze-all* cycles. Often these *freeze-all* cycles are done in conjunction with preimplantation genetic testing (preimplantation genetic testing for aneuploidy (PGT-A) or monogenic/single gene diseases (PGT-M)). In 2015, there were 354 *freeze-all* treatment cycles that used PGT-A and 407 treatment cycles that used PGT-M (6.7% and 7.7% of all treatment cycles that used autologous oocytes and did not have an embryo transfer, respectively). In comparison, in 2016 there were 1,459 *freeze-all* treatment cycles that used PGT-A and 598 treatment cycles that used PGT-M (22.4% and 9.2% of all treatment cycles that used autologous oocytes and did not have an embryo transfer, respectively). The significant rise in *freeze-all* cycles for PGT-A illustrates a change in clinical practice that has occurred over a relatively short time.

CARTR Plus has documented 31,430 clinical pregnancies with an overall clinical pregnancy rate per embryo transfer of 38.3%. The clinical pregnancy rate per embryo transfer cycle among IVF and FET cycles when autologous oocytes were used was comparable (39.3% and 37.2%, respectively). Fertility treatment cycles that used donor oocytes make up a small proportion of treatment cycles (IVF: 2,805; FET: 4,767). There was a substantial difference in the clinical pregnancy rate per embryo transfer cycle among IVF cycles that used donor oocytes (54.9%) compared with autologous oocytes. However, the clinical pregnancy rate per embryo transfer cycle among FET cycles that used donor oocytes was comparable to the IVF and FET cycles that used autologous oocytes (37.0%). Within CARTR Plus, treatment cycles can be linked by batches of oocytes retrieved, as well as by patient. This is important for evaluating the overall effect of fertility treatment, as opposed to success of a single stage of treatment. The Kaplan-Meier method was used to produce optimistic and conservative cumulative pregnancy rates using CARTR Plus data for all ART treatment cycles (2013–2016) [24]. After one egg retrieval cycle, the clinical pregnancy rate was 26.5% per patient. After two treatment cycles, the cumulative clinical pregnancy rate was 49.3% (optimistic estimate) and 41.5% (conservative estimate). After one treatment cycle, the cumulative pregnancy rate per batch of oocytes retrieved was 25.6% (IVF and FET cycles using autologous oocytes). As expected, after a second treatment cycle, the cumulative clinical pregnancy rate increased to 54.8% (optimistic estimate) and 36.4% (conservative estimate).

CARTR Plus also collects birth outcome information for all ART cycles performed in Canada. The database currently contains comprehensive birth outcomes from 2013 to 2015. Within these years, there were 18,394 pregnancies that resulted in a live birth (22.2% live birth rate per cycle start), of which the majority were singleton live births (87.0%). The miscarriage rate was 19.1% and the stillbirth rate was 0.78% among ongoing clinical pregnancies. As expected, there was a dramatic difference in the live birth rate when patient age was investigated at the time of oocyte retrieval. The live birth rate among younger patients (<35 years) was significantly higher (IVF: 40.5%; FET 32.4%) than among patients with very advanced maternal age (≥43 years (IVF: 6.27%; FET: 10.7%)).

Data Output

Through the BORN Information System, Canadian clinics have near real-time access to their data, as well as to a variety of comparative reports (annual summary, clinical and demographic reports). These reports were designed to assist clinics with day-to-day reporting. A clinic is able to view its data by self-determined time periods. Clinics are also able to view and compare their results with aggregated national data. A clinic only has access to its own data. Clinics are not publicly identified in CARTR Plus. Additionally, data from CARTR Plus are used for research and to inform public policy. Two major initiatives that CARTR Plus data helped to inform are (1) reducing the multiple pregnancy rate among IVF conceptions; and (2) public funding of fertility treatment in Ontario. Reducing the multiple pregnancy rate among Canadian IVF pregnancies was multifactorial. The Canadian Fertility and Andrology Society (CFAS) developed and published a position statement with decreasing targets from 2012 through 2015 [25]. CFAS aimed to reduce the multiple pregnancy rate to 25% by 2012 and to 15% by 2015. Additionally, in 2010, Quebec started publicly funding IVF treatment cycles (2010–2015). The majority of these publicly funded cycles required single embryo transfers (patients >38 years of age were allowed to have a maximum of two embryos transferred), which resulted in a decreased multiple pregnancy rate. In December 2015, Ontario began funding IVF treatment cycles with a similar directive of transferring only a single embryo. As a result, the Canadian Fertility and Andrology Society targets were met and surpassed. In 2012, the multiple pregnancy rate per ongoing clinical pregnancy was 17.4%, and in 2015 it was 11.4%. This decreasing trend has continued. In 2016, only 9.7% of ART treatment cycles in Canada were multiple pregnancies per ongoing clinical pregnancy (697 multiple pregnancies), of which only 26 were triplet or higher-order pregnancies. This has directly translated to a decreased multiple live birth rate (9.7% per ongoing clinical pregnancy).

Assuring Data Quality

The CARTR Plus database uses a variety of validation rules to enhance the quality of data that are entered into the database. These validation rules assist in making sure that only clinically appropriate responses are entered into the database (i.e. for fresh IVF cycles, oocyte retrieval date is <60 days from cycle start date). Additionally, the CARTR Plus database has been validated through a medical chart reabstraction project. A subset of Canadian fertility clinics was selected through a purposive sampling method to ensure that multiple geographic regions of Canada were represented. The sampling strategy also included the method of data entry (electronic medical record/manual entry) and the volume of fertility treatment cycles performed annually at each clinic. Twenty-five data elements were selected for this validation study. There was a high level of percentage agreement and validity found for the majority of variables that were examined. The results of the CARTR Plus validation study strengthen the notion of using these data for future ART surveillance, policy development and research.

Successes, Challenges and Future Plans

CARTR Plus has enabled the reporting of accurate and reliable ART data in Canada. Commitment from the Canadian IVF Medical Directors and the Canadian Fertility and Andrology Society has enhanced CARTR Plus. Aggregating data from fertility clinics across Canada strengthens the conclusions that can be determined from these data, given the proportionately smaller number of ART treatment cycles that are performed annually in Canada. Comprehensive data collection has allowed for evidence-based decision making to inform legislation and programs (e.g. the Ontario Fertility Program). It has also produced unbiased comparison reports for clinics to compare various data elements, including their markers of success (e.g. clinical pregnancy rate, singleton pregnancy rate). There are many benefits when using administrative health data (e.g. inexpensive, large number of subjects, ease of access); however, there are also limitations. These data were not collected for the purpose of a research or health policy question. Misclassification of data elements may be present, which has the potential to produce bias when used in analyses. Furthermore, the techniques used in ART change rapidly. The modifications that are often needed to amend CARTR Plus require a technical design and development period prior to implementation. As a result, there is a lag between the use of a new ART technique and the capture of this technique in CARTR Plus. Additionally, CARTR Plus does not currently collect information on intrauterine insemination treatment cycles; however, the database was designed so that intrauterine insemination treatment cycles could be added at a later date.

Nevertheless, CARTR Plus is a robust and reliable source of ART data. These data are presented annually at the Canadian Fertility and Andrology Society meeting. Additionally, CARTR Plus was designed to ensure that its data are comparable to other international ART registries. Data from CARTR Plus and its predecessor, CARTR, have been used for the International Committee Monitoring Assisted Reproductive Technologies (ICMART) world report, as well as numerous data requests and research projects. Canadian ART data have enabled high-quality national surveillance, valuable research and evidence-based decision making in the area of ART and infertility. The significance of the new ART database (CARTR Plus) will truly begin to show its value in the upcoming years when multiple years of fertility treatment data and birth outcomes data have been collected.

ART Surveillance in Mexico

On 24 February 1988, the first baby conceived with the help of assisted reproductive technology (specifically, gamete intrafallopian transfer) was born in Mexico [26]. Currently, more than 50 fertility clinics are offering a wide variety of infertility services in Mexico [27]. While Mexico does not require fertility clinics to report their ART outcomes, over half of ART clinics in Mexico voluntarily participate in a Latin American Registry of Assisted Reproduction (REDLARA), which was established in 1995. Before 2010, clinics reported aggregate outcomes; in 2010, they began collecting cycle-specific outcomes. There is no requirement to prospectively report, so some initiated but subsequently cancelled cycles are likely absent from the database. The collection system is web based and has been modified several times to capture changing practice patterns. In the last year reported (2014), 31 Mexican clinics reported 9,221 total cycles, of which 4,862 were IVF, 1,499 FET, 2,016 fresh donor egg and 744 were frozen donor egg [28]. See more information about REDLARA in Chapter 19, ART Surveillance in Latin America.

Acknowledgements

We would like to acknowledge Dr Vanessa Bacal and BORN Ontario for the work that they did validating the CARTR Plus database.

References

1. Edwards RG, Steptoe PC, Purdy JM. Clinical aspects of pregnancies established with cleaving embryos grown in vitro. *Br J Obstet Gynaecol.* 1980;**87**:757–68.

2. Jones HW Jr, Jones GS, Andrews MC, Acosta A, Bundren C, Garcia J, et al. The program for in vitro at Norfolk. *Fertil Steril.* 1982;**38**:14–21.

3. Jones HW Jr, Gosden RG, Veeck Gosden LL. *In Vitro Fertilization Comes to America: Memoir of a Medical Breakthrough.* Williamsburg, VA: Jamestowne Bookworks; 2014.

4. Toner JP. Progress we can be proud of: U.S. trends in assisted reproduction over the first 20 years. *Fertil Steril.* 2002;**78**(5):943–50.

5. Fertility Clinic Success Rate and Certification Act of 1992, Pub. L. No. 102–493 (1992).

6. Adashi EY, Wyden R. Public reporting of clinical outcomes of assisted reproductive technology programs: implications for other medical and surgical procedures. *JAMA.* 2011;**306**(10):1135–6.

7. CDC; American Society for Reproductive Medicine; Society for Assisted Reproductive Technology; RESOLVE. *1995 Assisted Reproductive Technology Success Rates.* Atlanta, GA: US Department of Health and Human Services; 1997.

8. Asch RH, Ellsworth LR, Balmaceda JP, Wong PC. Pregnancy after translaparoscopic gamete intrafallopian transfer. *Lancet.* 1984;**2**:1034.

9. Devroey P, Braeckmans P, Smitz J, van Waesberghe L, Wisanto A, vanSteirteghem A, et al. Pregnancy after translaparoscopic zygote intrafallopian transfer on a patient with sperm antibodies. *Lancet.* 1986;**1**:1329.

10. Malter HE, Cohen J. Partial zona dissection of the human oocyte: a nontraumatic method using micromanipulation to assist zona pellucida penetration. *Fertil Steril.* 1989;**51**:139.

11. Fishel S, Jackson P, Antinori S, Johnson J, Grossi S, Versaci C. Subzonal insemination for the alleviation of infertility. *Fertil Steril.* 1990;**54**:828.

12. Lanzendorf S, Maloney M, Ackerman S, Acosta A, Hodgen G. Fertilizing potential of acrosome-defective sperm following microsurgical injection into eggs. *Gamete Res.* 1988;**19**:329–37.

13. Palermo G, Joris H, Devroey P, van Steirteghem AC. Pregnancies after intracytoplasmic injection of single spermatozoon into an oocyte. *Lancet.* 1992;**340**:17–18.

14. Public Health Service Act of 1944, Pub. L. No. 78-410 (1944).

15. Kulkarni AD, Jamieson DJ, Jones HW Jr, Kissin DM, Gallo MF, Macaluso M, et al. Fertility treatments and multiple births in the United States. *N Engl J Med.* 2013;**369**(23):2218–25.

16. Williams RS, Doody KJ, Schattman GL, Adashi EY. Public reporting of assisted reproductive technology outcomes: past, present, and future. *Am J Obstet Gynecol.* 2015;**212**(2):157–62.

17. Kissin DM, Boulet SL, Jamieson DJ; Assisted Reproductive Technology Surveillance and Research Team. Fertility treatments in the United States: improving access and outcomes. *Obstet Gynecol.* 2016;**128**(2):387–90.

18. Centers for Disease Control and Prevention. *National Public Health Action Plan for the Detection, Prevention, and Management of Infertility.* Atlanta, GA: Centers for Disease Control and Prevention; 2014.

19. Gunby J, Bissonnette F, Librach C, Cowan L. Assisted reproductive technologies (ART) in Canada: 2006 results from the Canadian ART register. *Fertil Steril.* 2010;**93**(7):2189–201.

20. Gunby J, Bissonnette F, Librach C, Cowan L. Assisted reproductive technologies (ART) in Canada: 2007 results from the Canadian ART register. *Fertil Steril.* 2011;**95**(2):542–7.

21. Min J, Hughes E, Young D. Elective single embryo transfer following in vitro fertilization. *J Obstet Gynaecol (Lahore).* 2010(241):363–77.

22. Assisted Human Reproduction Canada. *Making a Difference: AHRC Annual Report 2010–2011.* AHRC; 2011.

23. Statistics Canada. Crude birth rate, age-specific fertility rates and total fertility rate (live births). Table 13-10-0418-91 (formerly CANSIM 1024505). Stat. Canada. 2017. Available at: www.statcan.gc.ca/tables-tableaux/sum-som/l01/cst01/hlth85a-eng.htm, accessed 20 March 2018.

24. Malizia BA, Hacker MR, Penzias AS. Cumulative live-birth rates after in vitro fertilization. *N Engl J Med.* 2009;**360**(3):236–43.

25. Canadian Fertility and Andrology Society. *Reduction of Multiple Pregnancy Risk Associated with IVF/ICSI IVF Medical Directors of Canada Position Statement 2012.* Canadian Fertility and Andrology Society; 2012.

26. Hernández Ayup S, Santos Haliscak R, García Martínez M, Morales Caballero F, Loret de Mola Gutiérrez R, Galache Vega P. GIFT: reproductive reality for the sterile couple. *Ginecol Obstet Mex.* 1989;**57**:315–19.

27. Gonzalez-Santos, SP. From esterilología to reproductive biology: the story of the Mexican assisted reproduction business. *Reprod Biomed Online.* 2016;**2**,116–27.

28. Zegers-Hochschild F, Schwarze JE, Crosby JA, Musri C, Urbina MT. Assisted reproductive techniques in Latin America: the Latin American registry, 2014. *JBRA Assist Reprod.* 2017;**21**(3):164–75.

Chapter

19

ART Surveillance in Latin America

Fernando Zegers-Hochschild, Javier A. Crosby and Juan Enrique Schwarze

On behalf of the Latin American Network of Assisted Reproduction

A Brief History of ART in Latin America

After Robert Edwards and Patrick Steptoe announced the birth via assisted reproductive technology (ART) of Louise Brown in the United Kingdom (UK), back in 1978, several groups in Australia and the United States (US) were already working in this area of research. The magnitude of biomedical and social transformations triggered by this revolutionary and unexpected discovery in human reproduction can be appreciated by the time it took to achieve success in other parts of the world. It took a few years after the birth of Louise Brown for the first birth to occur in Australia; it took four years in the US and six years to succeed in Latin America. It was in 1984 that almost simultaneously a group in Colombia led by Dr E. Lucena et al. and in Chile by Dr A. Costoya et al. reported the birth of their first baby born after in vitro fertilization (IVF) [1]. In the following years, births from IVF were reported in Argentina, Brazil and Mexico.

The global impact of this revolution is also reflected by its rapid spread around the globe. In less than 40 years, almost every country in the world has established IVF programs and approximately 8 million babies have been born so far. The contribution of Latin America to these 8 million is unfortunately very small. In the last report by the International Committee Monitoring Assisted Reproductive Technologies (ICMART), Latin America represented only 4 to 5% of the approximately 400,000 babies born each year [2]. Although the main barrier to IVF utilization is that the majority of patients must pay out of their pocket, the strong and permanent opposition of the Catholic Church has also been a difficult barrier to overcome, both for persons requiring treatment and for the establishment of public policies in favour of the right of persons to establish a family free of undue interference in their private lives. IVF technology has allowed for the development of other new techniques. For example, intracytoplasmic sperm injection (ICSI) was first communicated by

Palermo et al. in 1992 [3], and in 1994 more than 600 ICSI cases were reported for the first time in the Latin American Registry of Assisted Reproduction (RLA) (www.redlara.com).

Today, centres in the region are able to conduct virtually any type of in vitro fertilization procedure, using either autologous or donated gametes (both oocytes and sperm); preimplantation genetic testing both for aneuploidy (PGTa) and for single gene mutation (PGTm) is reported together as PGT. The use of gestational carriers is rarely practised, and in only a few countries, and is not reported by RLA.

Very little is known on outcome and procedures performed from 1984 to 1990, because there was neither regulation nor an organized reporting system. It was in 1990, with the birth of the Latin American registry of ART (RLA), that the first regional registry was established and data could be registered and examined systematically on a regional basis. Later, in 1995 centres reporting to RLA decided to enlarge their scope in order to include education and other regional activities, and the Latin American Network of ART (REDLARA) was established; RLA remained as one of its pillars. RLA and REDLARA will be referred to interchangeably.

ART in Latin America as Seen through the Latin American Registry (RLA)

The RLA is a large ART registry, which currently includes 662,875 initiated cycles, 183,453 clinical pregnancies and the birth of 180,840 babies (Fig. 19.1). It began in 1990, when 19 IVF centres from 12 countries began this voluntary initiative. Almost 30 years later, the registry has expanded, and a vast proportion of centres (>75%) performing ART in Latin America voluntarily report their data to RLA every year.

The RLA is a voluntary registry that collects and publishes a summary of regional data on a yearly basis. Throughout the years, the main objective of

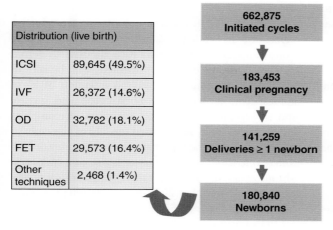

Distribution (live birth)	
ICSI	89,645 (49.5%)
IVF	26,372 (14.6%)
OD	32,782 (18.1%)
FET	29,573 (16.4%)
Other techniques	2,468 (1.4%)

662,875 Initiated cycles

183,453 Clinical pregnancy

141,259 Deliveries ≥ 1 newborn

180,840 Newborns

Figure 19.1 Number of initiated cycles and newborns in the past 25 years in Latin America. RLA 1990–2015.

RLA has been to disseminate information on ART procedures performed in Latin America. RLA often serves as an external quality control to be used by institutions performing ART in the region and for other regions of the world. The regional database is also used to monitor outcomes as well as trends in safety and efficacy, which contributes to developing better health interventions and appropriate public policies. Having access to an objective and external database is often well received by infertile persons when deciding whether to undergo treatment and when and what type of treatment should be undertaken. The RLA database is also used for epidemiological studies.

The first step in developing the database was to create standardized forms and distribute them among participating centres. During the 1990s, the forms for data collection were adapted from those developed by the International Working Group for Registers in Assisted Reproduction, today's International Committee Monitoring Assisted Reproductive Technologies (ICMART). Throughout the years, the forms have been further refined according to regional interests and the uninterrupted advancement of science and technology.

Initially, data were collected using printed forms that were sent by mail or fax. In 1990, special software was developed for the electronic collection of data. Although it had a built-in system to check for inconsistencies, it still required extensive interaction between the administrative office in Santiago, Chile, and each individual centre. Today, participating institutions enter their data directly online at www.redlara.com. The administrative office, still located in Santiago, periodically extracts and analyzes the data for consistency. Once all the information is cleared, and the centre is checked as accredited by the Latin American Network on Assisted Reproduction (REDLARA), the data are included and published as part of RLA's yearly report.

Prior to 2010, participating centres reported summary data. In 2010, RLA's personnel implemented a case-by-case register, and it became the first multinational cycle-based registry. The software used was field-tested in several institutions belonging to REDLARA. In order to implement this new method, workshops were held in different countries as part of the education programs organized by REDLARA. This modification in the reporting system represented huge efforts by all clinics and the professionals working in RLA.

The terminology used in the registry corresponds to the glossary developed and published in 2009 by ICMART and the World Health Organization (WHO) [4, 5], translated and published in Portuguese and Spanish [6] in compliance with WHO regulations. The glossary used today corresponds to the newest version of the International Glossary on Infertility and Fertility Care, 2017, led by ICMART together with all international regional organizations involved in fertility care and infertility [7].

Because RLA is a multinational registry and no reporting laws are or can be enforced, centres are not obliged to report a case as soon as a cycle is initiated (stimulated or monitored for IVF). Some centres report immediately, others do so retrospectively at monthly intervals or at the end of the reporting year. Today, an algorithm has been developed to follow each individual case until all aspirations and transfers have been completed. Thus, it is now possible to examine cumulative delivery rates in a large subset of cases that use a standard registration number.

The registration and reporting system has built-in software that allows every centre to look at and graphically display their own data and that of their home country. Because of this initiative, today every participating country in Latin America has the possibility of reporting their national ART database with information analyzed, verified and summarized by the RLA. After approval of the participating centres, national data are also sent to ICMART for inclusion in the publication of the world report [2].

Latin American reports corresponding to the years 1990 to 2004 were published as booklets and distributed among participating institutions and to attendees at several national and regional conferences held in the region. (Registries corresponding to years 2005 to 2009 are downloadable from www.redlara.com.) Starting with the registries corresponding to 2010, publications are available at REDLARA's official journal, *JBRA Assisted Reproduction*, and since 2012, it has been simultaneously published by RBM Online, thus reaching a much broader audience. There is an agreement with every reporting institution that the registry will never disclose or make available its individual data. All formal publications report regional data except for access/utilization where individual countries are identified when necessary.

Any member of a centre belonging to REDLARA can have access to RLA's database for scientific purposes. The provision of data is well regulated. Clinical and statistical support for several speakers at national and regional conferences is frequently provided and very well received. Policy makers have used the RLA data for the development of laws regulating ART; this has been the case in Argentina, Uruguay and later Costa Rica. Furthermore, the Inter-American Court of Human Rights used much of the information available in RLA in its ruling against Costa Rica in 2012. Costa Rica's Constitutional Court established in 2010 that IVF represented an attempt against the right to life of the human embryos that were generated by this technique and were subsequently discarded. It then established that given that embryos bear rights similar to those of persons, embryo life must be protected in equal terms; therefore, IVF was banned. After unsuccessful attempts to reverse this mandate, the case was taken before the Inter-American Commission on Human Rights. In 2012, it finally reached the Inter-

American Court of Human Rights (ICHR), the first time that the ICHR ruled in a matter of reproductive rights. In its ruling against the decision by the Constitutional Court of Costa Rica, the ICHR referred to data generated and presented on behalf of REDLARA showing there was no intention of harm nor a specific harm done to embryos generated in vitro; and embryonic death was not the result of manipulation but principally represented the fate of any embryo generated after either spontaneous procreation or IVF (*Inter-American Court of Human Rights case of Artavia Murillo et al. ('in vitro fertilization') v. Costa Rica* judgement of 28 November 2012; www.corteidh.or.cr/docs/casos/articulos/seriec_257_esp.pdf).

In this way, data collected and regular publications by the RLA are used for scientific purposes as well as for the establishment of evidence-based public policies in the region.

Accreditation Program of the Latin American Network of Assisted Reproduction (REDLARA)

In order to have their data published by RLA, all new centres are obliged to undergo accreditation, a process that is re-assessed every 5 years. The accreditation program started in 1985, but it was only in 2004, with the help of members of the College of American Pathologists and other volunteer biologists, that a professionalized accreditation committee was organized with clinicians and biologists from different countries. This committee had as main objectives to enhance the accreditation and re-accreditation procedures; unify criteria between evaluators with courses and workshops; check accreditation and re-accreditation results given by the visiting professionals and provide results to the board of directors for the final decision. It is also their role to recommend corrective actions or even sanctions to centres reporting non-verifiable results or the lack of rigour in reporting their data. The accreditation program is seen today not only as a guarantee for minimum standards of performing and reporting ART procedures; it is also seen as an external quality control program that helps institutions look at their results and introduce changes when necessary.

Process of Accreditation

Only a handful of countries in Latin America have established their own accreditation processes for

quality control assessment of clinical and laboratory activities. For this reason, the majority of ART centres in the region work with the accreditation protocol established by REDLARA to regulate the practice of ART in their countries. The accreditation process is initiated with a visit to the centre by a clinician and an embryologist acting as evaluators. The certifying bodies are members of already accredited, distinguished centres with a working experience of at least 5 years. Evaluators must be from a country different from that of the centre they are evaluating and must sign a form of non-disclosure of the data concerning a particular centre. They must also acknowledge absence of conflict of interest.

It is mandatory that during the accreditation visit the clinical and laboratory directors be present and available for questions and a final discussion. The visit includes a tour of the facilities to see the working areas and equipment; review of the clinical and laboratory procedures/protocols and manuals; review of the quality control procedures of the laboratory; verification of accuracy in the data reported to the Latin American Registry; and review of the informed consents signed by all patients. The forms used in the accreditation program can be found at www.redlara.com.

Global Access to ART Procedures in Latin America

Although the number of initiated cycles reported has increased steadily, reaching 75,121 initiated cycles in 2015 (Fig. 19.2), the utilization of ART procedures in the region is still far from the threshold of 1,500 cycles per annum per million inhabitants, proposed by the ESHRE Capri Group, in order to fulfil the theoretical ART needs of a population [8]. Using the same measurement, the utilization of ART procedures in the region reached only 133 per million in 2015, which is much lower than developed regions such as most of Europe and, recently, Japan, as well as Australia and New Zealand, which report more than 2,500 cycles per million (Table 19.1).

There are important differences between countries, explained mainly by each country's reimbursment policy. In recent years, three countries in Latin America have developed laws regulating universal access to ART. This began in Argentina in 2013, followed by Uruguay in 2015. The ICHR compelled Costa Rica to develop a law for universal access, which was accomplished in 2017. Other countries in the region have different forms of regulation. In Brazil, the Federal Council of Medicine establishes standards that are concerned mainly with laboratory and tissue-handling procedures. In Chile, the Minister of Health established infertility as a disease and recognized in a decree that ART procedures could be performed in infertile women as well as in persons with other forms of reproductive inability leading to disability. Other countries have regulatory bodies established by their reproductive societies, but most of them have been copied from what was developed in Latin America. It is therefore reasonable to say that the majority of countries, either directly or indirectly, follow guidelines developed or influenced by REDLARA.

Laws in Argentina and Uruguay are quite straightforward both for homologous and heterologous reproduction; however, the 2017 law enacted in Costa Rica had to accommodate the Constitutional Court, run by the extreme conservative party and bound to the Catholic Church. Thus, the law as passed is quite restrictive, both in the language used and parameters established for ART procedures, especially concerning embryo cryopreservation and PGT. Furthermore, in countries without legal regulation, there seems to be more freedom to perform ART, but access is restricted to those who can pay.

As we shall see, the way assisted reproduction is performed is very much influenced by the difficulty or ease of access to treatment. The mean number of embryos transferred in countries with universal access to ART is in general lower than the number of embryos transferred in countries with out-of-pocket funding. The pressure that patients exert for immediate success influences medical decisions and the way patients evaluate the risks and benefits with which they are confronted.

Description of and Trends in ART Procedures Reported to the Latin American Registry

Fertilization Procedure

Since its introduction in Latin America in 1994, ICSI has become the preferred method of insemination. Since 2008, more than 80% of inseminations used ICSI, and it has remained so in spite of the fact that only 25% of couples have a primary diagnosis of male factor infertility. Meanwhile, gamete intrafallopian transfer (GIFT) represented

Table 19.1 Assisted reproductive technology procedures reported to RLA and access in 2015

	Centres	FP	FRESH	FET	OD	Other	Total	Access*
Argentina	29	655	10,003	3,638	3,247	245	17,788	409
Bolivia	3	2	483	47	151	5	688	64
Brazil	58	1,510	18,058	8,407	2,255	986	31,216	153
Chile	10	268	2,262	1,101	644	194	4,469	255
Colombia	11	28	1,101	259	431	38	1,857	40
Dominican Rep.	2	0	162	8	89	0	259	25
Ecuador	5	4	328	106	149	3	590	37
Guatemala	1	4	119	36	31	0	190	13
Mexico	31	164	5,433	1,746	2,780	179	10,302	85
Nicaragua	1	0	131	0	24	0	155	26
Panama	3	17	482	142	118	24	783	214
Paraguay	1	3	87	24	15	4	133	20
Peru	11	531	1,835	622	1,353	459	4,800	158
Uruguay	2	13	335	80	78	4	510	153
Venezuela	7	33	828	193	322	5	1,381	45
Total	175	3,232	41,647	1,6409	1,1687	2,146	75,121	133

FP, fertility preservation; FRESH, initiated IVF/ICSI cycles; FET, initiated frozen autologous embryo cycles; OD, initiated cycles for transfer of fresh or frozen embryos using donated oocytes; Other, frozen oocyte–embryo transfer (FOT) etc.

* Number of initiated cycles in the country per million population in 2015 (World Population Data Sheet, World Bank).

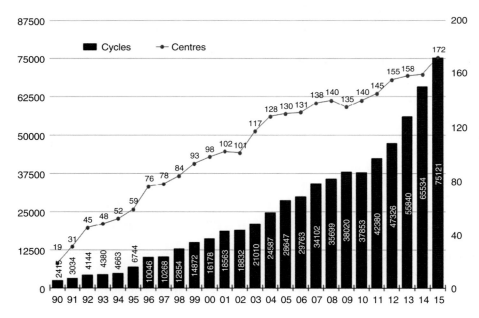

Figure 19.2 Number of initiated cycles and ART centres that report in Latin America. RLA 1990–2015.

30% of procedures performed in 1990 when the first report was published. Since then, its use has decreased, and in 2011 it was no longer registered because very few cases were reported in the region. Trends of fertilization type over time can be seen in Figure 19.3.

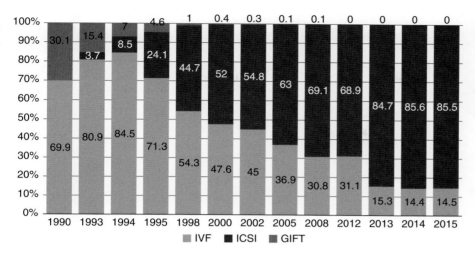

Figure 19.3 Trends in type of fertilization: retrievals. RLA 1990–2015. IVF, in vitro fertilization; ICSI, intracytoplasmic sperm injection; GIFT, gamete intrafallopian transfer. A colour version of this figure is provided in the plate section.

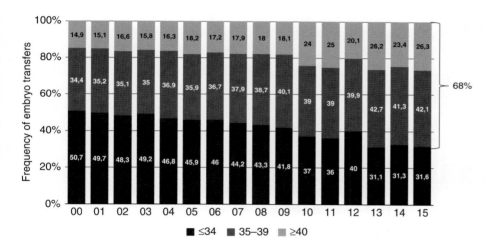

Figure 19.4 Frequency of embryo transfers in IVF/ICSI according to a woman's age. RLA 2000–2015. A colour version of this figure is provided in the plate section.

Age Distribution of Women Treated in Latin America

In the first registry published in 1990, 67% of procedures were performed in women ≤34 years; in 2015, this group represented only 31.6% of fresh autologous embryo transfers (Fig. 19.4). In 2015, the mean age of women undergoing IVF/ICSI was 36.2 (standard deviation (SD) 4.6). The majority of cycles were performed in women aged 35 to 39 years (42.1%), followed by women aged 40 and older (26.3%), which means that 68.4% of women using autologous ART were ≥35 years. This is important to consider when comparing results across continents. The tendency in Latin America is to treat older women. This of course influences the mean number of embryos transferred as well as the results of each treatment.

Use of Oocyte Donations in Latin America

In the case of transfer of embryos generated by the insemination of donated oocytes, in 1990, 23 transfers were reported, reaching a 43.5% clinical pregnancy rate. Ten years later, 1,363 embryo transfers were reported, reaching a 33.5% clinical pregnancy rate. In 2015, there were 9,503 embryo transfers, reaching a 46.0% clinical pregnancy rate. This is slightly lower than the 49.8% reported by the European IVF Monitoring (EIM) Consortium [9].

The mean age of women undergoing fresh oocyte donation (OD) was 41.0 years (SD 5.3); and 41% of the cycles were performed in women of 42 years and older. As expected, the delivery rate per embryo transfer decreased with advancing age in the case of autologous IVF/ICSI, but not in OD (Fig. 19.5).

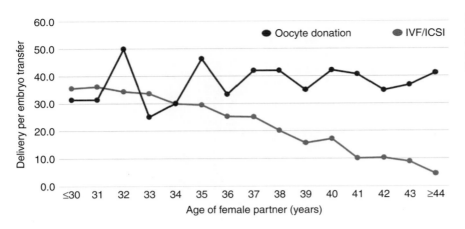

Figure 19.5 Delivery rate per embryo transfer in IVF/ICSI and OD cycles. RLA 2015. A colour version of this figure is provided in the plate section.

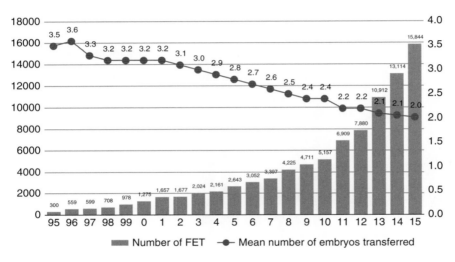

Figure 19.6 Mean number of embryos transferred and number of FET cycles. RLA 1995–2015. A colour version of this figure is provided in the plate section.

Frozen Embryo Transfers

The first cycles of frozen embryo transfers (FETs) were reported by four centres in 1992, and in the mid-1990s, the clinical pregnancy rate reached 18.5% (www.redlara.com). Ten years later, it increased to 27.6%, and in our latest registry [10], pregnancy rate reached 27.8% for FET cycles performed after a fresh transfer and 30% in embryo transfer cycles preceded by total embryo freezing.

The increasing success rates with FET are not the only important change over time. The number of FET cycles has increased every year with an inverse correlation with the number of embryos transferred. The fewer embryos transferred, the more the tendency for embryo freezing increases (Fig. 19.6).

Number of Embryos Transferred in Latin America

The mean number of embryos transferred has decreased over time – in the case of IVF/ICSI, from more than three embryos in the early 1990s to two in 2015. More important, the proportion of three and more embryos transferred dropped from 60% in 1990 to 19% in 2015. In the latest registry, the proportion of two embryos transferred reached 60.9%; however, it is very alarming that in 2015 even in patients with good prognosis, e.g. patients under 35 years undergoing fresh IVF/ICSI or patients undergoing OD cycles, three or more embryos were transferred in 13.1% and 17.4% of ET, respectively. This might be explained by a false belief of both physicians and patients that transferring three embryos will improve the outcome of any given cycle in its first attempt. As shown in Figure 19.7,

Table 19.2 Perinatal mortality according to gestational order in 2015

Assisted reproductive technology procedure	Singletons			Twins			≥Triplets		
	Live birth	Stillbirth	Early neonatal birth	Live birth	Stillbirth	Early neonatal death	Live birth	Still birth	Early neonatal birth
FET	3,542	11	14	1,579	2	15	117	2	7
IVF/ICSI	5,151	20	33	2,516	13	35	177	3	6
OD	2,450	16	25	1,892	22	18	104	3	4
Other	362	2	1	226	3	5	15	0	0
Total	11,505	49	73	6,213	40	73	413	8	17
Perinatal mortality *	10.5			17.9			57.1		

FET, frozen embryo transfer; IVF, in vitro fertilization; ICSI, intracytoplasmic sperm injection; OD, oocyte donation

* Proportion of stillbirth plus early neonatal death per 1,000 newborns

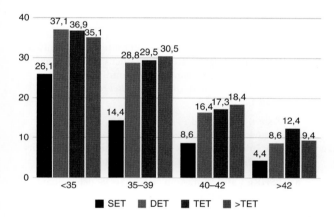

Figure 19.7 Delivery rate according to the number of embryos transferred by age of women in IVF/ICSI. RLA 2015. DET, double embryo transfer; SET, single embryo transfer; TET, triple embryo transfer. A colour version of the figure is provided in the plate section.

transferring two embryos instead of only one significantly increases the chance of birth. Transferring three and more embryos, however, does not increase the birth rate; it only contributes to high-order multiple births and perinatal morbidity and mortality.

It is reasonable to ask whether Latin America has improved its outcome in the past 15 years. In 2000, the proportion of two and three or more embryos reached 18.6% and 70.5%, respectively, and there was a delivery rate per OPU of 18.1%. Furthermore, the proportions of twins and triplets in 2000 were 23.5% and 7.7%, respectively. Fifteen years later, the proportion of two embryos increased to 60.7% but the proportion of three or more embryos dropped to 19.4%. Thus, the proportion of twins remained at 19.6%, while triplets and more dropped to 0.9%. Hence, in spite of decreasing the number of ET and a significant rise in the age of women, DR/OPU increased from 18.1% to 21.8%, with fewer high-order multiple births.

Perinatal Mortality

As seen in Table 19.2, perinatal mortality in 18,191 births in 2015 increased from 10.5 per thousand in singletons to 17.9 in twins and then there was a sharp rise to 57.1 per thousand in triplets and more. This has remained consistent over the years.

Conclusions

It has been 28 years since the RLA began a voluntary collection of ART data from Latin American centres. Five years after that, clinicians and biologists from each of the 21 centres then reporting decided to use this network to accomplish other regional activities such as the development of a continuous education program and a strict regional accreditation program in order to help institutions reach a minimum standard of good quality practice and also ensure that the data reported were sound. With these premises in mind, the Latin American Network of Assisted Reproduction (REDLARA) was initiated in 1995 and the registry (RLA) became the main activity of this broader organization. Today, Latin America can look back and examine trends on how reproductive decisions have evolved over the years and influenced our practice. We believe we are well equipped to look forward to adopting new procedures as they develop and also helping other regions build their own reporting systems, as we have recently done in South Africa and with ANARA, the African network of ART.

Latin America is moving in the same direction as the rest of the world, trying to balance efficacy and safety by reducing the number of embryos transferred. The mean number of embryos transferred in 2015 was 2.0, with 23% of women ≤40 years of age, and more than 80% of treatments paid for with out-of-pocket funding. These two conditions, age and source of funding, determine to a great extent the way ART is practised in Latin America.

It is very unlikely that Latin America will follow in the same direction as the Nordic countries or Australia, with a majority of single embryo transfers; but there is no doubt that, at its own pace, Latin America is moving in the right direction, maintaining efficacy in spite of drastic reductions in the number of multiple births.

References

1. Costoya A, Schmitt JM, Rey M, Dujovne S, Sánchez MI, Gadán A. Pregnancy obtained by in vitro fertilization and embryo transfer. *Rev Chil Obstet Ginecol.* 1984;**49**(3):206–16.

2. Dyer S, Chambers GM, de Mouzon J, Nygren KG, Zegers-Hochschild F, Mansour R, et al. International Committee for Monitoring Assisted Reproduction Technologies world report: assisted reproductive technology 2008, 2009 and 2010. *Hum Reprod.* 2016;**31**(7):1588–609.

3. Palermo G, Joris H, Devroey P, Van Steirteghem AC. Pregnancies after intracytoplasmic injection of single spermatozoon into an oocyte. *Lancet.* 1992;**340**:17–18.

4. Zegers-Hochschild F, Adamson GD, de Mouzon J, Ishihara O, Mansour R, Nygren K, et al., on behalf of ICMAT and WHO. The International Committee for Monitoring Assisted Reproductive Technology (ICMART) and the World Health Organization (WHO) revised glossary on art terminology, 2009. *Hum Reprod.* 2009;**24**(11):2683–7.

5. Zegers-Hochschild F, Adamson GD, de Mouzon J, Ishihara O, Mansour R, Nygren K, et al., on behalf of ICMAT and WHO. International Committee for Monitoring Assisted Reproductive Technology (ICMART) and the World Health Organization (WHO) revised glossary on art terminology, 2009. *Fertil Steril.* 2009;**92**(5):1520–4.

6. Zegers-Hochschild F, Adamson GD, de Mouzon J, Ishihara O, Mansour R, Nygren K, et al., on behalf of ICMAT and WHO. Glosario de terminología en Técnicas de Reproducción Asistida (TRA). Versión revisada y preparada por el International Committee for Monitoring Assisted Reproductive Technology (ICMART) y la Organización Mundial de la Salud (OMS), 2010. *JBRA Assist Reprod.* 2010;**14**(2):19–23.

7. Zegers-Hochschild F, Adamson GD, Dyer S, Racowsky C, de Mouzon J, Sokol R, et al. The International Glossary on Infertility and Fertility Care. *Fertil Steril.* 2017;**108**(3):393–406.

8. ESHRE Capri Workshop Group. Social determinants of human reproduction. *Hum Reprod.* 2001;**16**(7):1518–26.

9. Calhaz-Jorge C, De Geyter C, Kupka MS, de Mouzon J, Erb K, Mocanu E, et al., and the European IVF-monitoring (EIM) Consortium for the European Society of Human Reproduction and Embryology (ESHRE). Assisted reproductive technology in Europe, 2013: results generated from European registers by ESHRE. *Hum Reprod.* 2017;**32**(10):1957–73.

10. Zegers-Hochschild F, Schwarze JE, Crosby J, Musri C, Urbina MT, Latin American Network of Assisted Reproduction (REDLARA). Assisted reproduction techniques in Latin America: the Latin American Registry, 2015. *Reprod Biomed Online*, in press.

Chapter

20

The Importance of Non-ART Fertility Treatments in Public Health

Christine Wyns, Diane de Neubourg and Eli Y. Adashi

Introduction

Non-assisted reproductive technology (ART) treatments form a group of specific interventions to enhance fertility with no intention of performing ART (Table 20.1), such as surgery for endometriosis and for congenital or acquired conditions of the reproductive system, ovarian stimulation for ovulatory disorders and infertility treatment with intrauterine insemination (IUI) for various indications. This chapter intends to focus on the latter.

IUI is often the first intervention offered for unexplained or mild to moderate male infertility with the aim to improve fertility by bringing sperm closer to the oocyte for fertilization at the appropriate time. IUI can be associated with ovarian stimulation (OS) to increase the number of mature oocytes available for fertilization. This results in a multiple pregnancy rate of 9 to 15% of ongoing pregnancies [1, 2, 3], with an increase of 6%, 14% and 10%, respectively, in the case of 2, 3 or 4 follicles and a pregnancy rate (PR) of 15% for multifollicular growth.

IUI with the husband's sperm is the most common non-ART infertility treatment and is applied worldwide. However, its utilization is not often documented and is difficult to evaluate based on registries such as the European IVF Monitoring Consortium of the European Society of Human Reproduction and Embryology (EIM-ESHRE), as these have not always had full reporting coverage of fertility services [4]. However, in some countries where registration is mandatory, as in Denmark, IUI accounts for more than half of all fertility treatments [4, 5]. A survey on utilization of fertility-related services in the United States (US) in 2002 showed that among 1.1 million women seeking medical help for infertility, 13.1% underwent IUI whereas 2.9% used ART [6].

IUI utilization has also been influenced over time by the 2013 modification of the United Kingdom's (UK) National Institute for Health and Care

Excellence (NICE) guidelines, which disputed its effectiveness, suggesting that in vitro fertilization (IVF) should be the first-line treatment. This recommendation led to a huge debate among physicians [7, 8]. Access factors such as health care coverage, affordability and availability of services also have an impact on IUI utilization. In some settings, the choice of IVF over IUI with OS mainly depends on the out-of-pocket cost for the patient, but as IVF is more invasive and expensive for the patient and health care system, there is an urgent need for trials aiming at resolving the question of the most appropriate treatment.

Offering a First-Line Treatment of Infertility with IUI

IUI Prior to IVF

Indications

IUI is generally accepted as a first choice of infertility treatment except when there is a major tubal factor or severe male infertility, and in many countries IUI with OS is the first-line treatment in couples presenting with unexplained infertility. IUI also appears to be a safe method by which to prevent HIV transmission in serodiscordant couples [9].

The latest Cochrane systematic review and meta-analysis evaluating IUI for unexplained infertility did not find a difference in live birth rates (LBRs) for most of the comparisons, i.e. for IUI compared with timed intercourse (TI) both with and without OS, except for IUI in natural cycle versus TI, or expectant management (EM) in stimulated cycles (increase in LBR for IUI: odds ratio (OR) = 1.95, confidence interval (CI) 1.10–3.44, based on 1 randomized controlled trial with $n = 342$), although all evidence was of moderate quality [10].

Regarding male subfertility, there is no consensus reached on specific cut-off values of sperm parameters

Table 20.1 Non-ART interventions to improve fertility, including surgery, medical therapy or other interventions

Surgical interventions for congenital or acquired conditions of the reproductive system	Drug therapies for follicular development and ovulation induction	Other non-ART interventions
- Hydrosalpinges - Endometriosis - Myoma - Uterine polyps - Intrauterine synechia - Pelvic adhesions - Uterine malformation, i.e. vaginal/uterine septum	- Ovarian stimulation with recombinant gonadotropins - Ovarian stimulation with human menopausal gonadotropins - Ovarian stimulation with oral agents, i.e. clomiphene citrate, aromatase inhibitors - Ovulation induction with human chorionic gonadotropin	- Intra-cervical insemination - Intrauterine insemination - Fallopian tube sperm perfusion - Cycle monitoring for timed intercourse - Tubal flushing

to perform IUI and there is no clear definition of mild, moderate or severe male infertility that correlates with IUI outcome. However, the total motile sperm count appears to have a consistent direct relationship with the pregnancy rate (PR) per IUI [11, 12, 13]. The delivery rate per couple was also significantly reduced when the number of progressive motile spermatozoa recovered after semen preparation was less than 1 million or 2 million [14, 15]. Similar thresholds were also observed by others [11, 16, 17].

A number of studies aimed at evaluating whether first-line IVF rather than IUI could be a better option for couples with unexplained or mild male infertility. An initial pilot randomized controlled trial suggested that three cycles of IUI-OS might be as effective in terms of PR as one attempt of IVF with elective single embryo transfer (eSET) in couples with unexplained infertility [18]. The effectiveness of IUI with OS for unexplained and mild male infertility was also suggested in a larger comparative trial where the number of couples who delivered a healthy child was similar for IVF-SET, IVF in a modified natural cycle and IUI-OS [19]. Markers to select couples who would have a higher chance of live birth from immediate IVF instead of IUI could thus far not be identified from the Bensdorp trial [20]. Another study showed that singleton LBR with three cycles of IUI-OS was also not significantly different from one IVF cycle in couples treated for unexplained infertility [21]. However, the effectiveness of both three cycles of IUI and one IVF cycle may be jeopardized because it assumes that IUI is superior to no treatment and that IVF also has added value over EM in this population [22]. Unfortunately, the most recent Cochrane meta-

analysis could not add concluding evidence to shed light on this matter [10].

With regard only to unexplained infertility, 5.9 to 27% ongoing PRs were reported without intervention [23, 24] and no significant difference was found in LBR when IUI was compared with expectant management [25]. A recent pragmatic open-label, randomized, controlled, two-centre trial comparing IUI with OS to expectant management for unexplained infertility did show that IUI with OS is a safe and effective treatment for those women who had an unfavourable prognosis for natural conception [26]. In addition, a shorter median time to pregnancy was observed with an accelerated approach involving clomiphene citrate (CC) plus IUI followed by IVF compared with a stepwise strategy including CC plus IUI, gonadotropins plus IUI and IVF [27].

Ovarian Stimulation

The development of bifollicular IUI cycles potentially increases the chance of achieving a pregnancy by 3.4-fold compared with unifollicular cycles [28]. This was further confirmed in a review including 1,038 cycles where the strongest predictive factor for pregnancy after IUI was ovulation stimulation enabling the recruitment of at least two follicles measuring 16 mm or more [29]. However, in the sole randomized controlled trial comparing IUI with OS versus EM, no significant difference in ongoing PR was observed, but it is of note that 58% of cycles showed a monofollicular development and that cancellation rates were as high as 14% owing to protocol requirements [23]. The benefit of OS in IUI cycles was further investigated in a prospective multicentre observational study where delivery rates significantly increased with the number of mature follicles ≥15 mm [30]. However, this should be put into balance with the risk of multiple pregnancies estimated to be increased by 6%, 14% and 10% when 2, 3 or 4 follicles developed, respectively [3]. Furthermore, a spontaneous luteinizing hormone (LH) rise was reported in 20% of IUI cycles stimulated with CC or gonadotropins [13]. The use of a gonadotropin-releasing hormone (GnRH) antagonist to prevent an LH surge at an inappropriate time was also associated with an improvement of clinical pregnancy rates (from 11 to 23% compared with controls), although its benefit was solely demonstrated when at least two mature follicles were obtained [31]. While some trials evaluating the benefit of an antagonist in IUI cycles showed controversial results, no other large prospective studies separately reported data for multifollicular growth. However, a multicentre double-blind, placebo-controlled, randomized trial concluded in the absence of a benefit in terms of delivery rates and the pooled data of available randomized controlled trials did not show any difference in the PR per couple [32].

The type of medication used for OS may also influence the IUI outcome, although so far there is little evidence for the preference of one method of ovarian stimulation over another during IUI in terms of pregnancy or live birth rates. Ovarian stimulation with low-dose gonadotropins has been proven to be associated with better reproductive outcomes and lower cancellation rates per IUI cycle than with CC [33, 34]. In addition, there was no evidence that CC was more effective than no treatment or placebo for clinical pregnancy with IUI (OR = 0.79, with CI 0.70–8.19) [35].

Number of Attempts

The latest World Health Organization (WHO) recommendation suggests that at least three IUI cycles be performed [36], and it is generally accepted that IUI should be limited to four to six cycles and that IVF should be recommended in the event of failure. The correlation between the number of IUI attempts and pregnancy rates has been shown in a number of studies [37, 38]. It has been reported that cumulative PRs of 39.2% versus 48.5% were reached after three and six IUI-OS cycles, respectively [39], and that 97% of pregnancies were obtained during the first four cycles of IUI, with the highest rate for the first cycle [40]. Corroborating this figure, 91.4% of LBs (as the primary outcome measure of the retrospective cohort

study) occurred within the first two IUI-OS attempts [41]. Moreover, an odds ratio of LB per additional IUI-OS cycle of 0.76 was reported after adjustment for age, previous parity, length of time trying to conceive, basal follicle-stimulating hormone (FSH) level and aetiology of infertility. A significant difference for LBR between attempt one and three was also observed [41].

Providing Quality of Care in IUI

Effectiveness: Success, Prognostic Factors

Data from the European Society of Human Reproduction and Embryology showed that the PR per cycle after IUI has remained stable for years at 12.4%, as did delivery rates of 9.2% in women <40 years using the husband's sperm [42].

Factors influencing IUI results may be related to the infertile couple (such as age, infertility duration, smoking and body mass index (BMI)), the procedure or the cycle. The female age-related effect on fertility is well known and also appeared to be the strongest predictor of IUI success. Threshold ages for successful IUI were reported from 35 or less to 40 or less [13, 43, 44]. Some studies have evaluated the possibility that ovarian stimulation could compensate for or counteract the age effect on pregnancy rates and found a benefit of OS after 40 years of age [45]. Thijssen et al. [46] analyzed 1,401 IUI cycles in 556 couples and concluded that clinical pregnancy rates after homologous IUI are significantly influenced by female age, male smoking and primary and secondary infertility. In the multivariate analysis, female obesity was not a prognostic variable.

For other prognosis factors of IUI success, conclusions reached in different studies may be discrepant, e.g. for the duration of infertility or parity, as inclusion criteria of IUI programs may vary [13, 28, 37, 40, 41, 47, 48]. The same applies for the ovarian reserve, although a secondary analysis of data from two randomized controlled trials found that the group of patients with levels of basal FSH between 10 and 15 international units per litre (IU/L) and of oestradiol at 40 picograms per millilitre (pg/mL) or above had no LB during IUI compared with a 33% LBR for IVF regardless of age [49].

Concerning the procedure and cycle, the timing of IUI in a natural cycle is an important determinant of the clinical pregnancy rate [50]. Literature on the appropriate timing to perform IUI revealed more LBs when a human chorionic gonadotropin (hCG) to IUI interval of 34–36 hours was used compared with a shorter interval of 24 hours, although the difference was not significant (for review, see [51]). Moreover, no difference in clinical PR was observed between a 34- to 36-hour interval versus none [52]. Furthermore, there is no evidence to support the use of double versus single IUI [53].

Safety

Literature on perinatal outcomes of pregnancies resulting from IUI is scarce. Increased risks compared with spontaneous conceptions have been described [54, 55, 56]. Data on comparison with IVF are also limited and point to similar or lower perinatal risks [57, 58, 59]. Perinatal morbidities and mortality were evaluated in a retrospective cohort study showing IUI to be at lower risk (compared with IVF and ICSI) for prematurity (OR = 2.35 vs 5.95), for low birth weight (OR = 2.38 vs 5.54) and for mortality (insignificant vs OR = 4.33) [60].

Multiple pregnancies are responsible for most perinatal morbidities and are dependent on the aggressiveness of OS protocols, although when a strict protocol is applied for the number of follicles on the day of hCG trigger (with potential follicle aspiration or cycle cancellation when more than two follicles are present), a cumulative multiple pregnancy rate over three cycles of 5.5% and no high-order multiple pregnancies were observed [41]. However, the contribution of non-ART treatments to multiple births may also increase with improved affordability of fertility treatments, as is the case in some states in the US [61, 62].

Patient Centredness

As reproductive medicine provides treatments of varying invasiveness, not only are professionals' treatment decisions important, but also patients' treatment preferences should be considered when choosing the right option [63]. Among therapeutic dimensions influencing these choices, effectiveness appeared the most important followed equally by safety and cost, and burden seemed the least important [64]. However, while it is clear that the patient's central role is crucial in the infertility treatment framework, no studies have so far explored the patient's experience of 'burden' in IUI cycles.

Moreover, aspects considered as burdensome may differ between patients and professionals, pointing to the need to perform studies taking this into account [65].

Cost Efficiency

Cost efficiency appears to be influenced by the indication, the associated medication for OS and perinatal complications mainly related to multiple pregnancies.

With regard to male subfertility, Moolenaar et al. found the cost per LB for IUI to be dependent on the pre-wash total motile sperm count (TMSC) (€40,203 for a TMSC of 1 million and €5,833 for TMSC of 10 million) [66]. Furthermore, IUI-OS had a lower cost per LB compared with IVF if the pre-wash TMSC was above 3 million.

A number of studies addressed comparisons of costs of treatment strategies with or without IUI. Different settings, e.g. with or without health care coverage and different levels of success rates, may influence costs of these strategies. In addition, cost estimates may also vary in different countries, as discontinuation rates may vary with social security coverage or the amount of patients' out-of-pocket payments. The economical costs of sick leave or absence from work and travel also need to be taken into account. While it has been calculated that only 1% of the total costs of couples were due to costs of the health care system [27], health care costs related to multiple pregnancies have a bigger impact in settings with high rates of multiples.

In the US, the fast track and standard treatment (FASTT) trial concluded that primary treatment with IVF would be more cost-effective than IUI with 150 IU FSH followed by IVF [27]. In a retrospective study, one IVF cycle also appeared to be more effective, although costlier, than two cycles of IUI-OS [67]. In Europe, health economics and cost-effectiveness have been calculated for the two randomized trials comparing IUI with IVF [18, 19], where it was shown that IVF-eSET was less cost-effective. Van Rumste et al. [68] evaluated the costs of the multicentre randomized pilot trial comparing one cycle of IVF-eSET followed by one cryocycle and three cycles of IUI-OS with clomiphene citrate or 50–75 IU recombinant FSH within a time frame of 4 months starting from the initial treatment cycle [18]. They evaluated the costs including clinical and laboratory costs, specialist fees and medication up to an ongoing pregnancy of 12 weeks or end of follow-up period and this was in a health care system with full coverage for couples with unexplained and mild male subfertility. Considering that 10% of IUI cycles were cancelled for risk of high-order multiple pregnancies (more than 3 follicles >18 mm), they found additional costs per ongoing pregnancy of €2,456 and per couple of €915 for IVF-eSET. While equivalent costs for eSET-IVF and IUI-OS would have been reached for use of 1,522 IU FSH per IUI, the mean use of FSH in IUI cycles was 580 IU [68].

A cost-effectiveness analysis of the Bensdorp trial [19] was also performed from a health care perspective, focusing on direct medical costs during treatment, excluding indirect costs generated by transportation or productivity loss. These authors found the mean cost per couple to be significantly higher for IVF strategies than for IUI-OS with comparable LBR [69].

With regard to the OS, when comparing one IUI treatment with human menopausal gonadotropin (hMG) and clomiphene citrate, the average direct costs per clinical pregnancy from a health care payer perspective and practice in a Belgian university setting were €6,152 and €8,312, respectively, as hMG appeared to be more expensive per cycle but led to higher pregnancy rates per cycle [70]. When an antagonist was associated with OS, the cost of the treatment evaluated in a French health care system increased from €500 to €700, but as the efficiency with antagonist use was higher, the cost per delivery was lower (€5,280 vs €4,565) [30].

Compared with ART, non-ART singleton births were associated with diminished costs because of shorter hospital stays at birth (1.8 days) and a 20% reduced risk of being readmitted during the first five years of life [71].

New developments such as blastocyst transfer or embryo vitrification and selection might possibly make IVF the more favourable approach, although this should be demonstrated in future randomized controlled trials.

Equity (in Access to Treatment)

Several factors determine access to IUI treatment, such as health care coverage, affordability and availability of services, presence of tubal factor or severe male factor infertility. In some settings, the choice of IVF over IUI with OS depends mainly on the out-of-pocket cost for the patient. For these reasons, equity in access to IUI treatment is very difficult to compare and has not been studied in depth to our knowledge.

Conclusion

There is increasing evidence that IUI may still be proposed as a first-line infertility therapy unless there is a major tubal or severe male factor infertility involved. Some important determinants of IUI success in terms of delivery rates have been put forward such as association with OS using low-dose gonadotropins or a GnRH antagonist. While currently IUI with OS was shown to be cost-effective, further studies are needed to confirm this in settings with advanced ART techniques including optimized cryopreservation programs and aiming at a single selected embryo transfer. Systematic registration of IUI and OS cycles with outcomes will further increase knowledge on their effectiveness and safety and pave the way for a global surveillance of non-ART treatments.

References

1. Steures P, van der Steeg JW, Hompes PG, van der Veen F, Mol BW. Intrauterine insemination in the Netherlands. *Reprod Biomed Online*. 2007;**14**(1):110–16.

2. Brandes M, Hamilton CJ, Bergevoet KA, de Bruin JP, Nelen WL, Kremer JA. Origin of multiple pregnancies in a subfertile population. *Acta Obstet Gynecol Scand*. 2010;**89**(9):1149–54. doi:10.3109/00016349.2010.498495.

3. Van Rumste MM, Custers IM, van der Veen F, van Wely M, Evers JL, Mol BW. The influence of the number of follicles on pregnancy rates in intrauterine insemination with ovarian stimulation: a meta-analysis. *Hum Reprod Update*. 2008;**14**(6):563–70. doi:10.1093/humupd/dmn034. Epub 2008 Aug 6.

4. European IVF-monitoring Consortium (EIM); European Society of Human Reproduction and Embryology (ESHRE), Calhaz-Jorge C, De Geyter C, Kupka MS, de Mouzon J, Erb K, Mocanu E, et al. Assisted reproductive technology in Europe, 2013: results generated from European registers by ESHRE. *Hum Reprod*. 2017;**32**(10):1957–73. doi:10.1093/humrep/dex264.

5. Nyboe Andersen A, Erb K. Register data on assisted reproductive technology (ART) in Europe including a detailed description of ART in Denmark. *Int J Androl*. 2006;**29**(1):12–16.

6. Vahratian A. Utilization of fertility-related services in the United States. *Fertil Steril*. 2008;**90**(4):1317–19. doi:10.1016/j.fertnstert.2007.10.034. Epub 2008 Mar 4.

7. Woodward B, Tomlinson M, Kirkman-Brown J. Replacing IUI with IVF for initial treatment of unexplained infertility: why this NICE recommendation is cause for concern. *Hum Fertil (Camb)*. 2016;**19**(2):

80–4. doi:10.1080/14647273.2016.1182220. Epub 2016 May 13.

8. National Institute for Health and Care Excellence. *Assessment and Treatment for People with Fertility Problems.* NICE Clinical Guideline 156; 2013.

9. Barnes A, Riche D, Mena L, Sison T, Barry L, Reddy R, et al. Efficacy and safety of intrauterine insemination and assisted reproductive technology in populations serodiscordant for human immunodeficiency virus: a systematic review and meta-analysis. *Fertil Steril.* 2014;**102**(2):424–34. doi:10.1016/j.fertnstert.2014.05.001. Epub 2014 Jun 18.

10. Veltman-Verhulst SM, Hughes E, Ayeleke RO, Cohlen BJ. Intra-uterine insemination for unexplained subfertility. *Cochrane Database Syst Rev.* 2016;**19**;2: CD001838. doi:10.1002/14651858.CD001838.pub5.

11. Lee VM, Wong JS, Loh SK, Leong NK. Sperm motility in the semen analysis affects the outcome of superovulation intrauterine insemination in the treatment of infertile Asian couples with male factor infertility. *BJOG.* 2002;**109**(2):115–20.

12. Akanji Tijani H, Bhattacharya S. The role of intrauterine insemination in male infertility. *Hum Fertil (Camb).* 2010;**13**(4):226–32. doi:10.3109/14647273.2010.533811.

13. Dinelli L, Courbière B, Achard V, Jouve E, Deveze C, Gnisci A, et al. Prognosis factors of pregnancy after intrauterine insemination with the husband's sperm: conclusions of an analysis of 2,019 cycles. *Fertil Steril.* 2014;**101**(4):994–1000. doi:10.1016/j.fertnstert.2014.01.009. Epub 2014 Feb 15.

14. Ombelet W, Vandeput H, Van de Putte G, Cox A, Janssen M, Jacobs P, et al. Intrauterine insemination after ovarian stimulation with clomiphene citrate: predictive potential of inseminating motile count and sperm morphology. *Hum Reprod.* 1997;**12**(7):1458–63.

15. Punjabi U, De Neubourg D, Van Mulders H, Cassauwers W, Peeters K. Validating semen processing for an intrauterine program should take into consideration the inputs, actions and the outputs of the process. *Andrologia.* 2018;e12977.

16. Wainer R, Albert M, Dorion A, Bailly M, Bergère M, Lombroso R, et al. Influence of the number of motile spermatozoa inseminated and of their morphology on the success of intrauterine insemination. *Hum Reprod.* 2004;**19**(9):2060–5. Epub 2004 Jul 8.

17. Ombelet W, Dhont N, Thijssen A, Bosmans E, Kruger T. Semen quality and prediction of IUI success in male subfertility: a systematic review. *Reprod Biomed Online.* 2014;**28**(3):300–9. doi:10.1016/j.rbmo.2013.10.023. Epub 2013 Nov 15.

18. Custers IM, König TE, Broekmans FJ, Hompes PG, Kaaijk E, Oosterhuis J, et al. Couples with unexplained subfertility and unfavorable prognosis: a randomized pilot trial comparing the effectiveness of in vitro fertilization with elective single embryo transfer versus intrauterine insemination with controlled ovarian stimulation. *Fertil Steril.* 2011;**96**(5):1107–11.e1. doi:10.1016/j.fertnstert.2011.08.005. Epub 2011 Sep 3.

19. Bensdorp AJ, Tjon-Kon-Fat RI, Bossuyt PM, Koks CA, Oosterhuis GJ, Hoek A, et al. Prevention of multiple pregnancies in couples with unexplained or mild male subfertility: randomised controlled trial of in vitro fertilisation with single embryo transfer or in vitro fertilisation in modified natural cycle compared with intrauterine insemination with controlled ovarian hyperstimulation. *BMJ.* 2015;**350**:g7771. doi:10.1136/bmj.g7771.

20. Tjon-Kon-Fat RI, Tajik P, Zafarmand MH, Bensdorp AJ, Bossuyt PMM, Oosterhuis GJE, et al.; INeS Study Group. IVF or IUI as first-line treatment in unexplained subfertility: the conundrum of treatment selection markers. *Hum Reprod.* 2017;**32**(5):1028–32. doi:10.1093/humrep/dex037.

21. Nandi A, Bhide P, Hooper R, Gudi A, Shah A, Khan K, et al. Intrauterine insemination with gonadotropin stimulation or in vitro fertilization for the treatment of unexplained subfertility: a randomized controlled trial. *Fertil Steril.* 2017;**107**(6):1329–35.e2. doi:10.1016/j.fertnstert.2017.03.028. Epub 2017 May 10.

22. Tjon-Kon-Fat RI, Bensdorp AJ, Scholten I, Repping S, van Wely M, Mol BW, et al. IUI and IVF for unexplained subfertility: where did we go wrong? *Hum Reprod.* 2016;**31**(12):2665–7. Epub 2016 Sep 22.

23. Steures P, van der Steeg JW, Hompes PG, Habbema JD, Eijkemans MJ, Broekmans FJ, et al.; Collaborative Effort on the Clinical Evaluation in Reproductive Medicine. Intrauterine insemination with controlled ovarian hyperstimulation versus expectant management for couples with unexplained subfertility and an intermediate prognosis: a randomised clinical trial. *Lancet.* 2006;**368**(9531):216–21.

24. Evers JL, de Haas HW, Land JA, Dumoulin JC, Dunselman GA. Treatment-independent pregnancy rate in patients with severe reproductive disorders. *Hum Reprod.* 1998;**13**(5):1206–9.

25. Bhattacharya S, Harrild K, Mollison J, Wordsworth S, Tay C, Harrold A, et al. Clomifene citrate or unstimulated intrauterine insemination compared with expectant management for unexplained infertility: pragmatic randomised controlled trial. *BMJ.* 2008;**337**:a716. doi:10.1136/bmj.a716.

26. Farquhar CM, Liu E, Armstrong S, Arroll N, Lensen S, Brown J. Intrauterine insemination with ovarian stimulation versus expectant management for unexplained infertility (TUI): a pragmatic, open-label, randomised, controlled, two-centre trial. *Lancet.*

2018;**391**(10119):441–50. doi:10.1016/S0140-6736(17)32406-6. Epub 2017 Nov 23.

27. Reindollar RH, Regan MM, Neumann PJ, Levine BS, Thornton KL, Alper MM, et al. A randomized clinical trial to evaluate optimal treatment for unexplained infertility: the fast track and standard treatment (FASTT) trial. *Fertil Steril.* 2010;**94**(3):888–99. doi:10.1016/j.fertnstert.2009.04.022. Epub 2009 Jun 16.

28. Tomlinson MJ, Amissah-Arthur JB, Thompson KA, Kasraie JL, Bentick B. Prognostic indicators for intrauterine insemination (IUI): statistical model for IUI success. *Hum Reprod.* 1996;**11**(9):1892–6.

29. Merviel P, Heraud MH, Grenier N, Lourdel E, Sanguinet P, Copin H. Predictive factors for pregnancy after intrauterine insemination (IUI): an analysis of 1038 cycles and a review of the literature. *Fertil Steril.* 2010;**93**(1):79–88. doi:10.1016/j.fertnstert.2008.09.058. Epub 2008 Nov 8.

30. Monraisin O, Chansel-Debordeaux L, Chiron A, Floret S, Cens S, Bourrinet S, et al. Evaluation of intrauterine insemination practices: a 1-year prospective study in seven French assisted reproduction technology centers. *Fertil Steril.* 2016; **105**(6):1589–93. doi:10.1016/j.fertnstert.2016.01.039. Epub 2016 Feb 23.

31. Gómez-Palomares JL, Acevedo-Martín B, Chávez M, Manzanares M, Ricciarelli E, Hernández ER. Multifollicular recruitment in combination with gonadotropin-releasing hormone antagonist increased pregnancy rates in intrauterine insemination cycles. *Fertil Steril.* 2008;**89**(3):620–4. Epub 2007 Aug 6.

32. Cantineau AE, Cohlen BJ, Klip H, Heineman MJ; Dutch IUI Study Group Collaborators. The addition of GnRH antagonists in intrauterine insemination cycles with mild ovarian hyperstimulation does not increase live birth rates–a randomized, double-blinded, placebo-controlled trial. *Hum Reprod.* 2011;**26**(5):1104–11. doi:10.1093/humrep/der033. Epub 2011 Feb 20.

33. Cantineau AE, Cohlen BJ, Heineman MJ. Ovarian stimulation protocols (anti-oestrogens, gonadotrophins with and without GnRH agonists/antagonists) for intrauterine insemination (IUI) in women with subfertility. *Cochrane Database Syst Rev.* 2007;**18**(2): CD005356.

34. Peeraer K, Debrock S, De Loecker P, Tomassetti C, Laenen A, Welkenhuysen M, et al. Low-dose human menopausal gonadotrophin versus clomiphene citrate in subfertile couples treated with intrauterine insemination: a randomized controlled trial. *Hum Reprod.* 2015;**30**(5):1079–88. doi:10.1093/humrep/dev062. Epub 2015 Mar 18.

35. Hughes E, Brown J, Collins JJ, Vanderkerchove P. Clomiphene citrate for unexplained subfertility in women. *Cochrane Database Syst Rev.* 2010;(1): CD000057. doi:10.1002/14651858.CD000057.pub2.

36. Cohlen B, Bijkerk A, Van der Poel S, Ombelet W. IUI: review and systematic assessment of the evidence that supports global recommendations. *Hum Reprod Update.* 2018;**24**(3):300–19. doi:10.1093/humupd/dmx041.

37. Steures P, van der Steeg JW, Mol BW, Eijkemans MJ, van der Veen F, Habbema JD, et al.; CECERM (Collaborative Effort in Clinical Evaluation in Reproductive Medicine). Prediction of an ongoing pregnancy after intrauterine insemination. *Fertil Steril.* 2004;**82**(1):45–51.

38. Custers IM, Steures P, Hompes P, Flierman P, van Kasteren Y, van Dop PA, et al. Intrauterine insemination: how many cycles should we perform? *Hum Reprod.* 2008;**23**(4):885–8. doi:10.1093/humrep/den008. Epub 2008 Feb 8.

39. Aboulghar M, Mansour R, Serour G, Abdrazek A, Amin Y, Rhodes C. Controlled ovarian hyperstimulation and intrauterine insemination for treatment of unexplained infertility should be limited to a maximum of three trials. *Fertil Steril.* 2001;**75** (1):88–91.

40. Nuojua-Huttunen S, Tomas C, Bloigu R, Tuomivaara L, Martikainen H. Intrauterine insemination treatment in subfertility: an analysis of factors affecting outcome. *Hum Reprod.* 1999;**14** (3):698–703

41. Geisler ME, Ledwidge M, Bermingham M, McAuliffe M, McMenamin MB, Waterstone JJ. Intrauterine insemination – no more Mr. N.I.C.E. guy? *Eur J Obstet Gynecol Reprod Biol.* 2017;**210**:342–7. doi:10.1016/j.ejogrb.2017.01.016. Epub 2017 Jan 18.

42. Ferraretti AP, Nygren K, Nyboe Andersen A, de Mouzon J, Kupka M, Calhaz-Jorge C, et al., the European IVF-Monitoring Consortium (EIM), for the European Society of Human Reproduction and Embryology (ESHRE). Trends over 15 years in ART in Europe: an analysis of 6 million cycles. *Hum Reprod Open.* 2017(2):1–10 doi:10.1093/hropen/hox012.

43. Ashrafi M, Rashidi M, Ghasemi A, Arabipoor A, Daghighi S, Pourasghari P, et al. The role of infertility etiology in success rate of intrauterine insemination cycles: an evaluation of predictive factors for pregnancy rate. *Int J Fertil Steril.* 2013;**7**(2):100–7. Epub 2013 Jul 31.

44. Sicchieri F, Silva AB, Silva ACJSRE, Navarro PAAS, Ferriani RA, Reis RMD. Prognostic factors in intrauterine insemination cycles. *JBRA Assist Reprod.* 2018;**22**(1):2–7. doi:10.5935/1518-0557.20180002.

45. Gomez R, Schorsch M, Steetskamp J, Hahn T, Heidner K, Seufert R, et al. The effect of ovarian stimulation on the outcome of intrauterine

insemination. *Arch Gynecol Obstet.* 2014;**289**(1):181–5. doi:10.1007/s00404-013-2952-3. Epub 2013 Jul 14.

46. Thijssen A, Creemers A, Van der Elst W, Creemers E, Vandormael E, Dhont N, et al. Predictive value of different covariates influencing pregnancy rate following intrauterine insemination with homologous semen: a prospective cohort study. *Reprod Biomed Online.* 2017;**34**(5):463–72. doi:10.1016/j.rbmo.2017.01.016. Epub 2017 Feb 24.

47. Stone BA, Vargyas JM, Ringler GE, Stein AL, Marrs RP. Determinants of the outcome of intrauterine insemination: analysis of outcomes of 9963 consecutive cycles. *Am J Obstet Gynecol.* 1999;**180**(6 Pt 1):1522–34.

48. Erdem A, Erdem M, Atmaca S, Korucuoglu U, Karabacak O. Factors affecting live birth rate in intrauterine insemination cycles with recombinant gonadotrophin stimulation. *Reprod Biomed Online.* 2008;**17**(2):199–206.

49. Kaser DJ, Goldman MB, Fung JL, Alper MM, Reindollar RH. When is clomiphene or gonadotropin intrauterine insemination futile? Results of the Fast Track and Standard Treatment Trial and the Forty and Over Treatment Trial, two prospective randomized controlled trials. *Fertil Steril.* 2014;**102**(5):1331–7.e1. doi:10.1016/j.fertnstert.2014.07.1239. Epub 2014 Sep 16.

50. Blockeel C, Knez J, Polyzos NP, De Vos M, Camus M, Tournaye H. Should an intrauterine insemination with donor semen be performed 1 or 2 days after the spontaneous LH rise? A prospective RCT. *Hum Reprod.* 2014;**29**(4):697–703. doi:10.1093/humrep/deu022. Epub 2014 Feb 18.

51. Cantineau AE, Janssen MJ, Cohlen BJ, Allersma T. Synchronised approach for intrauterine insemination in subfertile couples. *Cochrane Database Syst Rev.* 2014;(**12**):CD006942. doi:10.1002/14651858. CD006942.pub3.

52. Aydin Y, Hassa H, Oge T, Tokgoz VY. A randomized study of simultaneous hCG administration with intrauterine insemination in stimulated cycles. *Eur J Obstet Gynecol Reprod Biol.* 2013;**170**(2):444–8. doi:10.1016/j.ejogrb.2013.07.022. Epub 2013 Aug 6.

53. Arab-Zozani M, Nastri CO. Single versus double intrauterine insemination (IUI) for pregnancy: a systematic review and meta-analysis. *Eur J Obstet Gynecol Reprod Biol.* 2017;**215**:75–84. doi:10.1016/j.ejogrb.2017.05.025. Epub 2017 May 26.

54. Ombelet W, Martens G, De Sutter P, Gerris J, Bosmans E, Ruyssinck G, et al. Perinatal outcome of 12,021 singleton and 3108 twin births after non-IVF-assisted reproduction: a cohort study. *Hum Reprod.* 2006;**21**(4):1025–32. Epub 2005 Dec 8.

55. Gaudoin M, Dobbie R, Finlayson A, Chalmers J, Cameron IT, Fleming R. Ovulation induction/

intrauterine insemination in infertile couples is associated with low-birth-weight infants. *Am J Obstet Gynecol.* 2003;**188**(3):611–16.

56. Yılmaz NK, Sargın A, Erkılınç S, Özer İ, Engin-Üstün Y. Does ovulation induction and intrauterine insemination affect perinatal outcomes in singletons? *J Matern Fetal Neonatal Med.* 2018;**31**(1):14–17. doi:10.1080/14767058.2016.1223033. Epub 2017 Jun 19.

57. Nuojua-Huttunen S, Gissler M, Martikainen H, Tuomivaara L. Obstetric and perinatal outcome of pregnancies after intrauterine insemination. *Hum Reprod.* 1999;**14**(8):2110–15.

58. De Sutter P, Veldeman L, Kok P, Szymczak N, Van der Elst J, Dhont M. Comparison of outcome of pregnancy after intra-uterine insemination (IUI) and IVF. *Hum Reprod.* 2005;**20**(6):1642–6. Epub 2005 Mar 24.

59. Malchau SS, Loft A, Henningsen AK, Nyboe Andersen A, Pinborg A. Perinatal outcomes in 6,338 singletons born after intrauterine insemination in Denmark, 2007 to 2012: the influence of ovarian stimulation. *Fertil Steril.* 2014;**102**(4):1110–16.e2. doi:10.1016/j.fertnstert.2014.06.034. Epub 2014 Jul 23.

60. Poon WB, Lian WB. Perinatal outcomes of intrauterine insemination/clomiphene pregnancies represent an intermediate risk group compared with in vitro fertilisation/intracytoplasmic sperm injection and naturally conceived pregnancies. *J Paediatr Child Health.* 2013;**49**(9):733–40. doi:10.1111/jpc.12257. Epub 2013 Jun 12.

61. Kulkarni AD, Adashi EY, Jamieson DJ, Crawford SB, Sunderam S, Kissin DM. Affordability of fertility treatments and multiple births in the United States. *Paediatr Perinat Epidemiol.* 2017;**31**(5):438–48. doi:10.1111/ppe.12383. Epub 2017 Aug 1.

62. Kulkarni AD, Jamieson DJ, Jones HW Jr, Kissin DM, Gallo MF, Macaluso M, et al. Fertility treatments and multiple births in the United States. *N Engl J Med.* 2013;**369**(23):2218–25.

63. Mulley AG, Trimble C, Elwyn G. Stop the silent misdiagnosis: patients' preferences matter. *BMJ.* 2012;**345**:e6572. doi:10.1136/bmj.e6572.

64. Dancet EA, D'Hooghe TM, Spiessens C, Sermeus W, De Neubourg D, Karel N, et al. Quality indicators for all dimensions of infertility care quality: consensus between professionals and patients. *Hum Reprod.* 2013;**28**(6):1584–97. doi:10.1093/humrep/det056. Epub 2013 Mar 18.

65. Dancet EA, D'Hooghe TM, van der Veen F, Bossuyt P, Sermeus W, Mol BW, et al. 'Patient-centered fertility treatment': what is required? *Fertil Steril.* 2014;**101**(4):924–6. doi:10.1016/j.fertnstert.2013.12.045. Epub 2014 Feb 4. Erratum in: *Fertil Steril.* 2014;**102**(5):1499.

66. Moolenaar LM, Cissen M, de Bruin JP, Hompes PG, Repping S, van der Veen F, et al. Cost-effectiveness of assisted conception for male subfertility. *Reprod Biomed Online*. 2015;**30**(6):659–66. doi:10.1016/j.rbmo.2015.02.006. Epub 2015 Feb 24.

67. Chambers GM, Sullivan EA, Shanahan M, Ho MT, Priester K, Chapman MG. Is in vitro fertilisation more effective than stimulated intrauterine insemination as a first-line therapy for subfertility? A cohort analysis. *Aust N Z J Obstet Gynaecol*. 2010;**50**(3):280–8. doi:10.1111/j.1479-828X.2010.01155.x.

68. Van Rumste MM, Custers IM, van Wely M, Koks CA, van Weering HG, Beckers NG, et al. IVF with planned single-embryo transfer versus IUI with ovarian stimulation in couples with unexplained subfertility: an economic analysis. *Reprod Biomed Online*. 2014;**28**(3):336–42. doi:10.1016/j.rbmo.2013.10.021. Epub 2013 Dec 1.

69. Tjon-Kon-Fat RI, Bensdorp AJ, Bossuyt PM, Koks C, Oosterhuis GJ, Hoek A, et al. Is IVF – served two different ways – more cost-effective than IUI with controlled ovarian hyperstimulation? *Hum Reprod*. 2015;**30**(10):2331–9. doi:10.1093/humrep/dev193. Epub 2015 Aug 12.

70. Peeraer K, Luyten J, Tomassetti C, Verschueren S, Spiessens C, Tanghe A, et al. Cost-effectiveness of ovarian stimulation with gonadotrophin and clomiphene citrate in an intrauterine insemination programme for subfertile couples. *Reprod Biomed Online*. 2018;**36**(3):302–10. doi:10.1016/j.rbmo.2017.12.007. Epub 2017 Dec 27.

71. Chambers GM, Hoang VP, Lee E, Hansen M, Sullivan EA, Bower C, et al. Hospital costs of multiple-birth and singleton-birth children during the first 5 years of life and the role of assisted reproductive technology. *JAMA Pediatr*. 2014;**168**(11):1045–53. doi:10.1001/jamapediatrics.2014.1357.

Chapter 21

Non-ART Surveillance

Markus S. Kupka and Anja Bisgaard Pinborg

Non-ART Surveillance

Defining Non-ART Fertility Treatments

According to the second revision of the International Glossary on Infertility and Fertility Care from the International Committee Monitoring Assisted Reproductive Technologies (ICMART), medically assisted reproduction (MAR) is defined as "reproduction brought about through various interventions, procedures, surgeries and technologies to treat different forms of fertility impairment and infertility. These include ovulation induction, ovarian stimulation, ovulation triggering, all ART procedures, uterine transplantation and intra-uterine, intra-cervical and intravaginal insemination with semen of husband/partner or donor" [1]. Assisted reproductive technology (ART) is defined as "all interventions that include the in vitro handling of both human oocytes and sperm or of embryos for the purpose of reproduction. This includes, but is not limited to, IVF and embryo transfer ET, intracytoplasmic sperm injection ICSI, embryo biopsy, preimplantation genetic testing PGT, assisted hatching, gamete intrafallopian transfer GIFT, zygote intrafallopian transfer, gamete and embryo cryopreservation, semen, oocyte and embryo donation, and gestational carrier cycles. Thus, ART does not, and ART-only registries do not, include assisted insemination using sperm from either a woman's partner or a sperm donor" [1].

According to the ICMART glossary, ART encompasses all treatments that involve in vitro treatment (i.e. outside the body) using egg cells, sperm cells or embryos with the aim of assisting reproduction. This includes, but is not limited to, in vitro fertilization (IVF) and embryo transfer procedures. Hence, intrauterine insemination (IUI) is not by definition an ART method, though this distinction is inconsequently used in practice.

Insemination and cycle monitoring (timed intercourse) are included only in a limited few cases in large national and international data collection on MAR.

Further, the definition of non-ART treatment is not clear, but we suggest it to be MAR treatments not included in ART. For surveillance purposes, non-ART treatment is in general defined as all fertility treatments that do not involve oocytes and embryos being handled outside the female body. Homologous and heterologous IUI cycles with or without ovarian stimulation are often the only non-ART procedures that are being recorded in MAR-registries. In some countries, for example, the use of clomiphene citrate (CC) is not included in an overarching definition of treatment with ovarian stimulation, as this frequently refers only to the subcutaneous administration of gonadotropins; however, for safety reasons CC should also be included.

The Importance of Monitoring Non-ART Fertility Treatments

ART treatments are burdensome to the patients, expensive and time-consuming and treatment-related risks are greater, while non-ART treatments such as mild ovarian stimulation and/or insemination are more patient friendly, cheaper and safer. Fertility treatment needs tailoring to the specific infertility diagnosis; hence, anovulatory patients should not start with ART, but rather with ovulation induction and insemination. Further, IUI programs have been shown to be efficient in patients with unexplained infertility and mild male factor infertility. For these patient groups, ART should not be the first-choice treatment, although this is the case in many settings. As with ART, monitoring of non-ART is necessary to secure efficacy and safety. Therefore, it is of utmost importance that IUI cycles are also included in the monitoring of fertility treatments. Kulkarni et al. showed that from 2004 and onwards, non-ART fertility treatments including ovarian stimulation (OS) and IUI became the most highly associated treatment procedure with triplets and other high-order births in the United States (US) [2]. As Kulkarni et al. used the data from the National ART Surveillance System (NASS) and National Vital Statistics System (NVSS) of the Centers for Disease Control and Prevention (CDC), this is an example of very useful information on the contribution of non-ART treatment to multiple births that can be implemented in future strategies to diminish MAR-related risks. The risk of multiple gestations is still an obstacle in IUI, and low multiple birth rates are reached only with mild ovarian stimulation, in particular with gonadotropin stimulation, sufficient ultrasound surveillance and reasonable cancellation criteria in case of multifollicular growth. A requirement in an efficient and safe IUI program is low multiple birth rates.

In a multicentre randomized controlled trial, couples with unexplained or mild male subfertility and an unfavourable prognosis for natural conception were randomly allocated to IVF-SET (single embryo transfer) (201 couples) and IUI-OS (ovarian stimulation) (207 couples) [3, 4]. The authors predefined the following baseline characteristics as potential treatment selection markers: female age, ethnicity, smoking status, type of subfertility (primary/secondary), duration of subfertility, body mass index (BMI), pre-wash total motile count and Hunault prediction score [5, 4]. For each potential treatment selection marker, they explored the association with the chances of a healthy child after IVF-SET and IUI-OS and tested to see whether there was an interaction with treatment. The authors could not identify couples with unexplained or mild male subfertility who would have had higher chances of a healthy child from immediate IVF-SET than from IUI-OS. As in the original trial, IUI-OS had similar effectiveness and was cheaper compared with IVF-SET. The authors concluded that IUI-OS should remain the preferred first-line treatment in these couples [3, 4]. These reports have shown that IUI-OS is the most cost-effective strategy for mild male factor or unexplained infertility with a poor prognosis of natural conception. In a very recent review on IUI, the same conclusion regarding the benefit of IUI for specific causes for infertility was emphasized [6]. To facilitate the implementation of this strategy, recording IUI cycles in national and international databases is essential, as well as in registries to surveil that IUI is used as first-line treatments for these diagnoses.

	Cycles	Pregnancies	%
IUI-H < 40	105 214	12 641	12.0
IUI-H > 40	12 953	892	6.9
Total*	171 722	20 112	11.7
IUI-D < 40	33 327	6 148	18.4
IUI-D > 40	5 999	523	8.7
Total*	43 003	7 439	17.3

* Totals differ from the sum of the age categories as for some countries the age stratification is missing

Figure 21.1 Pregnancy rates per cycle for homologous and heterologous insemination in Europe, 2006–2015. H = husband, D = donor.

Source: De Geyter C, Calhaz-Jorge C, Wyns C, Kupka MS, Mocanu E, Motrenko T, et al. Presentation of the preliminary results 2015 of the European IVF-Monitoring Consortium (EIM), for the European Society of Human Reproduction and Embryology (ESHRE), ESHRE conference, July 2018, Barcelona.

Monitoring Non-ART Fertility Treatments in International Registries (ICMART, EIM)

The worldwide IVF registry from ICMART includes information on non-ART treatments. The European registry for reproductive medicine (European IVF Monitoring (EIM) Consortium) also contains this information, and to a considerable extent, based on a historical development, traceable to the data collection process for this registry (Fig. 21.1).

This process involves working in modules that relate to different treatment concepts, such as egg donation, preimplantation genetic diagnosis, cross-border patient couples and the like. From the start of the EIM data collection in 1997, it established a module for homologous and heterologous insemination. For historical reasons, too, a distinction was made between women aged > or <40 (Fig. 21.2).

Monitoring Non-ART Fertility Treatments in National Registries

Thirty-eight European countries are currently participating in data collection for the EIM [7]. In terms of

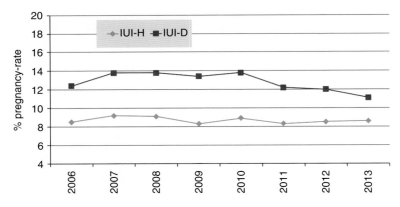

Figure 21.2 Pregnancy rates per cycle for homologous and heterologous insemination in Europe, 2015.
Source: De Geyter C, Calhaz-Jorge C, Wyns C, Kupka MS, Mocanu E, Motrenko T, et al. Presentation of the preliminary results 2015 of the European IVF-Monitoring Consortium (EIM), for the European Society of Human Reproduction and Embryology (ESHRE), ESHRE conference, July 2018, Barcelona.
H = husband, D = donor.

insemination treatments, information on homologous inseminations was available from 27 countries for the 2014 analysis year. Twenty-one countries were also able to report on treatments using donor sperm. The reason for this uniform approach is that the structure of the national registries is very heterogeneous. There are both voluntary and obligatory registries. There are registries that collect information cycle by cycle, and registries that collect only cumulative data already compiled. Financing systems also play a role in some countries. For example, in Austria the IVF registry is responsible only for those that come under the country's statutory health insurance. In many countries, national authorities attempt to pool the data from this field by, for example, making approval for the respective laboratories dependent on participation. For larger countries, e.g. the US and India, no information is available in official registries for non-ART treatments.

However, national ART databases in some countries include IUI cycles. An example of a country with a very high number of IUI cycles performed is Iran, where the first national report published on Iranian ART centres presented a summary of the status of ART in Iran during 2011. They stated that a total of 52 centres reported treatment cycles and performed approximately 29,000 intrauterine inseminations (IUIs), in addition to 35,000 in vitro fertilizations (IVFs) and intracytoplasmic sperm injection (ICSI) cycles [8]. The authors concluded that the considerable

potential to provide IVF services for both Iranians as well as other nationalities throughout the region proved the need for a national centre that will implement a registry system.

IUI is a simple and non-invasive technique applicable in poor-income countries where ART is not accessible for the majority of the population owing to the expensive infrastructure and equipment needed for ART [9]. Thus, IUI is probably one of the most used MAR worldwide, but only a very small proportion of IUI cycles is reported.

Variables Collected in Non-ART Registries

Significantly, fewer fields per dataset are generally required for data collection of non-ART treatments compared with ART treatments. For these data, information on patient age, natural or stimulated cycles and the use of ovarian hormone drug treatment, including type of ovulation trigger, fallopian tube function and quality of ejaculate, is of particular importance. However, demographics, BMI, smoking, infertility diagnosis and pregnancy should also be recorded for non-ART. Obviously, donor-IUI cycles also account for an important segment, including information on heterosexual and homosexual couples and single women. As is the case for all modern registries, the end date for data collection in this case is not the end of clinical pregnancy, but rather the live birth that should optimally be included in the registry.

The information that is available by the European registry includes these reference values [10]. The following countries are able to provide information on birth rates for non-ART treatments: Belarus, Belgium, Bulgaria, Croatia, Denmark, Finland, France, Greece, Ireland, Italy, Kazakhstan, Latvia, Lithuania, Moldova, Montenegro, Norway, Poland, Portugal, Romania, Russia, Serbia, Slovenia, Ukraine and the UK. In principle, pregnancy rates from inseminations are lower than they are after ART, which holds true across the board for the aforementioned countries.

The most effective data collection method is digital. Within this, there are different concepts, such as nationally universal, web-based systems, which are easy to use and maintain because the data entry is via an Internet browser. However, working with such systems demonstrates that doctors feel a need to 'benefit' in some way if these data are to be published online by them. The motivation for practitioners to carry out data entry is either the use of penalties, such as not renewing licences to continue offering these treatments, or the use of incentives, such as insurance companies making payments for services rendered only where evidence can be provided that the data have been fully entered up to a given end date.

Use of Non-ART Treatment Data

To date, there is evidence that there is no separate recording of non-ART-treatments, but rather an established IVF registry appends these as extra records. In many countries, general gynaecologists not working in the field of reproductive medicine perform the IUI cycle monitoring. These medical practices must also be given the chance and/or be required to collect the data. There are no stringent regulations concerning this, however, in any country. Flexible online registration systems will, of course, enhance this process.

Treatments with donor sperm will experience far-reaching changes, as European legislation should include a comprehensive requirement of a uniform code for semen samples. This uniform semen coding system is necessary, as semen samples need traceability regarding their origin. In some countries, e.g. Germany, there have been changes in the law so that data must additionally be passed on to a central data collection point to allow children conceived by the means of treatments with donor sperm to be able to identify who their genetic father is. Hence, cycles

with the use of donor sperm may attract more attention and need to be included in MAR surveillance programs. The hope is that cycles with the use of homologous semen will also be part of the registration.

Surveillance of Quality and Safety of Non-ART Treatments

Surveillance of non-ART treatments is necessary for monitoring of success rates, quality and safety to evaluate treatment strategies. In particular, countries with a fertility treatment program involving IUI are obliged to survey IUI treatments to offer patients the most cost-effective treatment strategy. As part of the national treatment program in Denmark, ovulation induction and up to six IUI cycles have been offered to patients with anovulatory infertility, and three IUI cycles have been offered as the primary treatment strategy for couples suffering from unexplained or mild to moderate male factor infertility. This is also included in the Danish national guideline provided by the Danish Fertility Society. This treatment strategy was assessed based on national data on IUI that have been collected since IUI cycles were included in the Danish IVF registry beginning in 2007. The cumulative live birth rate including data on a full treatment course of IUI showed that for heterosexual couples referred for IUI treatment, 35% achieved a live birth after the national program of three IUI treatments was fulfilled [11]. Thus, even though the live birth rate per IUI cycle was 12.9% in 2017 according to the Danish Fertility Society (www.fertilitetsselskab.dk), more than one in three couples had a live birth after three IUI cycles [11]. In the optimal setting, data should be available both on pregnancy and live birth rates per cycle but cumulative live birth rates after 3–6 cycles and 1, 2 and 5 years of follow-up should also be available.

Perinatal Outcomes

Perinatal outcomes after non-ART treatment can be added if the MAR registry includes a link to the Medical Birth Registry or if data can be cross-linked by a personal identification number of the mother. This is the optimal scenario for both non-ART and ART treatments.

The results of a large Belgian study showed a significantly higher incidence of prematurity (<32 and <37 weeks), low and very low birth weight, transfer to the neonatal intensive care unit and most neonatal morbidity parameters for singletons conceived by ovarian stimulation with or without IUI [12].

National registry data on IUI assessing perinatal outcomes of the children compared with children conceived after ART or spontaneous conception, showed that IUI children have perinatal risks, somewhere in between ART and spontaneously conceived children [13]. Long-term child health outcomes of children conceived by non-ART are monitored by using national surveillance data, as in a Danish study on fertility treatment and risk of childhood and adolescent mental disorders [14], Bay et al. [14], reported that children born after ovulation induction with or without insemination had low but significantly increased risks of any mental disorder (hazard ratio (HR) 1.20, 95% CI 1.11–1.31; absolute risk 4.1%) and autism spectrum disorders (HR 1.20, 95% CI 1.05–1.37; 1.5%). The increased risks were related to ovulation induction and anovulatory infertility and not the IUI procedure itself.

Conclusions

After many years of participation in the EIM Consortium, the economic pressure, which in many European countries relates to the reimbursement in the field of non-ART fertility treatment, leads to less invasive forms of fertility treatment being devalued. Therefore, utilization of appropriate data analysis tools is necessary to assess the probability of success attributed from each non-ART treatment.

Because of the lack of registration of non-ART treatments and linkage to maternal and child health outcomes, data on indications, success rates and risks associated with IUI are limited and in most countries nonexistent. We recommend that non-ART treatments should be part of national surveillance registries to secure a sufficient, cost-effective and safe fertility treatment program. Countries should improve their monitoring of non-ART cycles by including non-ART in the already established registries, or, in the case of no national MAR database, countries should start the process of establishing one that includes non-ART cycles.

References

1. Zegers-Hochschild F, Adamson GD, Dyer S, Racowsky C, de Mouzon J, Sokol R, et al. The International Glossary on Infertility and Fertility Care, 2017. *Hum Reprod.* 2017;**32**:1786–801.

2. Kulkarni AD, Jamieson DJ, Jones HW Jr, Kissin DM, Gallo MF, Macaluso M, et al. Fertility treatments and multiple births in the United States. *N Engl J Med.* 2013;**369**:2218–25.

3. Bensdorp AJ, Tjon-Kon-Fat RI, Bossuyt PM, Koks CA, Oosterhuis GJ, Hoek A, et al. Prevention of multiple pregnancies in couples with unexplained or mild male subfertility: randomised controlled trial of in vitro fertilisation with single embryo transfer or in vitro fertilisation in modified natural cycle compared with intrauterine insemination with controlled ovarian hyperstimulation. *BMJ.* 2015;**350**:g7771.

4. Tjon-Kon-Fat RI, Tajik P, Zafarmand MH, Bensdorp AJ, Bossuyt PMM, Oosterhuis GJE, et al.; INeS Study Group. IVF or IUI as first-line treatment in unexplained subfertility: the conundrum of treatment selection markers. *Hum Reprod.* 2017;**32**:1028–32.

5. Hunault CC, Habbema JD, Eijkemans MJ, Collins JA, Evers JL, te Velde ER. Two new prediction rules for spontaneous pregnancy leading to live birth among subfertile couples, based on the synthesis of three previous models. *Hum Reprod.* 2004;**19**:2019–26.

6. Cohlen B, Bijkerk A, Van der Poel S, Ombelet W. IUI: review and systematic assessment of the evidence that supports global recommendations. *Hum Reprod Update.* 2018;**24**:300–19.

7. European IVF-monitoring Consortium (EIM); European Society of Human Reproduction and Embryology (ESHRE); Calhaz-Jorge C, De Geyter C, Kupka MS, de Mouzon J, Erb K, Mocanu E, et al. Assisted reproductive technology in Europe, 2013: results generated from European registers by ESHRE. *Hum Reprod.* 2017;**32**:1957–73.

8. Abedini M, Ghaheri A, Omani Samani R. Assisted reproductive technology in Iran: the First National Report on Centers, 2011. *Int J Fertil Steril.* 2016;**10**:283–9.

9. Ombelet W, Cooke I, Dyer S, Serour G, Devroey P. Infertility and the provision of infertility medical services in developing countries. *Hum Reprod Update.* 2008;**14**:605–21.

10. Ferraretti AP, Nygren K, Nyboe Andersen A, de Mouzon J, Kupka MS, Calhaz-Jorge C, et al.; The European IVF-Monitoring Consortium (EIM), for the European Society of Human Reproduction and Embryology (ESHRE). Trends over 15 years in ART in Europe: an analysis of 6 million cycles. *Hum Reprod Open.* 2017;**2**:1–10.

11. Malchau SS, Henningsen AA, Loft A, Rasmussen S, Forman J, Nyboe Andersen A, et al. The long-term prognosis for live birth in couples initiating fertility treatments. *Hum Reprod.* 2017;**32**:1439–49.

12. Ombelet W, Martens G, De Sutter P, Gerris J, Bosmans E, Ruyssinck G, et al. Perinatal outcome of 12,021 singleton and 3108 twin births after non-IVF-assisted reproduction: a cohort study. *Hum Reprod.* 2006;**21**:1025–32.

13. Malchau SS, Loft A, Henningsen AK, Nyboe Andersen A, Pinborg A. Perinatal outcomes in 6,338 singletons born after intrauterine insemination in Denmark, 2007 to 2012: the influence of ovarian stimulation. *Fertil Steril.* 2014;**102**:1110–16.

14. Bay B, Mortensen EL, Hvidtjørn D, Kesmodel US. Fertility treatment and risk of childhood and adolescent mental disorders: register based cohort study. *BMJ.* 2013;**347**:f3978.

Appendix A   ART Surveillance System Variables and Definitions

Patient demographic information	Date of cycle reporting Patient identifier Optional patient identifier(s) (as needed by clinic to identify a patient, not reported) Patient's date of birth Patient's gender (female, male) Patient's residency (country, city, state/province, zip/postal code)
Cycle information: Intended cycle information	Intended type of cycle (IVF, GIFT, ZIFT, oocyte or embryo banking) 　If oocyte banking, source and type of oocytes (donor or autologous, fresh or frozen) 　If embryo banking, duration of banking (short term [<12 months] or long term [≥12 months] 　　If short-term banking, reason (delay of transfer to obtain genetic information or other reasons) 　　If long-term banking, reason (banking for fertility preservation prior to gonadotoxic medical treatments or other reasons) Intended embryo source (patient, donor) Intended embryo state (fresh, frozen) Intended oocyte source (patient, donor) Intended oocyte state (fresh, frozen) Intended sperm source (partner, donor, patient, unknown) Pregnancy carrier (patient, gestational carrier, none [for banking only])
Cycle information: Actual cycle information	Actual type of cycle (IVF, GIFT, ZIFT, oocyte or embryo banking) 　If oocyte banking, source and type of oocytes (donor or autologous, fresh or frozen) 　If embryo banking, duration of banking (short term [<12 months] or long term [≥12 months] 　　If short-term banking, reason (delay of transfer to obtain genetic information or other reasons) 　　If long-term banking, reason (banking for fertility preservation prior to gonadotoxic medical treatments or other reasons) Actual embryo source (patient, donor) Actual embryo state (fresh, frozen) Actual oocyte source (patient, donor) Actual oocyte state (fresh, frozen)
Patient medical evaluation: Reason(s) for ART	Male Infertility (yes, no) 　If male infertility, type (medical condition, genetic or chromosomal abnormality, abnormal sperm parameters, or other) 　　If abnormal sperm parameters, specify (obstructive azoospermia, non-obstructive azoospermia, severe oligospermia, moderate oligospermia, low motility, low morphology) History of endometriosis (yes, no) Tubal ligation for contraception (yes, no) Current or prior hydrosalpinx 　If hydrosalpinx, type (communicating, occluded, unknown) Other tubal disease (not current or historic hydrosalpinx) (yes, no) Ovulatory disorders (yes, no) 　If ovulatory disorders, specify (polycystic ovaries, other ovulatory disorders) Diminished ovarian reserve (yes, no) Uterine factor (yes, no) Preimplantation genetic diagnosis (including aneuploidy screening) as primary reason for ART (yes, no) Oocyte or embryo banking as reason for ART (yes, no) Indication for use of gestational carrier (yes, no) 　If gestational carrier is indicated, reason (absence of uterus, significant uterine anomaly, medical contraindication to pregnancy, recurrent pregnancy loss, unknown)

(cont.)

	Recurrent pregnancy loss (yes, no) Other reasons related to infertility (specify) Other reasons not related to infertility (specify) Unexplained infertility (yes, no)
Female patient history and physical	Height Weight History of smoking History of prior pregnancies (full term, preterm, stillbirth, spontaneous abortion, ectopic pregnancies) Months attempting pregnancy History of prior ART (fresh and frozen cycles) If prior ART cycles, live births after ART (yes, no) Maximum FSH level (value [mIU/mL]) Most recent AMH level (value [ng/mL] and date)
Oocyte source information (if not female patient)	Date of Birth Race (White, Black, Asian, Native Hawaiian/Pacific Islander, American Indian or Alaska Native) Ethnicity (Hispanic, non-Hispanic, refused, unknown) Height Weight History of smoking History of prior pregnancies (full term, preterm, stillbirth, spontaneous abortion, ectopic pregnancies) Months attempting pregnancy History of prior ART (fresh and frozen cycles) If prior ART cycles, live births after ART (yes, no) Maximum FSH level (value [mIU/mL]) Most recent AMH level (value [ng/mL] and date)
Gestational carrier information (if not female patient)	Date of Birth Race (White, Black, Asian, Native Hawaiian/Pacific Islander, American Indian or Alaska Native) Ethnicity (Hispanic, non-Hispanic, refused, Unknown)
Sperm source information	Sperm source (partner, donor, male patient) Date of Birth Race (White, Black, Asian, Native Hawaiian/Pacific Islander, American Indian or Alaska Native) Ethnicity (Hispanic, non-Hispanic, refused, unknown)

Stimulation and medications	Stimulation for follicular development (yes, no)
	   Minimal stimulation cycle (yes, no)
	   Aromatase inhibitor/oestrogen receptor modulator (clomiphene and letrozole dosage)
	   FSH medication (short-acting, long-acting, dosage)
	   LH/hCG medication
	   Gonadotropin-releasing hormone protocol (none, GnRH agonist suppression, GnRH agonist flare, GnRH antagonist suppression)

Cycle cancellation	Cancelled cycle (yes, no)
	   Cycle cancelled prior to retrieval (yes, no)
	   Date of cancelled cycle
	   Reason for cancelled cycle (low ovarian response, high ovarian response, inadequate endometrial response, concurrent illness, withdrawal for personal reasons, other)

Oocyte retrieval	Date of retrieval Number of oocytes retrieved Use of retrieved oocytes (for this cycle, oocytes frozen for future use, oocytes shared with other patients, embryos frozen for future use) Number of fresh oocytes frozen for future use
Complications of ovarian stimulation or oocyte retrieval	Complications of ovarian stimulation or oocyte retrieval (yes, no) Complications (infection, haemorrhage requiring transfusion, ovarian hyperstimulation requiring intervention or hospitalization, medication side effect, anesthetic complication, thrombosis, death of patient, other) Complication(s) required hospitalization (yes, no)
Sperm retrieval	Sperm status (fresh, thawed, mix of fresh and thawed) Sperm source utilized (ejaculated, epididymal, testis, electroejaculation, retrograde urine, donor, unknown)

(cont.)

Laboratory information	Intracytoplasmic sperm injection (ICSI) performed on oocytes (all oocytes, some oocytes, no oocytes, unknown)
	  If ICSI performed, indication for ICSI (prior failed fertilization, poor fertilization, preimplantation genetic diagnosis (PGD) or PGS, abnormal semen parameters on day of fertilization, low oocyte yield, laboratory routine, frozen oocyte, rescue ICSI, other)
	In vitro maturation (IVM) performed on oocytes (all oocytes, some oocytes, no oocytes, unknown)
	Preimplantation genetic diagnosis or screening (PGS) performed on embryos (yes, no, unknown)
	  Total number of 2PN
	  Reason for PGD or PGS (either genetic parent is a known carrier of a gene mutation or a chromosomal abnormality, aneuploidy screening of the embryos, elective gender determination, other screening of the embryos)
	  Technique used for PGD or PGS (polar body biopsy, blastomere biopsy, blastocyst biopsy, unknown)
	Assisted hatching performed on embryos (all embryos, some embryos, no embryos, unknown)
	Research cycle (yes, no)
	  If research cycle, study type (device study, protocol study, pharmaceutical study, laboratory technique, other research)
	  Approval code

Transfer information	Transfer attempted (yes, no)
	  If transfer not attempted, primary reason (low ovarian response, high ovarian response, failure to survive oocyte thaw, inadequate endometrial response, concurrent illness, withdrawal only for personal reasons, unable to obtain sperm specimen, insufficient embryos, other)
	  If transfer performed, date of transfer
	  Endometrial thickness at trigger (mm)

Fresh embryo transfer information	Number of fresh embryos available on day of transfer Number of fresh embryos transferred to uterus If only one fresh embryo was transferred to the uterus, was this an elective single embryo transfer (yes, no) Quality of each transferred embryo (good, fair, poor, unknown) Date of oocyte retrieval for each transferred embryo Number of fresh embryos cryopreserved
Frozen embryo transfer information	Number of frozen-thawed embryos available on day of transfer Number of thawed embryos transferred to uterus If only one thawed embryo was transferred to the uterus, was this an elective single embryo transfer (yes, no) Quality of each transferred embryo (good, fair, poor, unknown) Date of oocyte retrieval for each transferred embryo Number of thawed embryos cryopreserved (re-frozen)
GIFT/ZIFT/TET transfer information	Number of oocytes or embryos transferred to the fallopian tube

Outcome of transfer	Outcome of treatment cycle (not pregnant, biochemical only, clinical intrauterine gestation, ectopic, heterotopic, unknown)
	  If clinical intrauterine gestation, maximum number of fetal hearts on ultrasound performed before 7 weeks or prior to reduction
	    If ultrasound performed before 7 weeks or prior to reduction, ultrasound date
	  Any monochorionic twins or multiples (yes, no, unknown)

Outcome of pregnancy	Outcome of pregnancy (live birth, spontaneous abortion, stillbirth, induced abortion, maternal death prior to birth, outcome unknown)
	Date of pregnancy outcome
	Source of information confirming pregnancy outcome (verbal confirmation from patient, written confirmation from patient, verbal confirmation from physician or hospital, written confirmation from physician or hospital)
	  If live birth or stillbirth, number of infants born
	  Method of delivery (vaginal, caesarean, unknown)

Birth information (for each infant)	Birth status (live born, stillborn, unknown) Gender (male, female, unknown) Birth weight Birth defects (cleft lip/palate, genetic defect/chromosomal abnormality, neural tube defect, cardiac defect, limb defect, other defect, birth defects unknown, none)

Source: United States National ART Surveillance System, 2018 (www.cdc.gov/ART).

Appendix B The International Glossary on Infertility and Fertility Care

(Source: Zegers-Hochschild F, Adamson GD, Dyer S, Racowsky C, de Mouzon J, Sokol R, Rienzi L, Sunde A, Schmidt L, Cooke ID, Simpson JL, van der Poel S. The International Glossary on Infertility and Fertility Care, 2017. *Hum Reprod.* 2017;32(9):1786–801. By permission of Oxford University Press.)

Acrosome: A membrane-bound structure covering the anterior of the sperm head that contains enzymes necessary to penetrate the zona pellucida of the oocyte.

Adenomyosis: A form of endometriosis marked by the presence of endometriosis-like epithelium and stroma outside the endometrium in the myometrium.

Adhesions: Bands of fibrous scar tissue that may bind the abdominal and pelvic organs, including the intestines and peritoneum, to each other. They can be dense and thick or filmy and thin.

Age specific fertility rate (ASFR): The number of live births per woman in a particular age group in a specific calendar year expressed per 1,000 women in that age group.

Agglutination: Clumping of spermatozoa in the ejaculate.

Andrology: The medical practice dealing with the health of the male reproductive system.

Aneuploidy: An abnormal number of chromosomes in a cell. The majority of embryos with aneuploidies are not compatible with life.

Anti-sperm antibodies: Antibodies that recognize and bind to antigens on the surface of the spermatozoon.

Aspermia: Lack of external ejaculation.

Assisted hatching: An ART procedure in which the zona pellucida of an embryo is either thinned or perforated by chemical, mechanical or laser methods.

Assisted reproductive technology (ART): All interventions that include the in vitro handling of both human oocytes and sperm or of embryos for the purpose of reproduction. This includes, but is not limited to, IVF and embryo transfer ET, intracytoplasmic sperm injection ICSI, embryo biopsy, preimplantation genetic testing PGT, assisted hatching, gamete intrafallopian transfer GIFT, zygote intrafallopian transfer, gamete and embryo cryopreservation, semen, oocyte and embryo donation, and gestational carrier cycles. Thus, ART does not, and ART-only registries do not, include assisted insemination using sperm from either a woman's partner or a sperm donor. (See broader term, medically assisted reproduction, MAR.)

Asthenoteratozoospermia: Reduced percentages of motile and morphologically normal sperm in the ejaculate below the lower reference limit. When reporting results, the reference criteria should be specified.

Asthenozoospermia: Reduced percentage of motile sperm in the ejaculate below the lower reference limit. When reporting results, the reference criteria should be specified.

Azoospermia: The absence of spermatozoa in the ejaculate.

Binucleation: The presence of two nuclei in a blastomere (cell).

Biochemical pregnancy: A pregnancy diagnosed only by the detection of beta hCG in serum or urine.

Birth (single): The complete expulsion or extraction from a woman of a fetus after 22 completed weeks of gestational age, irrespective of whether it is a live birth or stillbirth, or, if gestational age is unknown, a birth weight more than 500 grams. A single birth refers to an individual newborn; and a delivery of multiple births, such as a twin delivery, would be registered as two births.

Blastocoele: Fluid-filled central region of the blastocyst.

Blastocyst: The stage of preimplantation embryo development that occurs around day 5–6 after insemination or ICSI. The blastocyst contains a fluid-filled central cavity (blastocoele), an outer layer of cells (trophectoderm) and an inner group of cells (inner cell mass).

Blastomere: A cell in a cleavage stage embryo.

Blastomere symmetry: The extent to which all blastomeres are even in size and shape.

Bleeding after oocyte aspiration: Significant bleeding, internal or external, after oocyte aspiration retrieval requiring hospitalization for blood transfusion, surgical intervention, clinical observation or other medical procedure.

Cancelled ART cycle: An ART cycle in which ovarian stimulation or monitoring has been initiated with the intention to treat, but which did not proceed to follicular aspiration or in the case of a thawed or warmed embryo did not proceed to embryo transfer.

Childlessness: A condition in which a person, voluntarily or involuntarily, is not a legal or societally recognized parent to a child, or has had all children die.

Chimerism: Presence in a single individual of two or more cell lines, each derived from different individuals.

Cleavage stage embryos: Embryos beginning with the 2-cell stage and up to, but not including, the morula stage.

Clinical fertility: The capacity to establish a clinical pregnancy.

Clinical pregnancy: A pregnancy diagnosed by ultrasonographic visualization of one or more gestational sacs or definitive clinical signs of pregnancy. In addition to intra-uterine pregnancy, it includes a clinically documented ectopic pregnancy.

Clinical pregnancy rate: The number of clinical pregnancies expressed per 100 initiated cycles, aspiration cycles or embryo transfer cycles. When clinical pregnancy rates are recorded, the denominator (initiated, aspirated or embryo transfer cycles) must be specified.

Clinical pregnancy with fetal heart beat: A pregnancy diagnosed by ultrasonographic or clinical documentation of at least one fetus with a discernible heartbeat.

Cohort total fertility rate (CTFR): The observed average number of live born children per woman applied to a birth cohort of women as they age through time. This is obtained from data on women after completing their reproductive years.

Compaction: The process during which tight junctions form between juxtaposed blastomeres resulting in a solid mass of cells with indistinguishable cell membranes.

Complex aneuploidies: Two or more aneuploidies involving different chromosomes in the embryo. When autosomes are involved, this condition is not compatible with human life.

Congenital anomalies: Structural or functional disorders that occur during intra-uterine life and can be identified prenatally, at birth or later in life. Congenital anomalies can be caused by single gene defects, chromosomal disorders, multifactorial inheritance, environmental teratogens and micronutrient deficiencies. The time of identification should be reported.

Congenital anomaly birth rate: The number of births exhibiting signs of congenital anomalies per 10,000 births. The time of identification should have been reported.

Congenital bilateral absence of the vasa deferentia (CBAVD): The absence, at birth, of both duct systems (vas deferentia) that connect the testes to the urethra and may be associated with cystic fibrosis transmembrane conductance regulator (CTFR) gene mutation. Although the testes usually develop and function normally, men present with azoospermia.

Conventional in vitro insemination: The co-incubation of oocytes with sperm in vitro with the goal of resulting in extracorporeal fertilization.

Corona radiata cells: The innermost cells of the cumulus oophorus.

Cross border reproductive care: The provision of reproductive health services in a different jurisdiction or outside of a recognized national border within which the person or persons legally reside.

Cryopreservation: The process of slow freezing or vitrification to preserve biological material (e.g. gametes, zygotes, cleavage stage embryos, blastocysts or gonadal tissue) at extreme low temperature.

Cryptorchidism: Testis not in scrotal position within the neonatal period and, up to but not limited to, 1 year post birth. If the testis has not descended into the scrotum, this condition can cause primary testicular failure and increased risk of testicular cancer development.

Cumulative delivery rate per aspiration/initiated cycle with at least one live birth: The number of deliveries with at least one live birth resulting from one initiated or aspirated ART cycle, including all cycles in which fresh and/or frozen embryos are transferred, until one delivery with a live birth occurs or until all embryos are used, whichever occurs first. The delivery of a singleton, twin, or other multiples is registered as one delivery. In the absence of complete data, the cumulative delivery rate is often estimated.

Cumulus oophorus: The multilayered mass of granulosa cells surrounding the oocyte.

Cytoplasmic maturation: The process during which the oocyte acquires the capacity to support nuclear maturation, fertilization, pronuclei formation, syngamy and subsequent early cleavage divisions until activation of the embryonic genome.

Cytoplasmic transfer: A procedure that can be performed at different stages of an oocyte's development to add to or replace various amounts of cytoplasm from a donor egg.

Decreased spermatogenesis: A histological finding in which spermatogenesis is present with few cells in the seminiferous tubules, resulting in a decreased number or absence of sperm in the ejaculate.

Delayed ejaculation: A condition in which it takes a man an extended period of time to reach orgasm and ejaculation.

Delayed embryo transfer: A procedure in which embryo transfer is not performed within the time frame of the oocyte aspiration cycle but at a later time.

Delivery: The complete expulsion or extraction from a woman of one or more fetuses, after at least 22 completed weeks of gestational age, irrespective of whether they are live births or stillbirths. A delivery of either a single or multiple newborn is considered as one delivery. If more than one newborn is delivered, it is often recognized as a delivery with multiple births.

Delivery rate: The number of deliveries expressed per 100 initiated cycles, aspiration cycles, or embryo transfer cycles. When delivery rates are recorded, the denominator (initiated, aspirated or embryo transfer cycles) must be specified. It includes deliveries that resulted in the birth of one or more live births and/or stillbirths. The delivery of a singleton, twin or other multiple pregnancy is registered as one delivery. If more than one newborn is delivered, it is often recognized as a delivery with multiple births.

Delivery rate after fertility treatment per patient: The number of deliveries with at least one live birth or stillbirth, expressed per 100 patients, after a specified time and following all treatments.

Delivery with multiple births after fertility treatments: A single delivery with more than one newborn, following all fertility treatments.

Diandric oocytes: An oocyte with an extra set of haploid chromosomes of paternal origin.

Digynic oocytes: An oocyte with an extra set of haploid chromosomes of maternal origin.

Diminished ovarian reserve: A term generally used to indicate a reduced number and/or reduced quality of oocytes, such that the ability to reproduce is decreased. (See ovarian reserve.)

Diploidy/euploidy: The condition in which a cell has two haploid sets of chromosomes. Each chromosome in one set is paired with its counterpart in the other set. A diploid embryo has 22 pairs of autosomes and two sex chromosomes, the normal condition.

Disomy: The normal number of chromosomes characterized by 22 pairs of autosomal chromosomes and one pair of sex chromosomes (XX or XY). The chromosome number in human cells is normally 46.

Donor insemination: The process of placing laboratory processed sperm or semen from a man into the reproductive tract of a woman who is not his intimate sexual partner, for the purpose of initiating a pregnancy.

Double embryo transfer (DET): The transfer of two embryos in an ART procedure. This may be elective (eDET) when more than two embryos of sufficient quality for transfer are available.

Early neonatal death/mortality: Death of a newborn within 7 days of birth.

Ectopic pregnancy: A pregnancy outside the uterine cavity, diagnosed by ultrasound, surgical visualization or histopathology.

Ejaculation: Co-ordinated contractions of the genitourinary tract leading to the ejection of spermatozoa and seminal fluid.

Ejaculation retardate: A condition resulting in an inability to ejaculate during vaginal intercourse.

Ejaculatory duct: The canal that passes through the prostate just lateral to the verumontanum where the vas deferens and the duct from the seminal vesicle coalesce.

Elective embryo transfer: The transfer of one or more embryos, selected from a larger cohort of available embryos.

Elective single embryo transfer (eSET): The transfer of one (a single) embryo selected from a larger cohort of available embryos.

Embryo: The biological organism resulting from the development of the zygote, until eight completed weeks after fertilization, equivalent to 10 weeks of gestational age.

Embryo bank: Repository of cryopreserved embryos stored for future use.

Embryo donation (for reproduction): An ART cycle, which consists of the transfer of an embryo to the uterus or fallopian tube of a female recipient, resulting from gametes that did not originate from the female recipient or from her male partner, if present.

Embryo fragmentation: The process during which one or more blastomeres shed membrane vesicles containing cytoplasm and occasionally whole chromosomes or chromatin.

Embryo recipient cycle: An ART cycle in which a woman's uterus is prepared to receive one or more cleavage stage embryos/blastocysts, resulting from gametes that did not originate from her or from her male partner, if present.

Embryo transfer (ET): Placement into the uterus of an embryo at any embryonic stage from day 1 to day 7 after IVF or ICSI. Embryos from day 1 to day 3 can also be transferred into the fallopian tube.

Embryo transfer cycle: An ART cycle in which one or more fresh or frozen/thawed embryos at cleavage or blastocyst stage are transferred into the uterus or fallopian tube.

Emission (semen): Co-ordinated contractions of the vas deferentia, seminal vesicles, and ejaculatory ducts leading to deposition of semen into the urethral meatus prior to ejaculation.

Endometriosis: A disease characterized by the presence of endometrium-like epithelium and stroma outside the endometrium and myometrium. Intrapelvic endometriosis can be located superficially on the peritoneum (peritoneal endometriosis), can extend 5 mm or more beneath the peritoneum (deep endometriosis) or can be present as an ovarian endometriotic cyst (endometrioma).

Epididymis: A convoluted, highly coiled duct that transports the spermatozoa from the testis via the efferent ducts to the vas deferens.

Erectile dysfunction: Inability to have and/or sustain an erection sufficient for intercourse.

Euploidy: The condition in which a cell has chromosomes in an exact multiple of the haploid number; in the human this multiple is normally two. Thus, a normal embryo that is euploid is also diploid.

Excessive ovarian response: An exaggerated response to ovarian stimulation characterized by the presence of more follicles than intended. Generally, more than 20 follicles >12 mm in size and/or more than 20 oocytes collected following ovarian stimulation are considered excessive, but these numbers are adaptable according to ethnic and other variables.

Expectant fertility management: Management of fertility problems including infertility without any specific active clinical or therapeutic interventions other than fertility information and advice, to improve natural fertility, based upon the probability of becoming pregnant.

Extremely low birth weight: Birth weight less than 1,000 g.

Extremely preterm birth: A birth that takes place after 22 but before 28 completed weeks of gestational age.

Fecundability: The probability of a pregnancy, during a single menstrual cycle in a woman with adequate exposure to sperm and no contraception, culminating in a live birth. In population-based studies, fecundability is frequently measured as the monthly probability.

Fecundity: Clinically defined as the capacity to have a live birth.

Female infertility: Infertility caused primarily by female factors encompassing: ovulatory disturbances; diminished ovarian reserve; anatomical, endocrine, genetic, functional or immunological abnormalities of the reproductive system; chronic illness; and sexual conditions incompatible with coitus.

Fertility: The capacity to establish a clinical pregnancy.

Fertility awareness: The understanding of reproduction, fecundity, fecundability, and related individual risk factors (e.g. advanced age, sexual health factors such as sexually transmitted infections, and life style factors such as smoking, obesity) and non-individual risk factors (e.g. environmental and work place factors); including the awareness of societal and cultural factors affecting options to meet reproductive family planning, as well as family building needs.

Fertility care: Interventions that include fertility awareness, support and fertility management with an intention to assist individuals and couples to realize their desires associated with reproduction and/or to build a family.

Fertility preservation: Various interventions, procedures and technologies, including cryopreservation of gametes, embryos or ovarian and testicular tissue to preserve reproductive capacity.

Fertilization: A sequence of biological processes initiated by entry of a spermatozoon into a mature oocyte followed by formation of the pronuclei.

Fetal loss: Death of a fetus. It is referred to as early fetal loss when death takes place between 10 and 22 weeks of gestational age; late fetal loss, when death takes place between 22 and 28 weeks of gestational age; and stillbirth when death takes place after 28 weeks' gestational age.

Fetus: The stages of development of an organism from eight completed weeks of fertilization (equivalent to 10 weeks of gestational age) until the end of pregnancy

Freeze-all cycle: An ART cycle in which, after oocyte aspiration, all oocytes and/or embryos are cryopreserved and no oocytes and/or embryos are transferred to a woman in that cycle.

Frozen-thawed embryo transfer (FET) cycle: An ART procedure in which cycle monitoring is carried out with the intention of transferring to a woman, frozen/thawed or vitrified/warmed embryo(s)/blastocyst(s). Note: A FET cycle is initiated when specific medication is provided or cycle monitoring is started in the female recipient with the intention to transfer an embryo.

Frozen-thawed oocyte cycle: An ART procedure in which cycle monitoring is carried out with the intention of fertilizing thawed/warmed oocytes and performing an embryo transfer.

Full-term birth: A birth that takes place between 37 and 42 completed weeks of gestational age.

Gamete intrafallopian transfer (GIFT): An ART procedure in which both gametes (oocytes and spermatozoa) are transferred into a fallopian tube(s).

Germinal vesicle (GV): The nucleus in an oocyte at prophase I.

Gestational age: The age of an embryo or fetus calculated by the best obstetric estimate determined by assessments which may include early ultrasound and the date of the last menstrual period and/or perinatal details. In the case of ART, it is calculated by adding two weeks (14 days) to the number of completed weeks since fertilization. Note: For frozen-thawed embryo transfer (FET) cycles, an estimated date of fertilization is computed by subtracting the combined number of days an embryo was in culture pre-cryopreservation and post-thaw/-warm, from the transfer date of the FET cycle.

Gestational carrier: A woman who carries a pregnancy with an agreement that she will give the offspring to the intended parent(s). Gametes can originate from the intended parent(s) and/or a third party (or parties). This replaces the term 'surrogate'.

Gestational sac: A fluid-filled structure associated with early pregnancy, which may be located inside or, in the case of an ectopic pregnancy, outside the uterus.

Globozoospermia: Describes spermatozoa with a reduced or absent acrosome.

Haploidy: The condition in which a cell has one set of each of the 23 single chromosomes. Mature human gametes are haploid, each having 23 single chromosomes.

Hatching: The process by which an embryo at the blastocyst stage extrudes out of, and ultimately separates from, the zona pellucida.

Heterotopic pregnancy: Concurrent pregnancy involving at least one embryo implanted in the uterine cavity and at least one implanted outside of the uterine cavity.

High-order multiple births: The complete expulsion or extraction from their mother of three or more fetuses, after 22 completed weeks of gestational age, irrespective of whether they are live births or stillbirths.

High-order multiple gestation: A pregnancy with three or more embryos or fetuses.

Hydrosalpinx: A distally occluded, dilated, fluid-filled fallopian tube.

Hypergonadotropic hypogonadism: Gonadal failure associated with reduced gametogenesis, reduced gonadal steroid production and elevated gonadotropin production.

Hyperspermia: High volume of ejaculate above the upper reference limit. When reporting results, the reference criteria should be specified.

Hypogonadotropic hypogonadism: Gonadal failure associated with reduced gametogenesis and reduced gonadal steroid production due to reduced gonadotropin production or action.

Hypospermatogenesis: Histopathological description of reduced production of spermatozoa in the testes.

Hypospermia: Low volume of ejaculate below the lower reference limit. When reporting results, the reference criteria should be specified.

Iatrogenic testicular failure: Damage to testicular function after radiation, chemotherapy or hormone treatment; or devascularization as a consequence of hernia surgery.

Immature oocyte: An oocyte at prophase of meiosis I (i.e. an oocyte at the germinal vesicle (GV)-stage).

Implantation: The attachment and subsequent penetration by a zona-free blastocyst into the endometrium, but when it relates to an ectopic pregnancy, into tissue outside the uterine cavity. This process starts 5 to 7 days after fertilization of the oocyte usually resulting in the formation of a gestation sac.

Implantation rate: The number of gestational sacs observed divided by the number of embryos transferred (usually expressed as a percentage, %).

In vitro fertilization (IVF): A sequence of procedures that involves extracorporeal fertilization of gametes. It includes conventional in vitro insemination and ICSI.

In vitro maturation (IVM): A sequence of laboratory procedures that enable extracorporeal maturation of immature oocytes into fully mature oocytes that are capable of being fertilized with potential to develop into embryos.

Induced abortion: Intentional loss of an intrauterine pregnancy, through intervention by medical, surgical or unspecified means. (See induced embryo/fetal reduction.)

Induced embryo/fetal reduction: An intervention intended to reduce the number of gestational sacs or embryos/fetuses in a multiple gestation.

Infertility: A disease characterized by the failure to establish a clinical pregnancy after 12 months of regular, unprotected sexual intercourse or due to an impairment of a person's capacity to reproduce either as an individual or with his/her partner. Fertility interventions may be initiated in less than 1 year based on medical, sexual and reproductive history, age, physical findings and diagnostic testing. Infertility is a disease, which generates disability as an impairment of function.

Infertility counselling: A professional intervention with the intention to mitigate the physical, emotional and psychosocial consequences of infertility.

Initiated medically assisted reproduction cycle (iMAR): A cycle in which the woman receives specific medication for ovarian stimulation or in which cycle monitoring is carried out with the intention to treat, irrespective of whether or not insemination is performed, follicular aspiration is attempted in an ovarian stimulation cycle or whether egg(s) or embryo(s) are thawed or transferred in a frozen embryo transfer (FET) cycle.

Inner cell mass: A group of cells attached to the polar trophectoderm consisting of embryonic stem cells, which have the potential to develop into cells and tissues in the human body, except the placenta or amniotic membranes.

Intended parent(s): A couple or person who seek(s) to reproduce with the assistance of a gestational carrier or traditional gestational carrier.

Intra-cervical insemination: A procedure in which laboratory processed sperm are placed in the cervix to attempt a pregnancy.

Intracytoplasmic sperm injection (ICSI): A procedure in which a single spermatozoon is injected into the oocyte cytoplasm.

Intrauterine insemination: A procedure in which laboratory processed sperm are placed in the uterus to attempt a pregnancy.

Intrauterine pregnancy: A state of reproduction in which an embryo has implanted in the uterus.

Laparoscopic ovarian drilling: A surgical method for inducing ovulation in females with anovulatory or oligo-ovulatory polycystic ovarian syndrome, utilizing either laser or electrosurgery.

Large for gestational age: A birth weight greater than the 90th centile of the sex-specific birth weight for a given gestational age reference. When reporting outcomes, the reference criteria should be specified. If gestational age is unknown, then the birth weight should be registered.

Leukospermia: A high number of white blood cells in semen above the upper reference limit. When reporting results, the reference criteria should be specified.

Leydig cell: Type of testicular cell located in the interstitial space between the seminiferous tubules, that secretes testosterone.

Live birth: The complete expulsion or extraction from a woman of a product of fertilization, after 22 completed weeks of gestational age; which, after such separation, breathes or shows any other evidence of life, such as heartbeat, umbilical cord pulsation or definite movement of voluntary muscles, irrespective of whether the umbilical cord has been cut or the placenta is attached. A birth weight of 500 grams or more can be used if gestational age is unknown. Live births refer to the individual newborn; for example, a twin delivery represents two live births.

Live birth delivery rate: The number of deliveries that resulted in at least one live birth, expressed per 100 cycle attempts. In the case of ART/MAR interventions, they can be initiated cycles, insemination, aspiration cycles or embryo transfer cycles. When delivery rates are given, the denominator (initiated, inseminated, aspirated or embryo transfer cycles) must be specified.

Low birth weight: Birth weight less than 2,500 grams.

Luteal phase defect: A poorly defined abnormality of the endometrium presumably due to abnormally low progesterone secretion or action on the endometrium.

Luteal phase support: Hormonal supplementation in the luteal phase, usually progesterone.

Major congenital anomaly: A congenital anomaly that requires surgical repair of a defect, is a visually evident or life-threatening structural or functional defect, or causes death.

Male infertility: Infertility caused primarily by male factors encompassing: abnormal semen parameters or function; anatomical, endocrine, genetic, functional or immunological abnormalities of the reproductive system; chronic illness; and sexual conditions incompatible with the ability to deposit semen in the vagina.

Maternal spindle transfer: Transfer of the maternal spindle (including maternal chromosomes) from a patient's oocyte into a donated oocyte in which the maternal spindle with chromosomes has been removed.

Mature oocyte: An oocyte at metaphase of meiosis II, exhibiting the first polar body and with the ability to become fertilized.

Maturing oocyte: An oocyte that has progressed from prophase I but has not completed telophase I, thus does not exhibit the first polar body.

Medically assisted reproduction (MAR): Reproduction brought about through various interventions, procedures, surgeries and technologies to treat different forms of fertility impairment and infertility. These include ovulation induction, ovarian stimulation, ovulation triggering, all ART procedures, uterine transplantation and intrauterine, intra-cervical and intravaginal insemination with semen of husband/partner or donor.

Microdissection testicular sperm extraction (MicroTESE): A surgical procedure using an operating microscope to identify seminiferous tubules that may contain sperm to be extracted for IVF and/or ICSI.

Micromanipulation in ART: A micro-operative ART procedure performed on sperm, egg or embryo; the most common ART micromanipulation procedures are ICSI, assisted hatching and gamete or embryo biopsy for PGT.

Microsurgical epididymal sperm aspiration/extraction (MESA/MESE): A surgical procedure performed with the assistance of an operating microscope to retrieve sperm from the epididymis of men with obstructive azoospermia. In the absence of optical magnification, any surgical procedure to retrieve sperm from the epididymis should also be registered as MESE.

Mild ovarian stimulation: for IVF A protocol in which the ovaries are stimulated with gonadotropins, and/or other pharmacological compounds, with the intention of limiting the number of oocytes following stimulation for IVF.

Missed spontaneous abortion/missed miscarriage: Spontaneous loss of a clinical pregnancy before 22 completed weeks of gestational age, in which the embryo(s) or fetus(es) is/are nonviable and is/are not spontaneously absorbed or expelled from the uterus.

Modified natural cycle: An ART procedure in which one or more oocytes are collected from the ovaries during a spontaneous menstrual cycle. Pharmacological compounds are administered with the sole purpose of blocking the spontaneous LH surge and/or inducing final oocyte maturation.

Monosomy: The absence of one of the two homologous chromosomes in embryos. Autosomal monosomies in embryos are not compatible with life. Embryos with sex chromosome monosomies are rarely compatible with life.

Morula: An embryo formed after completion of compaction, typically 4 days after insemination or ICSI.

Mosaicism: A state in which there is more than one karyotypically distinct cell population arising from a single embryo.

Multinucleation: The presence of more than one nucleus in a cell.

Multiple birth: The complete expulsion or extraction from a woman of more than one fetus, after 22 completed weeks of gestational age, irrespective of whether it is a live birth or stillbirth. Births refer to the individual newborn; for example, a twin delivery represents two births.

Multiple gestation: A pregnancy with more than one embryo or fetus.

Natural cycle ART: An ART procedure in which one or more oocytes are collected from the ovaries during a menstrual cycle without the use of any pharmacological compound.

Necrozoospermia: The description of an ejaculate in which no live spermatozoa can be found.

Neonatal death/mortality: Death of a live born baby within 28 days of birth. This can be sub-divided into a) early, if death occurs in the first 7 days after birth; and b) late, if death occurs between 8 and 28 days after birth.

Neonatal mortality rate: Number of neonatal deaths (up to 28 days) per 1,000 live births.

Neonatal period: The period which commences at birth and ends at 28 completed days after birth.

Non-obstructive azoospermia: Absence of spermatozoa in the ejaculate due to lack of production of mature spermatozoa.

Nuclear maturation: The process during which the oocyte resumes meiosis and progresses from prophase I to metaphase II.

Obstructive azoospermia: Absence of spermatozoa in the ejaculate due to occlusion of the ductal system.

Oligospermia: A term for low semen volume now replaced by hypospermia to avoid confusion with oligozoospermia.

Oligozoospermia: Low concentration of spermatozoa in the ejaculate below the lower reference limit. When reporting results, the reference criteria should be specified.

Oocyte: The female gamete (egg).

Oocyte aspiration: Ovarian follicular aspiration performed with the aim of retrieving oocytes.

Oocyte bank: Repository of cryopreserved oocytes stored for future use.

Oocyte donation: The use of oocytes from an egg donor for reproductive purposes or research.

Oocyte donation cycle: An ART cycle in which oocytes are collected from an egg donor for reproductive purposes or research.

Oocyte cryopreservation: The freezing or vitrification of oocytes for future use.

Oocyte maturation triggering: An intervention intended to induce an oocyte in vitro or in vivo to resume meiosis to reach maturity (i.e. to reach metaphase II).

Oocyte recipient cycle: An ART cycle in which a woman receives oocytes from a donor, or her partner if in a same sex relationship, to be used for reproductive purposes.

Oolemma: The cytoplasmic membrane enclosing the oocyte.

Ooplasm: The cytoplasm of the oocyte.

Ovarian hyperstimulation syndrome (OHSS): An exaggerated systemic response to ovarian stimulation characterized by a wide spectrum of clinical and laboratory manifestations. It may be classified as mild, moderate or severe according to the degree of abdominal distention, ovarian enlargement and respiratory, haemodynamic and metabolic complications.

Ovarian reserve: A term generally used to indicate the number and/or quality of oocytes, reflecting the ability to reproduce. Ovarian reserve can be assessed by any of several means. They include: female age; number of antral follicles on ultrasound; anti-Müllerian hormone levels; follicle stimulating hormone and estradiol levels; clomiphene citrate challenge test; response to gonadotropin stimulation, and oocyte and/or embryo assessment during an ART procedure, based on number, morphology or genetic assessment of the oocytes and/or embryos.

Ovarian stimulation (OS): Pharmacological treatment with the intention of inducing the development of ovarian follicles. It can be used for two purposes: (1) for timed intercourse or insemination; (2) in ART, to obtain multiple oocytes at follicular aspiration.

Ovarian tissue cryopreservation: The process of slow-freezing or vitrification of tissue surgically excised from the ovary with the intention of preserving reproductive capacity.

Ovarian torsion: Partial or complete rotation of the ovarian vascular pedicle that causes obstruction to ovarian blood flow, potentially leading to necrosis of ovarian tissue.

Ovulation: The natural process of expulsion of a mature egg from its ovarian follicle.

Ovulation induction (OI): Pharmacological treatment of women with anovulation or oligo-ovulation with the intention of inducing normal ovulatory cycles.

Parthenogenetic activation: The process by which an oocyte is activated to undergo development in the absence of fertilization.

Parthenote: The product of an oocyte that has undergone activation in the absence of the paternal genome, with (induced) or without (spontaneous) a purposeful intervention.

Percutaneous epididymal sperm aspiration (PESA): A surgical procedure in which a needle is introduced percutaneously into the epididymis with the intention of obtaining sperm.

Perinatal death/mortality: Fetal or neonatal death occurring during late pregnancy (at 22 completed weeks of gestational age and later), during childbirth, or up to seven completed days after birth.

Perinatal mortality rate: The number of perinatal deaths per 1,000 total births (stillbirths plus live births).

Period total fertility rate (PTFR): The estimated average number of live born children per woman that would be born to a cohort of women throughout their reproductive years, if the fertility rates by age in a given period remained constant at the current age-specific fertility rate.

Perivitelline space: The space between the cytoplasmic membrane enclosing the oocyte and the innermost layer of the zona pellucida. (This space may contain the first and second polar bodies and extracellular fragments.)

Pituitary down-regulation: A medical or pharmacological method to prevent the release of gonadotropins (FSH, LH) from the pituitary gland.

Polar bodies: The small bodies containing chromosomes segregated from the oocyte by asymmetric division during telophase. The first polar body is extruded at telophase I and normally contains only chromosomes with duplicated chromatids (2 c); the second polar body is extruded in response to fertilization or in response to parthenogenetic activation and normally contains chromosomes comprising single chromatids (1 c).

Polycystic ovary syndrome (PCOS): A heterogeneous condition, which requires the presence of two of the following three criteria: (1) Oligoovulation or anovulation; (2) Hyperandrogenism (clinical evidence of hirsutism, acne, alopecia and/or biochemical hyperandrogenemia); (3) Polycystic ovaries, as assessed by ultrasound scan with more than 24 total antral follicles (2–9 mm in size) in both ovaries.

Polycystic ovary (PCO): An ovary with at least 12 follicles measuring 2–9 mm in diameter in at least one ovary (Rotterdam criteria). PCO may be present in women with PCOS, but also in women with normal ovulatory function and normal fertility.

Polyploidy: The condition in which a cell has more than two haploid sets of chromosomes: e.g. a triploid embryo has three sets of chromosomes and a tetraploid embryo has four sets. Polyploidy in a human embryo is not compatible with life.

Polyspermy: The process by which an oocyte is penetrated by more than one spermatozoon.

Poor ovarian responder (POR) in assisted reproductive technology: A woman treated with ovarian stimulation for ART, in which at least two of the following features are present: (1) Advanced maternal age (≥40 years); (2) A previous poor ovarian response (≤3 oocytes with a conventional stimulation protocol aimed at obtaining more than three oocytes); and, (3) An abnormal ovarian reserve test (i.e. antral follicle count 5–7 follicles or anti-Müllerian hormone 0.5–1.1 ng/mL (Bologna criteria); or other reference values obtained from a standardized reference population.)

Poor ovarian response (POR) to ovarian stimulation: A condition in which fewer than four follicles and/or oocytes are developed/obtained following ovarian stimulation with the intention of obtaining more follicles and oocytes.

Postimplantation embryo: An embryo at a stage of development beyond attachment to the endometrium to eight completed weeks after fertilization, which is equivalent to 10 weeks of gestational age.

Post-term birth: A live birth or stillbirth that takes place after 42 completed weeks of gestational age.

Posthumous reproduction: A process utilizing gametes and/or embryos from a deceased person or persons with the intention of producing offspring.

Pregnancy: A state of reproduction beginning with implantation of an embryo in a woman and ending with the complete expulsion and/or extraction of all products of implantation.

Pregnancy loss: The outcome of any pregnancy that does not result in at least one live birth. When reporting pregnancy loss, the estimated gestational age at the end of pregnancy should be recorded.

Pregnancy of unknown location (PUL): A pregnancy documented by a positive human chorionic gonadotropin (hCG) test without visualization of pregnancy by ultrasound. This condition exists only after circulating hCG concentration is compatible with ultrasound visualization of a gestational sac.

Preimplantation embryo: An embryo at a stage of development beginning with division of the zygote into two cells and ending just prior to implantation into a uterus.

Preimplantation genetic testing (PGT): A test performed to analyze the DNA from oocytes (polar bodies) or embryos (cleavage stage or blastocyst) for HLA-typing or for determining genetic abnormalities. These include: PGT for aneuploidies (PGT-A); PGT for monogenic/single gene defects (PGT-M); and PGT for chromosomal structural rearrangements (PGT-SR).

Preimplantation genetic diagnosis (PGD) and screening (PGS): These terms have now been replaced by preimplantation genetic testing PGT. (See term PGT and its definitions.)

Premature ejaculation: A condition in which semen is released sooner than desired.

Premature ovarian insufficiency: A condition characterized by hypergonadotropic hypogonadism in women younger than age 40 (also known as premature or primary ovarian failure). It includes women with premature menopause.

Preterm birth: A birth that takes place after 22 weeks and before 37 completed weeks of gestational age.

Primary childlessness: A condition in which a person has never delivered a live child, or has never been a legal or societally recognized parent to a child.

Primary female infertility: A woman who has never been diagnosed with a clinical pregnancy and meets the criteria of being classified as having infertility.

Primary involuntary childlessness: A condition in a person with a child wish, who has never delivered a live child, or has never been a legal or societally recognized parent to a child. A major cause of primary involuntary childlessness is infertility.

Primary male infertility: A man who has never initiated a clinical pregnancy and meets the criteria of being classified as infertile.

Pronuclei transfer: Transfer of the pronuclei from a patient's zygote to an enucleated donated zygote.

Pronucleus: A round structure in the oocyte surrounded by a membrane containing chromatin. Normally, two pronuclei are seen after fertilization, each containing a haploid set of chromosomes, one set from the oocyte and one from the sperm, before zygote formation.

Recipient (ART): A person or couple who receives donated eggs, sperm or embryos for the purposes of initiating a pregnancy with the intention of becoming a legally recognized parent.

Recipient ART cycle: An ART cycle in which a woman receives zygote(s) or embryo(s) from donor(s) or a partner.

Recurrent spontaneous abortion/miscarriage: The spontaneous loss of two or more clinical pregnancies prior to 22 completed weeks of gestational age.

Reproductive surgery: Surgical procedures performed to diagnose, conserve, correct and/or improve reproductive function in either men or women. Surgery for contraceptive purposes, such as tubal ligation and vasectomy, are also included within this term.

Retrograde ejaculation: A condition that causes the semen to be forced backward from the ejaculatory ducts into the bladder during ejaculation.

Salpingectomy: The surgical removal of an entire fallopian tube.

Salpingitis isthmica nodosa (SIN): A nodular thickening of the proximal fallopian tube (where the tubes join the uterus), which can distort or occlude the tubes and increase the risk of ectopic pregnancy and infertility.

Salpingostomy: A surgical procedure in which an opening is made in the fallopian tube either to remove an ectopic pregnancy or open a blocked fluid-filled tube (hydrosalpinx).

Secondary female infertility: A woman unable to establish a clinical pregnancy but who has previously been diagnosed with a clinical pregnancy.

Secondary involuntary childlessness: A condition in a person with a child wish, who has previously delivered a live child, or is or has been a legal or societally recognized parent to a child. A major cause of secondary involuntary childlessness is infertility.

Secondary male infertility: A man who is unable to initiate a clinical pregnancy, but who had previously initiated a clinical pregnancy.

Semen analysis: A description of the ejaculate to assess function of the male reproductive tract. Characteristic parameters include volume, pH, concentration, motility, vitality, morphology of spermatozoa and presence of other cells.

Semen liquefaction: The process whereby proteolytic enzymes degrade proteins causing seminal plasma to liquefy.

Semen viscosity: The description of the relative fluidity of seminal plasma.

Semen volume: The amount of fluid in an ejaculate.

Semen/Ejaculate: The fluid at ejaculation that contains the cells and secretions originating from the testes and sex accessory glands.

Seminal plasma: The fluids of the ejaculate.

Sertoli cell: The non-germinal cell type in the seminiferous tubule that mediates the actions of testosterone and FSH in the testis, provides nutrients and proteins to the developing spermatogenic cells, creates the blood-testis barrier, and secretes Müllerian-inhibiting hormone.

Sertoli cell-only syndrome: A condition in which only Sertoli cells line the seminiferous tubules with usually a complete absence of germ cells; also referred to as germ cell aplasia. Spermatogenesis in isolated foci can be observed in rare cases.

Severe ovarian hyperstimulation syndrome (OHSS): A systemic response as a result of ovarian stimulation interventions that is characterized by severe abdominal discomfort and/or other symptoms of ascites, haemoconcentration (Hct > 45) and/or other serious biochemical abnormalities requiring hospitalization for observation and/or for medical intervention (paracentesis, other).

Single embryo transfer (SET): The transfer of one embryo in an ART procedure. Defined as elective (eSET) when more than one embryo of sufficient quality for transfer is available.

Slow-freezing: A cryopreservation procedure in which the temperature of the cell(s) is lowered in a step-wise fashion, typically using a computer controlled rate, from physiological (or room) temperature to extreme low temperature.

Small for gestational age: A birth weight less than the 10th centile for gestational age. When reporting results the reference criteria should be specified. If gestational age is unknown, the birth weight should be registered.

Sperm bank: Repository of cryopreserved sperm stored for future use.

Sperm concentration: The (measure of the) number of spermatozoa in millions per 1 mL of semen.

Sperm density: A measure of the mass/volume ratio (specific gravity) for spermatozoa.

Sperm isolation: A procedure that involves the separation of sperm through centrifugation and resuspension in culture media. It can be used to remove seminal plasma and infectious agents before IUI and ART procedures. This procedure has been shown to be effective in the removal of HIV. It may also be effective in removing other infectious particles but clinical safety and efficacy have to be established for each particular infection. This term is sometimes referred to as 'sperm washing'.

Sperm motility: The percentage of moving spermatozoa relative to the total number of spermatozoa.

Sperm recipient cycle: A MAR cycle in which a woman receives spermatozoa from a person who is not her sexually intimate partner. In the case of ART registry data, a sperm recipient cycle would only include data from cycles using ART procedures.

Sperm vitality: The percentage of live spermatozoa relative to the total number of spermatozoa.

Spermatogenic arrest: Failure of germ cells to progress through specific stages of spermatogenesis at onset or during meiosis.

Spermatozoon: The mature male reproductive cell produced in the testis that has the capacity to fertilize an oocyte. A head carries genetic material, a midpiece produces energy for movement, and a long, thin tail propels the sperm.

Spontaneous abortion/miscarriage: The spontaneous loss of an intrauterine pregnancy prior to 22 completed weeks of gestational age.

Spontaneous reduction/vanishing sac(s): The spontaneous disappearance of one or more gestational sacs with or without an embryo or fetus in a multiple pregnancy documented by ultrasound.

Sterility: A permanent state of infertility.

Stillbirth: The death of a fetus prior to the complete expulsion or extraction from its mother after 28 completed weeks of gestational age. The death is determined by the fact that, after such separation, the fetus does not breathe or show any other evidence of life, such as heartbeat, umbilical cord pulsation, or definite movement of voluntary muscles. Note: It includes deaths occurring during labour.

Stillbirth rate: The number of stillbirths per 1,000 total births (stillbirths plus live births).

Subfertility: A term that should be used interchangeably with infertility.

Syngamy: The process during which the female and male pronuclei fuse.

Teratozoospermia: A reduced percentage of morphologically normal sperm in the ejaculate below the lower reference limits. When reporting results, the reference criteria should be specified.

Testicular sperm aspiration/extraction (TESA/TESE): A surgical procedure involving one or more testicular biopsies or needle aspirations to obtain sperm for use in IVF and/or ICSI.

Thawing: The process of raising the temperature of slow-frozen cell(s) from the storage temperature to room/physiological temperature.

Time to pregnancy (TTP): The time taken to establish a pregnancy, measured in months or in numbers of menstrual cycles.

Time-lapse imaging: The photographic recording of microscope image sequences at regular intervals in ART, referring to gametes, zygotes, cleavage stage embryos or blastocysts.

Total delivery rate with at least one live birth: The total number of deliveries with at least one live birth resulting from one initiated or aspirated ART cycle, including all cycles in which fresh and/or frozen embryos are transferred, including more than one delivery from one initiated or aspirated cycle if that occurs, until all embryos are used. Notes: The delivery of a singleton, twin or other multiple pregnancy is registered as one delivery. In the absence of complete data, the total delivery rate is often estimated.

Total fertility rate (TFR): The average number of live births per woman. It may be determined in retrospect, observed data (Cohort Total Fertility Rate, CTFR) or as an estimated average number (Period Total Fertility Rate, PTFR).

Total sperm count: The calculated total number of sperm in the ejaculate (semen volume multiplied by the sperm concentration determined from an aliquot of semen).

Traditional gestational carrier: A woman who donates her oocytes and is the gestational carrier for a pregnancy resulting from fertilization of her oocytes either through an ART procedure or insemination. This replaces the term 'traditional surrogate'.

Trisomy: An abnormal number of chromosome copies in a cell characterized by the presence of three homologous chromosomes rather than the normal two. The majority of human embryos with trisomies are incompatible with life.

Trophectoderm: Cells forming the outer layer of a blastocyst that have the potential to develop into the placenta and amniotic membranes.

Tubal pathology: Tubal abnormality resulting in dysfunction of the fallopian tube, including partial or total obstruction of one or both tubes (proximally, distally or combined), hydrosalpinx and/or peri-tubal and/or peri-ovarian adhesions affecting the normal ovum pickup function. It usually occurs after pelvic inflammatory disease or pelvic surgery.

Unexplained infertility: Infertility in couples with apparently normal ovarian function, fallopian tubes, uterus, cervix and pelvis and with adequate coital frequency; and apparently normal testicular function, genito-urinary anatomy and a normal ejaculate. The potential for this diagnosis is dependent upon the methodologies used and/or those methodologies available.

Unisomy: The condition in a cell resulting from loss of a single chromosome yielding a single copy of that particular chromosome rather than the normal two. The majority of unisomies in human embryos are incompatible with life.

Vaginal insemination: A procedure whereby semen, collected from a non-lubricated condom or similar method, is deposited into the vaginal cavity of a female. An intervention that can be self-administered by a woman attempting pregnancy.

Varicocele: A venous enlargement in the testicular pampiniform plexus.

Varicocelectomy: Procedure to occlude or remove part of the internal spermatic vein in situations in which it has expanded into a varicocele.

Vasectomy: Procedure to occlude the vas deferens. It is usually carried out bilaterally in order to secure sterilization.

Very low birth weight: Birth weight less than 1500 grams.

Viscosity: The description of the relative fluidity of the semen.

Vitrification: An ultra-rapid cryopreservation procedure that prevents ice formation within a cell whose aqueous phase is converted to a glass-like solid.

Voluntary childlessness: A condition describing a person who does not have or has not had a child wish and does not have any biologically, legally or societally recognized children.

Warming (cells): The process of raising the temperature of a vitrified cell or cells from the storage temperature to room/physiological temperature.

Y-chromosome microdeletions: Missing segments of the genetic material on the Y-chromosome that are associated with abnormal spermatogenesis.

Zona pellucida: The glycoprotein coat surrounding the oocyte.

Zygote: A single cell resulting from fertilization of a mature oocyte by a spermatozoon and before completion of the first mitotic division.

Zygote intrafallopian transfer (ZIFT): An ART procedure in which one or more zygotes is transferred into the fallopian tube.

Appendix C ICMART Data Collection Form

World Report on ART, National Form, Reporting Year 2014

Form 1. Organization of National ART Registers

Country name		☐☐☐
Contact person:	Full name	
	Institution	
	Address	
	Tel. Fax	
	Email	
Number of ART clinics in the country:	Total (included or not) Number included in the report	☐☐☐ ☐☐☐
Size of all country ART clinics. Number of clinics included in the report with, per year:		
	<100 cycles	☐☐
	100 – 199 cycles	☐☐
	200 – 499 cycles	☐☐
	500 – 999 cycles	☐☐
	≥1000 cycles	☐☐
Estimation of the total number of cycles in your country for reporting year 2013 (included or not in the report). The number of cycles per year includes all the initiated ("intention to treat") cycles for the purpose of IVF, ICSI, FET and OD. (See instructions.)		☐☐☐☐☐☐
Reporting requirement: 1. Compulsory; 2. Voluntary; 3. Other (please describe)		☐
Responsibility for the data register: 1. National Health Authority; 2. Medical Organization; 3. Other (please describe) 4. Not applicable		☐
Reporting methods:		
Cycles: 1. Individual cycles; 2. Summaries of cycles reported by the clinics		☐
Deliveries: 1. Individual cycles; 2. Summaries of deliveries reported by the clinics		☐
Link to other registers		
Birth register:		☐ No ☐ Yes
Congenital anomalies register:		☐ No ☐ Yes
Cytogenetic register:		☐ No ☐ Yes
Pre-implantation Genetic Diagnosis (PGD) register:		☐ No ☐ Yes
Disease register:		☐ No ☐ Yes
Other register: Please describe:		☐ No ☐ Yes
Total numbers of deliveries in the same year 2014 (if available) in the country, ART and non ART		
Total numbers of babies born in the same year 2014 (if available) in the country, ART and non ART		

In your country IVF register (or in a linkable register), is information available on:

	In general,	By technique,	By multiplicity
- Prematurity	☐ No ☐ Yes	☐ No ☐ Yes	☐ No ☐ Yes
- Perinatal mortality	☐ No ☐ Yes	☐ No ☐ Yes	☐ No ☐ Yes
- Malformation	☐ No ☐ Yes	☐ No ☐ Yes	☐ No ☐ Yes

If Yes, would you be able to send such data to ICMART register?   ☐ No ☐ Yes
If Yes, we will contact you later.

Comments

Form 2. Number of Treatments and Pregnancies

2(a). General procedures

	Fresh cycles[*]			FET[**]	Thawed oocytes[***]
	IVF	ICSI	GIFT	all	Thawings
Initiated cycles					*Thawings*
Aspirations				*Thawings*	
Embryos freezing without transfers				----	----
Transfers					
Pregnancies					
Deliveries: Total					
With live birth					

* *Include: GIFT cycles and cycles for foreign patients. Exclude: PGD, PGS, OD and cycles with oocyte freezing. (PGD and PGS results will be reported in Forms 7a and 7b. OD results will be reported in Form 8.)*

** *Information of FET cycles regardless of the fertilization technique (IVF or ICSI), but exclude PGD, PGS and OD. Record the numbers of cycles where frozen embryos were thawed for use in the box for Aspirations.*

*** *Cycles specifically performed with thawed oocytes.*

Additional information

• *Assisted hatching and in vitro maturation have to be included in the column of the relevant fertilization technique (IVF or ICSI).*
• *Where both conventional (standard) IVF and ICSI were used, report the technique that resulted in the transferred embryos. If both types of embryos were transferred, count as ICSI. This will apply to all the forms when both IVF and ICSI are performed in a single cycle. If both fresh and frozen embryos are transferred in a single cycle, report as a fresh embryo transfer cycle.*
• *In countries where surrogacy is performed, report surrogacy cycles with the fertilization technique (IVF or ICSI) that was used, without specifying it on all the forms. There are specific questions regarding surrogacy at the bottom of Form 9.*

2(b). Report on oocyte freezing[*]

Total number of cycles[**]	Freezing during an ART cycle	Cycles performed for fertility preservation only	
		Medical reason[***]	Social reason

* *Only report the numbers of cycles with freezing*

** *Include both freezing for Fertility Preservation and during ART (non-fertility preservation)*

*** *Cancer or other major medical disease*

In Vitro Maturation	Aspirations	Transfers	Pregnancies	Deliveries

See instructions specific to this form and use ICMART/WHO definitions in glossary.

2(c). Cycles performed for cross-border patients*

a. Summary of cycles

	Woman's own oocytes				Oocyte Donation	
	IVF	ICSI	GIFT	PGD	Anonymous	Non anonymous
Initiated cycles						

b. Countries of patients' origin and main reasons for cross-border travel for treatment

Main Countries of origin**		
	Country	Cycles
1.		
2.		
3.		
4.		
5.		
6.	Others (total)	

	Reason	Cycles
Legal	Illegal technique in home country	
	Illegal patients characteristics***	
Access	Care more expensive in home country	
	Distance, waiting list	
Quality	Previous failures	
Other		

* Patients living in a different country from the one where they had ART.

** Indicate the 5 main countries of patients' origin and give the number of cycles for each of them. Give the total number of cycles for all others.

*** For example, age limitation, legal couple status, sexual orientation, etc.

See instructions specific to this form and use ICMART/WHO definitions in glossary.

Form 3. Results by Women's Age and ART Technique

3(a). Fresh cycles

Women's age	After IVF			After ICSI			After both IVF and ICSI		
	Aspirations	Pregnancies	Deliveries*	Aspirations	Pregnancies	Deliveries*	Aspirations	Pregnancies	Deliveries*
≤34									
35–39									
≥40									

Note: This table excludes PGD, PGS and OD, which should be reported in Forms 7a, 7b and 8, respectively.

3(b). Frozen embryos transfers

Women's age	After IVF			After ICSI			After both IVF and ICSI		
	Thaws	Pregnancies	Deliveries*	Thaws	Pregnancies	Deliveries*	Thaws	Pregnancies	Deliveries*
≤34									
35–39									
≥40									

Note: This table excludes PGD, PGS and OD, which should be reported in Forms 7a, 7b and 8, respectively.

Aspirations: Include attempted aspirations in which no eggs were recovered.

Pregnancy: Evidence of pregnancy by clinical or ultrasound parameters (visualization of a gestational sac). It includes ectopic pregnancy. Multiple gestational sacs in one patient are counted as one clinical pregnancy.

Delivery: The expulsion or extraction of one or more fetuses from the mother after 22 completed weeks of gestational age.

Form 4. Results by Number of Transferred Embryos

4(a). All IVF and/or ICSI fresh cycles

	Number of transferred embryos							
	1		2		3	4	≥5	Total
	All	Elective*	All	Elective*				
Transfer cycles								
Clinical pregnancies								
Pregnancy losses**								
Deliveries: Total								
Singleton								
Twin								
Triplet +								
Lost to Follow-up								

Note: This table excludes PGD, PGS and OD, which should be reported in Forms 7a, 7b and 8, respectively.

* If possible, indicate the number of elective single and double embryo transfers.

** Abortions (spontaneous and induced) and ectopic pregnancies.

4(b). All FET cycles (resulting from IVF and/or ICSI)

| | Number of transferred embryos | | | | | | | |
| | 1 | | 2 | | 3 | 4 | ≥5 | Total |
	All	Elective*	All	Elective*				
Transfer cycles								
Clinical pregnancies								
Pregnancy losses**								
Deliveries: Total								
Singleton								
Twin								
Triplet +								
Lost to Follow-up								

Note: This table excludes PGD, PGS and OD, which should be reported in Forms 7a, 7b and 8, respectively.

* If possible, indicate the number of elective single and double embryo transfers.

** Abortions (spontaneous and induced) and ectopic pregnancies.

Form 5. Gestational Age by Treatment and Multiple Deliveries

5(a). Fresh cycles (total aspiration cycles following IVF and/or ICSI)

| Deliveries* | Gestational age (calculated completed weeks of amenorrhoea) | | | | | | |
	All	22–27	28–32	33–36	37–41	42 +	Unknown
Singleton							
Twin							
Triplet							
Quadruplet or higher							
Unknown							
Total							

Note: This table excludes PGD, PGS and OD, which should be reported in Forms 7a, 7b and 8, respectively.

* Deliveries: the expulsion or extraction of one or more fetuses from the mother after 22 completed weeks of gestational age.

5(b). FET cycles (total transfer cycles using only frozen embryos following IVF and/or ICSI)

Deliveries*	Gestational age (calculated as completed weeks of amenorrhoea)						
	All	22–27	28–32	33–36	37–41	42 +	Unknown
Singleton							
Twin							
Triplet							
Quadruplet or higher							
Unknown							
Total							

Note: This table excludes PGD, PGS and OD, which should be reported in Forms 7a, 7b and 8, respectively.

* Deliveries: the expulsion or extraction of one or more fetuses from the mother after 22 completed weeks of gestational age.

Gestational age calculation

- *Fresh cycles:* calculate the number of days between oocyte collection and delivery, add 14 days, divide the sum by 7 and use the integer.

- *FET cycles:* calculate the number of days between transfer and delivery date, add the embryo age at transfer (generally 2 to 6 days), add 14 days, divide the sum by 7 and use the integer.

Form 6. Neonatal Outcome in Relation to Treatment

6(a). Fresh cycles (total aspiration cycles following IVF and/or ICSI)

Number of babies	Health Status in the Perinatal Period Number of neonates				
	Total	Stillbirths	Live births	Neonatal deaths	Unknown
Singleton					
Twin					
Triplet					
Quadruplet or higher					
Unknown					
Total					

Note: This table excludes PGD, PGS and OD, which should be reported in Forms 7a, 7b and 8, respectively.
* Deliveries: the expulsion or extraction of one or more fetuses from the mother after 22 completed weeks of gestational age.

6(b). FET cycles (total transfer cycles using only frozen embryos following IVF and/or ICSI)

Number of babies	Health Status in the Perinatal Period Number of neonates				
	Total	Stillbirths	Live births	Neonatal deaths	Unknown
Singleton					
Twin					
Triplet					
Quadruplet or higher					
Unknown					
Total					

Notes: This table excludes PGD, PGS and OD, which should be reported in Forms 7a, 7b and 8, respectively.

Forms 6a and 6b report number of neonates (2 for twins, 3 for triplets, etc.).

- Live births: ≥22 weeks

- Stillbirths: ≥28 weeks

- Neonatal deaths are all the deaths occurring after live birth, up to 7 completed days of life.

Form 7(a). Preimplantation Genetic Diagnosis

	Women's age				
	≤34	35–39	≥40	Unknown	Total
Initiated cycles					
Aspirations					
Transfers					
Embryos examined					
Embryos normal					
Embryos transferred					
Pregnancies, clinical					
Deliveries: Total					
Singleton					
Twin					
Triplet or higher					
Unknown					
Babies born: Total					
Stillbirths					
Live births					
Neonatal deaths					
Unknown					

Note: Regardless of fertilization technique.

- Live births: ≥22 weeks

- Stillbirths: ≥28 weeks

- Neonatal deaths are all the deaths occurring after live birth, up to 7 completed days of life.

- Preimplantation Genetic Diagnosis (PGD): analysis of polar bodies, blastomeres, or trophectoderm from oocytes, zygotes, or embryos for the detection of specific genetic, structural, and/or chromosomal alterations.

Form 7(b). Preimplantation Genetic Screening

	Women's age				
	≤34	35–39	≥40	Unknown	Total
Initiated cycles					
Aspirations					
Transfers					
Embryos examined					
Embryos normal					
Embryos transferred					
Pregnancies, clinical					
Deliveries: Total					
Singleton					
Twin					
Triplet or higher					
Unknown					
Babies born: Total					
Stillbirths					
Live births					
Neonatal deaths					
Unknown					

Note: Regardless of fertilization technique.

- Live births: ≥22 weeks

- Stillbirths: ≥28 weeks

- Neonatal deaths are all the deaths occurring after live birth, up to 7 completed days of life.

- Preimplantation Genetic Screening (PGS): analysis of polar bodies, blastomeres, or trophectoderm from oocytes, zygotes, or embryos for the detection of aneuploidy, mutation, and/or DNA rearrangement

Form 8. Oocyte Donation

8(a). Aspiration cycles (donor)

	Women's age (donor)				
	≤34	35–39	≥40	Unknown	Total
Initiated cycles					
Aspirations: Total					
Specific donors					
Egg sharing					

8(b). Oocyte donation transfer cycles in recipients (fresh cycles)

	Women's age (recipient)					
	≤34	35–39	40–44	≥45	Unknown	Total
Transfers, total						
1 Embryo						
2 Embryos						
3 Embryos						
4 Embryos						
≥5 Embryos						
Pregnancies, clinical						
Deliveries: Total						
Singleton						
Twin						
Triplet						
Quadruplet or higher						
Unknown number						
Babies born: Total						
Stillbirths						
Live births						
Neonatal deaths						
Unknown						

Note: Regardless of the fertilization technique.

- *Live births: ≥22 weeks*

- *Stillbirths: ≥28 weeks*

- *Neonatal deaths are all the deaths occurring after live birth, up to 7 completed days of life.*

8(c). Oocyte donation transfer cycles in recipients (FET cycles)

	Women's age (recipient)					Total
	≤34	35−39	40−44	≥45	Unknown	Total
Transfers: Total						
1 Embryo						
2 Embryos						
3 Embryos						
4 Embryos						
≥ 5 Embryos						
Pregnancies, clinical						
Deliveries: Total						
Singleton						
Twin						
Triplet						
Quadruplet or higher						
Babies born: Total						
Stillbirths						
Live births						
Neonatal deaths						
Unknown						

Note: Regardless of the fertilization technique.

- Live births: ≥22 weeks

- Stillbirths: ≥28 weeks

- Neonatal deaths are all the deaths occurring after live birth, up to 7 completed days of life.

Form 9. Complications of Treatment

9(a). Women's complications with admission to hospital or medical intervention

	Number of cases*
Hyperstimulation syndrome	
Complications of oocyte retrieval: All	
Bleeding**	
Infection***	
Maternal death (documented)	

* *If a woman had two occurrences of the same complication, in 2 different cycles, count her twice. If a woman had two different complications, count her in each of them.*

** *Report bleeding if patient required a blood transfusion and/or was hospitalized.*

*** *Report infection if patient required intravenous/intramuscular antibiotics and/or was hospitalized.*

9(b). Congenital anomalies

Technique	Number of neonates/fetuses with congenital anomalies*				
	Total**	Delivered***	Fetal losses		
			Spontaneous	Induced	Total
IVF fresh cycles					
ICSI fresh cycles					
FET (IVF and/or ICSI)					
Oocyte donation					
PGD					
PGS					
GIFT					
TOTAL					

* *Malformations and genetic abnormalities.*

** *Delivered neonates include stillbirths and those with unknown health status at birth.*

*** *Including stillbirths and those with unknown health status at birth.*

If possible, report individual information on each malformed neonate or fetus on Form 10.

Additional Questions

1. Is in vitro maturation performed in your country?	☐ No	☐ Yes
If yes, indicate the number of cycles.		
2. Is fetal reduction allowed in your country?	☐ No	☐ Yes
If yes, indicate the number performed for ART pregnancies.		
3. Is maternal surrogacy allowed in your country?	☐ No	☐ Yes
If yes, indicate the number of ART aspiration cycles for surrogacy.		
If yes, indicate the number of cycles with deliveries, with at least one live birth from surrogacy.		
4. Is sperm donation performed in your country?	☐ No	☐ Yes
If yes, indicate the number of cycles.		
5. Is embryo donation performed in your country?	☐ No	☐ Yes
If yes, indicate the number of cycles		

Form 10. List of Congenital Anomalies
(Malformations and Genetic Abnormalities)

Baby	Congenital anomalies (Describe all anomalies found in each baby)	Woman's Age*	ART Technique**	Semen/ sperm***	Gestational age at birth/abortion****	Status*****
1.						
2.						
3.						
4.						
5.						
6.						
7.						
8.						
9.						
10.						
11.						
12.						
13.						
14.						
15.						
16.						
17.						
18.						
19.						
20.						
21.						
22.						
23.						
24.						
25.						

* Woman's age at conception.

** ART technique: IVF, ICSI, FET (IVF or ICSI), oocyte donation, GIFT.

*** ART semen/sperm: ejaculated (spouse/donor), TESE, MESA, fresh or frozen.

**** Gestational age: completed weeks of amenorrhoea (see the comment on form 5).

***** Status: Spontaneous abortion (miscarriage), Induced abortion, Stillbirth, Live birth, Neonatal death.
    Copy and use additional pages as necessary.

Form 11. Intrauterine Insemination (IUI)

IUI-H (Husband/Partner Sperm)

	Woman <35 years	Woman 35–39 years	Woman ≥40 years	Total
Number of IUI-H cycles				
Pregnancies*				
Deliveries: Total				
Singleton				
Twin				
Triplet +				

* Includes all IUI with or without ovarian stimulation.

IUI-D (Donor Sperm)

	Woman <35 years	Woman 35–39 years	Woman ≥40 years	Total
Number of IUI-D cycles				
Pregnancies*				
Deliveries: Total				
Singleton				
Twin				
Triplet +				

* Includes all IUI with or without ovarian stimulation.

Comments

Index

References to figures are in *italics*; tables in **bold**

abdominal ultrasound, 5
acceptability, 29, 107–8, 112
accessibility, 15, 112
accreditation, 97, 129
    Australia, 142–5
    China, 133
    India, 136
    Latin America, 184–5
    United States, 70
accuracy, data *see* data quality
ACDC *see* Assisted Conception Data
    Collection
acrosomes, 209
adenomyosis, 209
adhesions, 209
adverse events, 26, 34, 61, **63–4**
    underreporting, 50
adverse reactions, 62
Africa, ART surveillance, 124
    challenges, 131
    data collection methodology, 128–9
    data scope, 129
    data validity, 129
    establishment, 127–8
    future directions, 131–2
    history, 124–5
    origins, 125–7
    success, 129–31
Africa, regional registry, 18
African Fertility Society (AFS), 125
African Network and Registry for ART
    (ANARA), 124, 127–9
    challenges, 131–2
    data scope, 129
    data validity, 129
    success, 129–31
age limits, 96, 139
age specific fertility rate (ASFR), 209
age-related statistics, 108, 193, **222, 224**
    Canada, 178
    Latin America, 187, *187*
    United States, 175
agglutination, 209
AHEC (Australian Health Ethics
    Committee), 143
ANARA (African Network and
    Registry for ART), 124, 127–9
    challenges, 131–2

data scope, 129
data validity, 129
success, 129–31
andrology, 209
aneuploidy, 111, 119, 182, 209
anonymity
    child, 35
    clinics, 97, 127
    donor, 120
    patients, 169
anti-sperm antibodies, 209
ANZARD *see* Australian and New
    Zealand Assisted Reproduction
    Database
ART *see* assisted reproductive
    technology
Asia
    ART surveillance, 133, 139–41
    regional registry, 139
aspermia, 209
assessment, pre-treatment, 119
Assisted Conception Data Collection
    (ACDC), 145, 147
assisted hatching, 6, 26, 209
assisted reproductive technology (ART)
    (general)
    Africa, *126*
    Australia, 142–7
    China, 133–4, *134*
    definitions, 81, 200, 209
    early history, 2–7
    ethical aspects, 116
    global policy overview, 119–21
    global trends, *7*
    global variations, 7–8, 107–8,
      120
    growth by region, *107*
    India, *137*
    Japan, *138*
    Latin America, *183*, **186**
    legal aspects, 8, 34, 119
    practices, 116
    quality assurance, 73
    reporting mechanisms, 117–19
    United States, 172–5
asthenoteratozoospermia, 209
asthenozoospermia, 209
auditing, data, 27, 35, 148

Australia, 142, 145–7
    governance, 142–5
    history of ART, 142
    national registry, 15–16, 38
    regional registry, 17
    surveillance, ART, 145–7
Australian and New Zealand Assisted
    Reproduction Database
    (ANZARD), 40, 142, 147–8, 150
    annual reports, 148–9
    clinics performance, 149
    data collection, 148, **149**
    data quality, 148
    research, 149–50
Australian Health Ethics Committee
    (AHEC), 143
autologous ART
    Australia, 142, *144*
    Canada, 178
azoospermia, 65, 209

Belgium, health outcomes, 203–4
benchmarking, 14
Bertarelli Foundation, 102
BESST (Birth Emphasizing a Successful
    Singleton at Term), 40
Better Outcomes Registry & Network
    (BORN), 177
biopsy, embryos, 7
biovigilance, 26, 60–1; *see also* safety
    monitoring
birth, extremely preterm, 211
Birth Emphasizing a Successful
    Singleton at Term (BESST), 40
birth rates
    cumulative, 14, 41
    per embryo transferred, 41, 95
    per oocyte collection, 41–2, 95
    per primary transfer, 42
    per subsequent transfer, 42
    per treatment cycle, 41, 95
birth weight, extremely low, 211
births, multiple *see* multiple
    pregnancies/births
blastocyst transfers, 49, 60
blastomeres, 209
bleeding after oocyte aspiration, 14,
    59–60, 209

blood transfusion, 33
bone marrow transplantation, 33
BORN (Better Outcomes Registry & Network), 177
Brave New World (novel), 3
Brown, Louise, 4, 48, 135, 172

Cameroon, 124, 127
Canada
    ART history, 177
    ART surveillance, 179–80
    data collection, 177–8
    data quality, 178–9
    primary infertility, 1
Canadian Assisted Reproductive Technologies Register (CARTR), 177–80
cancelled ART cycles, 176, 180, 209
cancer, risk from ART, 85, 87, 147, 176
cancer registries, 72, 86
cancers, gynaecological, 85
Carr, Elizabeth, 172
CARTR (Canadian Assisted Reproductive Technologies Register), 177
CARTR Plus, 177–80
CASS (cycle-based China ART surveillance system platform), 134–5
catheter designs, 4
Centers for Disease Control and Prevention (CDC), 23, 42; *see also* National ART Surveillance System
    annual reports, 69
    data access, 52
    data collection, 83–4, 172, **206–8**
    quality assurance, 73, 175–6
Chang, Min Chueh, 3, 3
childbearing, postponement, 2, 160–1
chimerism, 209
China, 107, 133, 135
    centre-based surveillance, 133–4
    cycle-based surveillance, 134–5
    infertility, 133
    national registry, 133
China ART surveillance system platform (CASS), 134–5
chromosome continuity, 2
cleavage stage embryos, 7, 51, 60, 209–10
clinical pregnancy, 95, 210
    with fetal heart beat, 177, 210
    rate, 40, 210
clinical research, 47, 53
    access to data, 52–3
    advantages, 50, **51**
    limitations, 50–2, **51**
    safety, 48–50
    success rates, 47–8

clinical trials, 31, 37, 93
clinics, performance
    ANZARD, 149
    claims, 97
    comparisons, 97
    cycle rates, 96
    results presentation, 96, 176
    service presentation, 96–7
    United States, 172, *175*
clomiphene/clomiphene citrate, 4, 81, 200
    intrauterine insemination, 192, 194, 195
cohort total fertility rate (CTFR), 210
collaboration, government and professional bodies, 24
Committee of Nordic Assisted Reproductive Technology and Safety (CoNARTaS), 49, 87
compaction, 210
complete cycles, success rates, 37, 40–1, 43
complex aneuploidies, 210
complications, 14–15, 31, 34, 49, 59–60, 158–9, *160*, **231**; *see also* multiple pregnancies/births; ovarian hyperstimulation syndrome
    data collection, 109, 167
    IVF, 56–7
    patient education, 93
    perinatal, 49
    pregnancy, 49, 82
    risk management, 61
    United States, 176
components, ART cycle, 26, 27–8, 176
confidentiality *see* data confidentiality
confounding by indication, **51**, 52
congenital anomalies, **233**, 12, 34, 210
    Australia, 147
    birth rate, 210
    major, 145, 147, 213
congenital bilateral absence of the vasa deferentia (CBAVD), 210
contamination
    safety monitoring, 65
    semen, 65
control charts, 75–8, *76*
control groups
    long-term outcomes, 82, 85
    sibling studies, 50
conventional in vitro insemination, *76*, 210
corona radiata cells, 210
correlation
    aggregate data, 168
    cycle-level data, **51**, 52, 188, 193
    gender inequality, 112
cost efficiency, intrauterine insemination, 194–5

Costa Rica, 184
counselling, infertility, 37, 44, 60, 94–5, 143, 213
couples *see* patients
cross-border fertility care, 34, 103, 210, **222**
    Europe, 153
    Middle East, 167
    North America, 103
cross-sectional data analysis, 32
cryopreservation, 6, 32, 37, 119, 210
    embryos, 81, 157–8
    Middle East, 165–6
    success rates, 40
cryotanks failures, 64
cryptorchidism, 210
culture media, 4, 63–4
cumulative birth rates, 41, 42, 48, 73
    Canada, 178
    Denmark, 48
    effectiveness, 108, *109*
    Europe, 61
    per aspiration/initiated cycle, 210
    per embryo transferred, 95
    Sweden, 48
    United Kingdom, 14
cumulative data recording, 33–4
cumulus oophorus, 210
cycle initiations, 26
cycle numbers, intrauterine insemination, 193
cycle rates, clinics, 96
cycle-based China ART surveillance system, 134–5
cycle-level data, 24–5, 107, 147
    correlation, 52
    Latin America, 182, 183
    United States, 176
cycles *see* complete cycles; hidden cycles; single cycles
cycle-specific ART data, 16
cytoplasmic maturation, 210
cytoplasmic transfer, 210

data auditing, 27, 35, 148
data collection, 12; *see also* registries
    ANZARD, 148, **149**
    ART safety, 49
    compulsory, **156**
    Human Fertilisation and Embryology Authority, 41–2
    inaccurate, 50–1
    incomplete, 50
    list of variables, **206–8**
    methodologies, 107
    Middle East, 165–8
    non-ART fertility treatments, 202–3
    quality, 13, 29, 33, 34–5, 117
data confidentiality, 28–9, 35, 52, 71
    Africa, 129

Australia and New Zealand, 145
Middle East, 164, 167, 168, 169
decreased spermatogenesis, 210
delayed ejaculation, 210
delayed embryo transfer, 32, 37, 210
demographic definitions, infertility, 1
demographics, patient, 25–6, 50, 109,
148, **149**
Denmark
children born by ART, 156
national registry, 48, 87, 203
denominators, ART success rate, 13
complete cycles, 40–1
embryo transfers, 40
initiated single cycles, 40
women/couples, 41
deterministic linkage, 82
diandric oocytes, 210
digynic oocytes, 210
diminished ovarian reserve, 210–11
diploidy/euploidy, 211
disomy, 211
donated embryos, 25
donated gametes, 25, 37, 69, 119, 187
donor characteristics, 25–6, 56
success rates, 178, *201*
donors
anonymity, 120
characteristics, 25–6, 56
health risks, 85
insemination, 211
sperm, 147, 203
double embryo transfers, 211

early neonatal death/mortality, 211
ectopic pregnancies, 211
Edwards, Robert, 3, 4
effectiveness/efficacy *see* performance
measures/indicators
eggs *see* oocytes
Egypt, 124, 126, 163, 165–7
EIM *see* European IVF Monitoring
Consortium
ejaculate/ejaculation, 211
delayed, 210
quality, 202
retardate, 211
ejaculatory duct, 211
elective embryo transfer, 211
elective single embryo transfer, 57,
58–9, 211
Europe, *58*
outcome metrics, 74
risk reduction, 159
embryonic cells, experimentation, 120
embryo(s)
bank, 85, 211
donations, 25, 211
double transfers, 211
fragmentation, 211

multiple transfers, 57, 109, 188, *189*
recipient cycles, 211
safety monitoring, 64–5
single transfers, 57, 109, 178–9
status, 120
transfer cycles, 211
transfers, 26, 31, 40, *58*, *110*, 211, **224**
transfers, Australia, *144*
transfers, Latin America, *188*
emission (semen), 211
endometriosis, 95, 191, 211
epidemiological definitions, infertility, 1
epididymis, 211
equipment, safety monitoring, 63
erectile dysfunction, 211
ESHRE *see* European Society of
Human Reproduction and
Embryology
estimates of success, 14
ethical aspects, 15, 119, 134–5, 143
euploidy, 211
Europe, regional registry, 17–18, 153
European IVF Monitoring (EIM)
Consortium, 14, 17–18, 24, 31,
153, 161
annual reports, **154**
ART success rates, 47
complications, ART, 158–9
data collection, 156–8
future directions, 159–61
non-ART fertility treatments, 201
participation, 153–6, *155*
European Society of Human
Reproduction and Embryology
(ESHRE), 17–18, 153
annual reports, 28, **154**, 193
European Union Standards and
Training for the Inspection of
Tissue Establishments
(EUSTITE) Project 186, 210
European Union Tissue and Cells
Directive (EUTCD), 61, 62, 63
excessive ovarian response, 26, 59, 211
expectant fertility management, 211
extremely low birth weight, 211
extremely preterm birth, 211

fecundability, 211
fecundity, 211
declining, 2
impaired, 1, **2**
female infertility, 2, 211; *see also*
infertility
FER *see* frozen embryo replacements/
transfers
fertility, definitions, 211–12
Fertility Clinic Success Rate and
Certification Act (FCSRCA), 42,
47, 172
fertility societies, Africa, 125

Fertility Treatment: Trends and Figures
report, 16
fertility treatments, non-ART, 191,
192, 200, 204
data access, 203
data collection, 202–3
definitions, 200
health outcomes, 203–4
monitoring, 200–1
national registries, 201–2
quality assurance, 203
regional registries, 201
fertilization, 2–3, 212; *see also* in vitro
fertilization
types, Latin America, *187*
FET *see* frozen embryo replacements/
transfers
fetal loss, 39, 212
flexibility, 29
fluorescence in situ hybridization
(FISH), 7
follicle stimulating hormone (FSH), 4
follow-up surveillance, 34
ART-conceived children, 82
ART-treated women, 82
France, 4, 5, 16, 18
freeze-all treatment cycles, 14, 48, 111,
142, 157, 178, 212
frozen embryo replacements/transfers
(FER/FET), 6, **223**, **230**
definition, 212
early history, 14
Europe, 156–7
health outcomes, **226**
Latin America, *188*
prediction models, 43
results, **224**, **225**
United States, 27
frozen-thawed oocyte cycles, 139, 212
FSH (follicle stimulating hormone), 4
full-term births, 212
funding, fertility treatments, 7–8

gamete intrafallopian transfer (GIFT),
81, 108, 212
Australia and New Zealand, 146
Latin America, 185–6
United States, 174
gametes
donated *see* donated gametes,
safety monitoring, 64–5
source, 25
transportation, 32
generalized estimating equations, 52
Germany
legal aspects, 203
national registry, 16, 56
germinal vesicle (GV), 212
gestational age, 17, 39, 49, 212
miscarriage, 105

gestational carriers, 5–6, 25–6, 37, 119, 212
  characteristics, 56
  Latin America, 182
  Middle East, 167
  traditional, 217
gestational sacs, 26–7, 212
gestations, multiple *see* multiple pregnancies/births
Ghana, 124, 127
GIERAF *see* Groupe Interafricain d'Etude, de Recherche et d'Application sur la Fertilité
GIFT (gamete intrafallopian transfer), 81, 108, 212
  Australia and New Zealand, 146
  Latin America, 185–6
  United States, 174
global access, 107–8
global ART glossary, ICMART, 105–6
global data collection, ICMART, 106
global registries, 16–17, 56
global reporting, challenges, 110–12
global trends, ART, 7, 108
globozoospermia, 212
glossaries, characteristics, 105
gonadotropins, 4
  doses, 8
  high-dose human menopausal, 4–5
  human menopausal, 4, 195
  low-dose, 193
Groupe Interafricain d'Etude, de Recherche et d'Application sur la Fertilité (GIERAF), 125, 127, 128
gynaecological cancers, 85

haploidy, 212
hatching, 212
  assisted, 6, 26, 209
health care, quality assurance, 71–2
health data transparency, 37
health outcomes, 37, 38, 43, 44, **225**
  ART-conceived children, 49
  children, 60
  clinical research, 47
  frozen embryo replacements/transfers, **226**
  long-term, 49
  non-ART fertility treatments, 203–4
  Nordic countries, 48
  public reporting, 93
healthy babies, success rates, 39–40
haemovigilance, 33, 72
heterologous insemination, success rates, *201, 202*
heterotopic pregnancy, 212
HFEA *see* Human Fertilisation and Embryology Authority
hidden cycles, 48

high-dose human menopausal gonadotropins, 4–5
high-order multiple births, 212
high-order multiple gestations, 212
HIV transmission, 191
homologous insemination, success rates, *201, 202*
Human Fertilisation and Embryology Authority (HFEA), 16, 27–8, 37
  annual reports, 65
  cumulative birth rates, 14
  data collection, 41–2
  Fertility Treatment Trends and Figures report, 16
  quality assurance, 69
  reporting requirements, 18, 27–8
Huxley, Aldous, 3
hydrosalpinx, 212
hypergonadotropic hypogonadism, 212
hyperspermia, 212
hypogonadotropic hypogonadism, 212
hypospermatogenesis, 212
hypospermia, 212

IAPO *see* International Alliance of Patients' Organisations
iatrogenic testicular failure, 212
ICMART *see* International Committee Monitoring Assisted Reproductive Technologies
ICSI *see* intracytoplasmic sperm injection
IFFS *see* International Federation of Fertility Societies
impaired fecundity, 1, **2**
implantation, 26–7, 212
  delayed, 32, 37, 210
  rates, 6, 39, 212
incidents, 61–2
India, 135–6, 137
  infertility, 135
  legislation, 136–7
  national registry, 136
  web-based registry, 136
Indian Society for Assisted Reproduction (ISAR), 136
induced abortion, 147, 213
induced embryo/fetal reduction, 213
industrial history, quality assurance, 70–1
infertility, 1, 8, 81, 213
  China, 133
  counselling, 37, 44, 60, 94–5, 143, 213
  definition, 108
  demographic definitions, 1
  epidemiological definitions, 1
  female, 2, 211
  global variations, ART, 7–8

India, 135
  prevalence, 1–2, **2**
  primary, 1
  secondary, 1, 216
  treatment, early history, 2–7
  unexplained, 191, 192, 217
information complexity, 93–4
initiated medically assisted reproduction cycle, 213
initiated single cycles, success rates, 40
inner cell mass, 213
insemination
  conventional in vitro, *76*, 210
  donor, 211
  intra-cervical, 213
  vaginal, 217
insemination and cycle-monitoring, 200
intended parents, 213
Inter American Court of Human Rights (ICHR), 184
International Alliance of Patients' Organisations (IAPO), 97
International Committee Monitoring Assisted Reproductive Technologies (ICMART), 13, 17, 101; *see also* International Working Group for Registers on Assisted Reproduction
  activities, 102–4
  Africa, 128–9
  ART success rates, 47
  Canada, 179
  Europe, 159
  formation and organization, 102
  global ART glossary, 105–6
  global reporting, 106–12
  global reports, future, 112–13
  glossary of terms, 95
  good practice, 112
  history, 101–2
  Middle East, 164, 165–6
  relationship with World Health Organization, 104–5
  useful data, 112
  value added, 112
International Federation of Fertility Societies (IFFS), 116, 121
  history, 116–17
  meetings, 101–2
  surveillance methodology, 117
  surveillance reports, 8
  triennial survey, 116–17, 119
International Working Group for Registers on Assisted Reproduction (IWGROAR), 16
  Africa, 126
  history, 101–2
  as predecessor to ICMART, 102
intra-cervical insemination, 200, 213

intracytoplasmic sperm injection
  (ICSI), 6, 26, 108, 213
  birth rates, 157
  China, 133
  global availability, 119
  Latin America, 185
  micromanipulation, 174
  Middle East, 166
intrauterine insemination (IUI), 191,
  195, 200, 213
  comparison with IVF, 191–2, 201
  cost efficiency, 194–5
  donor, *201*, *202*
  effectiveness/efficacy, 193–4
  equity in access, 195
  husband/partner, **234**
  number of attempts, 193
  ovarian stimulation, 192–3
  safety, 194
  success rates, *201*, *202*
in vitro fertilization and embryo
  transfer (IVF-ET)
  China, 133
  Japan, 137
in vitro fertilization (IVF), 212
  Australia, 142, 145–6
  birth rates, 157
  comparison with IUI, 191–2, 201
  health concerns, 12
  history, 1, 2–7
  India, 135–6
  Middle East, 163
  New Zealand, 142, 145–6
  United States, 172
  world report, 102
in vitro maturation (IVM), 212–13
Iran, national registry, 202
ISAR (Indian Society for Assisted
  Reproduction), 136
IUI *see* intrauterine insemination
IVF *see* in vitro fertilization
IWGROAR *see* International Working
  Group for Registers on Assisted
  Reproduction

Japan, 138
  national registry, 137–8, 139
  reporting mechanisms, 139
  web-based registry, 138–9
Japan Society of Obstetrics and
  Gynecology (JSOG), 137, 138

key performance indicators, 73
Kruger, Thinus, 124

laparoscopic ovarian drilling, 4, 213
large for gestational age, 213
Latin America, 189–90
  ART history, 182
  ART trends, 189

data access, 185
data quality, 184–5
legal aspects, 185
regional registry, 17, 182–4
religious influences, 182
statistics, *186*, **186**
Latin American Network of Assisted
  Reproductive Technology
  (REDLARA), 180, 182
  accreditation, 184–5
  annual reports, 184
  public policies, 184
Latin American Registry of Assisted
  Reproduction (RLA), 127, 129,
  131, 182
  ART success rates, 47
  history, 182–4
league tables
  birth rates, *74*, 97
  outcome metrics, 74
Lebanon, religious influences, 165
legal aspects
  ART, 8, 34, 119
  Germany, 203
  Latin America, 185
  reporting mechanisms, ART, 117–18
leukospermia, 213
Leydig cells, 213
LH (luteinizing hormone), 4
linkage, ART data, 25
linkage methodologies
  deterministic, 82
  probabilistic, 82
linked health data, 81–2
linking health databases, USA, 82–6
live births/deliveries, 13, 95, 213
  success rates, 25, 39, 73, 213
long-term outcomes, 49, 81–2, 88
  control groups, 82
  follow-up surveillance, 82
  linkage methodologies, 82
  population-based linkages, Nordic
    countries, 86–8
  population-based linkages, US, 82–6
  SART CORS, 52
long-term surveillance, 34
low birth weight, 49, 60, 146–7, 203–4,
  213
low-dose gonadotropins, 193
luteal phase
  defects, 213
  support, 213
luteinizing hormone (LH), 4

major congenital anomalies, 145, 147,
  213
male infertility, 2, 6, 213
  intrauterine insemination, 191–2
  Middle East, 166, 168
Mali, 124

manipulations, 26
maternal age, advancing, 2
maternal deaths, 60, 159
maternal risks
  immediate, 12
  long term, 12
maternal spindle transfer, 213
maternal surrogacy *see* gestational
  carriers
mature oocytes, 159, 191, 213
maturing oocytes, 213
Mauritius, 124
medical biotechnology vigilance, 61
medical surveillance *see* surveillance
medically assisted reproduction
  (MAR), 200, 213
  definitions, 200
medicine, quality assurance, 71–2
MEFS (Middle East Fertility Society),
  163–4
Mexico, ART surveillance, 179–80
microdissection testicular sperm
  extraction (MicroTESE), 213
micromanipulation, 6–7, 174, 213–14;
  see also intracytoplasmic sperm
  injection
microsurgical epididymal sperm
  aspiration/extraction (MESA/
  MESE), 214
Middle East, 163, 169
  ART history, 163
  ART surveillance, 168–9
  data collection, 165–7, 168
  data quality, 167–8
  regional registry, 126, 163–4
  regulation, 164–5
  religious influences, 163
Middle East Fertility Society (MEFS),
  163–4
mild ovarian stimulation, 200, 214
missed spontaneous abortion/missed
  miscarriage, 214
modified natural cycles, 13, 192, 214
monitoring *see* surveillance
monosomy, 214
morula, 214
mosaicism, 111, 214
motivations, data reporting, 28
Mukherjee, Dr S., 135
multinucleation, 214
multiple pregnancies/births, 39, 57–8,
  201, 214
  Australia and New Zealand, 146,
    147, 150
  Canada, 178–9
  Europe, 159
  gestational age, **224**
  high-order, 212
  intrauterine insemination, 194,
    200–1

Japan, 138
likelihood, 95–6
Middle East, 166–7
outcome metrics, 73
risks, 12, 39–40, 48, 87
safety monitoring, 42, 57–9, *110*
SART reports, 42
United States, 176

National ART Surveillance System
    (NASS), 23, 39–40, 47
  data access, 52
  data collection, 173–4
  linkage data, 82–3
  quality assurance, 69
National Health and Medical Research
    Council (NHMRC), 142–3
National Institute for Health and Care
    Excellence (NICE), 191
National Perinatal Epidemiology and
    Statistics Unit (NPESU), 142
national registries, 15–16, 31, 37, *220*
  annual reports, 56
  Asia, 140
  Australia and New Zealand, 38, 142,
    145
  Canada, 177
  China, 133
  Denmark, 48
  Egypt, 126, 163
  Europe, 61
  Germany, 16, 56
  India, 136
  Japan, 137–8
  non-ART fertility treatments, 201–2
  Nordic countries, 48, 49
  North America, 172
  patient information, 93
  South Africa, 127
  Sweden, 48
  Switzerland, 34
natural cycle ART, 214
natural cycle IVF, 4
near miss events, 61
necrozoospermia, 214
neonatal deaths/mortalities, 203–4,
    214
  rates, 214
neonatal intensive care units (NICU),
    138
neonatal outcomes, 12, 87, **225**
neonatal period, 214
New Zealand, 142, 145–7
  governance, 142–5
  history of ART, 142
  national registry, 38
  regional registry, 17
  surveillance, ART, 145–7
NHMRC (National Health and
    Medical Research Council), 142–3

Nigeria, 124
non-ART treatments *see* fertility
    treatments, non-ART
non-obstructive azoospermia, 214
Nordic countries; *see also* population-
    based linkages
  data access, 52–3
  long-term outcomes, 49
  national registries, 48
North America, 56, *58*, 172; *see also*
    Canada; United States
  cross-border fertility care, 103
  cumulative birth rates, 109
notification criteria, safety monitoring,
    62–3
Notify Library, **63–4**, 63, 65
nuclear maturation, 214
nulliparity, 1
numerators, ART success rate, 13
  healthy babies, 39–40
  implanted embryos, 39
  live deliveries, 39
  pregnancies, 39

obstructive azoospermia, 214
OHSS *see* ovarian hyperstimulation
    syndrome
oligospermia *see* hypospermia
oligozoospermia, 214
oncology, quality assurance, 72
oocytes, 214
  aspiration, 5, 159, 214
  bank, 214
  cryopreservation, 6, 214
  damage, 65
  donation, 5, 187, 214, **228**
  donation cycles, 214
  freezing, **221**
  maturation triggering, 214
  mature, 159, 191, 213
  maturing, 213
  pick up, 31
  recipient cycles, 214, **229**, **230**
  retrievals, 13, 26
  source, 25
  transfers, 26
  transvaginal retrievals, 5
  vitrification, 32
oolemma, 214
ooplasm, 214
ophthalmology, quality assurance, 73
organ transplantation, quality
    assurance, 72
outcome metrics; *see also* performance
    measures; success rates
  cumulative birth rates, 73
  league tables, 74
  live birth rates, 73
  multiple pregnancies/births, 73
  pregnancy rates, 73

outcome monitoring, global, 118
ovarian cancer, 12
ovarian hyperstimulation syndrome
    (OHSS), 12, 14–15, 26, 32, 214
  Europe, 159
  Middle East, 167
  milder regimes, 49
  multiple pregnancies/births, 60
  safety monitoring, 59
  Sweden, 48
ovarian reserve, 75, 193, 214
ovarian response, excessive, 211
ovarian stimulation (OS), 4, 40–1, 214
  intrauterine insemination, 192–3
  mild, 214
ovarian tissue cryopreservation, 34,
    159, 214
ovarian tissue, retransplantation, 32,
    159
ovarian torsion, 14, 214
ovaries, stimulated, 4
ovulation, 214–15
  induction, 81, 96, 200, 215

parameter definitions, ART success
    rate, 13
parthenogenetic activation, 215
parthenotes, 215
paternal age, advancing, 2
patients; *see also* maternal; paternal
  advocacy organizations, Africa, 125
  centredness, 194
  characteristics, 25–6
  clinics performance, 96–7
  demographics, 25–6, 109, 148, **149**
  expectations, 93
  information complexity, 93–4
  international organizations, 98
  licensing bodies, 98
  making informed decisions, 93, 97
  organizations, 97–8
  perspectives, 93, 98
  prediction calculators, 96
  predictive factors, 47
  predictors, 43–4
  success rates, 37, 41
  understanding success rates, 94–5
  useful questions, 95–6
peer review, quality assurance, 74–5
percutaneous epididymal sperm
    aspiration (PESA), 215
performance measures/indicators,
    13–14, 37–8, 44, 47–8, 108–9
  choice of denominators, 40
  choice of numerators, 38–9
  clinical research, 47–8
  intrauterine insemination, 193–4
  process metrics, **75**, 75, *76*
  quality assurance, 73
  registries, 38

perinatal mortality, 215
  Australia, 147
  Latin America, **189**
  multiple pregnancies/births, 60
  rates, 215
perinatal outcomes *see* health
    outcomes
period total fertility rate (PTFR), 215
perivitelline space, 6, 215
PGT *see* preimplantation genetic
    testing
pharmovigilance, 32–3
Pincus, Gregory, 2, *3*
pituitary down-regulation, 215
polar bodies, 215
polycystic ovary (PCO), 215
polycystic ovary syndrome (PCOS),
    215
polyploidy, 215
polyspermy, 215
poor ovarian response (POR), 215
population-based linkages, Nordic
    countries
  ART registries, 87
  consortium studies, 87
  future directions, 88
  limitations, 87–8
  national registries, 86–7
  personal identity numbers, 86
population-based linkages, USA
  future directions, 86
  limitations, 85–6
  SART CORS–PELL, 84–5
  SART CORS–State Vital Records, 85
posthumous reproduction, 119, 215
post-implantation embryo, 215
post-term birth, 215
prediction calculators, patients, 96
prediction models, 43–4
predictive value positive, 29
predictor tools, 43–4
pregnancy, 95
  definitions, 26–7, 215
  heterotopic, 212
  losses, 1, 145, 215
  outcomes, 27
  rates, 73
  recurrent loss, 1
  success rates, 39
  time to, 192, 217
  unknown location (PUL), 215
Pregnancy to Early Life Longitudinal
    (PELL) data system, *84*, 85
pregnancy-induced complications, 60
preimplantation embryos, 7, 215
preimplantation genetic testing (PGT),
    37, 39, 119
  definition, 215
  hidden cycles, 48
  outcome reporting, **228**, 111

premature births *see* preterm deliveries
premature ejaculation, 215
premature ovarian insufficiency,
    215–16
preterm deliveries, 34, 60, 216
  multiple pregnancies/births, 60
pre-treatment assessment, 119
primary childlessness, 216
primary infertility, 1, 216
primary involuntary childlessness, 216
private vs public health, 124
probabilistic linkage, 82
process metrics, performance
    indicators, 75
prognostic factors, ART success
    rates, 43
pronuclei, 216
pronuclei transfers, 216
prospective reporting, 27
protection, data *see* data confidentiality
public health surveillance, 23
public reporting, 38, 41–4

quality assurance, 69–70, 78–9
  assisted reproductive technology, 73
  haemovigilance, 72
  industrial history, 70–1
  medicine, 71–2
  oncology, 72
  ophthalmology, 73
  organ transplantation, 72
  outcome metrics, 73–5
  process metrics, 75–8
  rare diseases, 72–3
quality control, 69
quality improvement, *70*, 70, 78
quality management, 70, 71, 78

rabbits, IVF, 2–3
randomized controlled trials (RCT),
    31, 37
rapid alerts, 64
rare diseases, quality assurance, 72–3
RCTs (randomized controlled trials),
    31, 37
recipient cycles, 149, 216
recipients, 216
recombinant follicle stimulating
    hormone/luteinizing hormone, 5,
    194
recurrent pregnancy loss, 1, 216
REDLARA *see* Latin American
    Network of Assisted Reproductive
    Technology
regional registries
  Africa, 18
  Asia, 139
  Australia and New Zealand, 17
  Europe, 17–18, 153
  fertility treatments, non-ART, 201

  Latin America, 17, 182–4
  Middle East, 126, 163–4, 168–9
  non-ART fertility treatments, 201
  sub-Saharan Africa, 127–8
registries, 15, 31, 103
  clinical quality, 38
  future directions, 112–13
  global, 16–17, 106
  national, 15–16, 31, 37, 106–7
  performance measures, 38
  quality assurance, 69
  regional, 17–18, 106–7
  types, 106–7
religious influences
  Latin America, 182
  Lebanon, 165
  Middle East, 163
  Shiite Muslims, 164–5
  Sunni Muslims, 164
reporting mechanisms, ART
  governmental bodies, 118
  legislation, 117–18
  outcome monitoring, 118
  professional organizations, 118
representativeness, 29
reproductive potential
  extending, 37, 160–1
  measuring, 40, 43
  reduced, 111
reproductive surgery, 216
research *see* clinical research;
    randomized controlled trials
results presentation, clinics, 96
retinoblastomas, 15
retrograde ejaculation, 216
retrospective reporting, 27–8
risk management, 61
RLA *see* Latin American Registry of
    Assisted Reproduction

safety monitoring/safety, 14–15, 56–7,
    65–6, 109–10
  clinical research, 48–50
  complications of ART, 59–60
  contamination, 65
  cryotanks failure, 64
  culture media, 63–4
  equipment, 63
  Europe, 60–2
  gametes and embryos, 64–5
  intrauterine insemination, 194
  multiple pregnancies, 57–9
  notification criteria, 62–3
  obstetric and perinatal outcomes, 60
  ovarian hyperstimulation
    syndrome, 59
salpingectomy, 216
SART (Society for Assisted
    Reproductive Technology), 31,
    83, 172, 175

SART Clinical Outcomes Reporting System (CORS), 23–4, 37, 42, 47
  data access, 52
  data collection, 173
  linking health databases, 83–4
  quality assurance, 69
sea urchins, 2
secondary infertility, 1, 216
secondary involuntary childlessness, 216
semen, 216; see also sperm
  analysis, 216
  collection, 64–5
  contamination, 65
  liquefaction, 216
  quality, 2, 192
  viscosity, 216
  volume, 216
seminal plasma, 216
sensitivity, high, 29
serious adverse events (SAE), 62, 64, 65
serious adverse reactions (SAR), 62, 64, 65
Sertoli cell-only syndrome, 216
Sertoli cells, 216
service presentation, clinics, 96–7
SET see single embryo transfers
severe OHSS, 216
Shiite Muslims, religious influences, 164–5
sibling studies, 50
side effects, 56–7
simplicity, 29
single cycles, success rates, 37, 40
single embryo transfers (SET), 8, 48, 216; see also elective single embryo transfers
  Australia, 58
  Europe, 58
  Japan, 138, 139
  rates, 8
slow-freezing, 216
small for gestational age, 60, 216
SMART (States Monitoring ART) Collaborative, 83
social aspects, ART, 15
Society for Assisted Reproductive Technology see SART
SOHO V&S (Surveillance of Substances of Human Origin), 62
South Africa, 124
South African Registry for ART (SARA), 127
sperm; see also intracytoplasmic sperm injection; semen
  bank, 216
  concentration/count, 2, 192, 194, 216
  density, 216
  isolation, 216–17
  motility, 217
  recipient cycles, 217

source, 25, 203
total count, 217
vitality, 217
spermatogenic arrest, 217
spermatozoon, 217
spina bifida, 147
spontaneous abortions/miscarriages, 217
spontaneous reductions/vanishing sacs, 217
stability, 29
stakeholders, 15
States Monitoring ART (SMART) Collaborative, 83
statistical significance, 51
stem cell research, 120
Steptoe, Patrick, 3
sterility, 217
stillbirths, 39, 105, 217
  Australia and New Zealand, 147
  Canada, 178
  rates, 217
stimulated cycles, 4, 13, 14, 15, 157
stimulated ovaries, 4, 6
subfertility, 49–50, 85, 217
  male, 191–2, 194, 201
sub-Saharan Africa, regional registry, 127–8
success rates; see also performance measures
  age-related, 95
  clinical research, 47–8
  complete cycles, 37, 40–1, 43
  cryopreservation, 40
  Denmark, 203
  donated gametes (eggs or sperm), 178, 201
  good prognosis group, 96
  healthy babies, 39–40
  heterologous insemination, 201, 202
  homologous insemination, 201, 202
  infertility type, 95
  initiated single cycles, 40
  intrauterine insemination (IUI), 201, 202
  Latin America, 189
  live births/deliveries, 25, 39, 73, 213
  Middle East, 167
  patient information, 93, 94
  patients, 37, 41
  possible measures, 95
  pregnancy, 39
  public reporting, 41–4
  single cycles, 37, 40
  thawing cycles, 61, 157
  understanding by patients, 93–4
summary-level data, 24, 25
Sunni Muslims, religious influences, 164
surrogacy see gestational carriers
surveillance, ART, 12–13, 29–30; see also clinical research

comparisons, 32–3
confidentiality, 35
definitions, 23, 153
efficacy, 13–14
future directions, 31–2, 33–4
historical aspects, 15–18
methods, 28–9
ongoing trends, 32
owners, 23–4
performance measures, 37–8
quality, data, 34–5
report information, 25–7
safety, 14–15
society, 15
suppliers of data, 24
timelines, 27–8
types of data, 24–5
vigilance, 34
surveillance methodology, 117
Sweden
  blastocyst transfers, 49
  national registry, 48
Switzerland, national registry, 34
syngamy, 217

teratozoospermia, 217
test tube babies, 3
testicular sperm aspiration/extraction (TESA/TESE), 217
thawing, 6, 217
thawing cycles, 157
  success rates, 61, 157
therapeutic cloning research, 120–1
time to pregnancy, 192, 217
timed intercourse, 200
time-lapse imaging, 217
timelines, data reporting, 28
timeliness, reporting, 29, 112
Togo, 124, 127
total delivery rate with at least one live birth, 217
total fertility rate (TFR), 217
total sperm count, 217
traceability, 33, 35
traditional gestational carriers, 217
transplantation, quality assurance, 72
transportation, gametes, 32
transvaginal approach, oocyte retrieval, 5, 6
treatment cycles, 31; see also freeze-all treatment cycles
  birth rates, 41, 95
  single embryo, 32
  subsequent, 31–2
treatments (general); see also fertility treatments, non-ART
  early history, 2–7
  modalities, 14, 15, 156–7, 157
  outcomes, 221, 26–7
triennial survey, IFFS, 116–17

trisomy, 217
trophectoderms, 217
tubal pathology, 3, 166, 191, 195, 217

Uganda, 124
ultrasound, abdominal, 5
underreporting, 33
unexplained infertility, 191, 192, 217
unisomies, 217
United Kingdom
  birth weights, 49
  data collection, 41–2
  frozen embryo replacements/ transfers, 14
  haemovigilance, 72
  Human Fertilisation and Embryology Authority, 27–8, 69
  in vitro fertilization, 1
  National Institute for Health and Care Excellence (NICE), 191
  national registry, 16, 18, 56

ovarian hyperstimulation syndrome, 14–15
United States, 172–5; *see also* population-based linkages
  ART history, 172
  ART surveillance, 176–7
  data collection, 172–5
  data quality, 175–6
  national registry, 16
  regulation, 172

vaginal insemination, 217
varicocelectomy, 217
varicoceles, 217
vasectomy, 217
very low birth weight, 217
vigilance, 34, 161; *see also* haemovigilance; medical biotechnology vigilance; pharmovigilance
Vigilance and Surveillance of Substances of Human Origin (SOHO V&S), 62

viscosity, 218
vital records, 85, 86
vitrification, 33, 218; *see also* cryopreservation
  embryos, 6, 195
  oocytes, 32
voluntary childlessness, 218

warming (cells), 218; *see also* thawing
woman-based data collection, 147–8; *see also* patients
World Health Organization (WHO)
  health care data, 71
  infertility, 116
  patient involvement, 97–8
  surveillance, definition, 153

Y-chromosome microdeletions, 218

zona pellucida, 6, 218
zygote intrafallopian transfer (ZIFT), 81, 174
zygotes, 105, 218